Clinical Problems, Injuries, and Complications of Gynecologic Surgery

Second Edition

Clinical Problems, Injuries, and Complications of Gynecologic Surgery

SECOND EDITION

Edited by

David H. Nichols, M.D.

Professor and Chairman, Department of Obstetrics and Gynecology, Brown University, Obstetrician and Gynecologist-in-Chief, Department of Obstetrics and Gynecology, Women & Infants Hospital of Rhode Island. Surgeon-in-Chief, Department of Gynecology & Obstetrics, Rhode Island Hospital, Providence, Rhode Island. Lecturer in Obstetrics and Gynecology, Tufts University School of Medicine, Boston, Massachusetts.

with the assistance of

George W. Anderson, M.D.

Lecturer, Department of Obstetrics and Gynecology, Brown University, Providence, Rhode Island. Associate Professor of Obstetrics and Gynecology, Tufts University School of Medicine, Boston, Massachusetts.

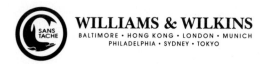

WILLIAMS & WILKINS
BALTIMORE • HONG KONG • LONDON • MUNICH
PHILADELPHIA • SYDNEY • TOKYO

Editor: Carol-Lynn Brown
Associate Editor: Victoria M. Vaughn
Copy Editor: Shelley Potler
Design: Saturn Graphics
Illustration Planning: Lorraine Wrzosek
Production: Raymond E. Reter
Cover Design: JoAnne Janowiak

Accurate indications, adverse reactions, and dosage schedules for drugs are provided
in this book, but it is possible that they may change. The reader is urged to review
the package information data of the manufacturers of the medications mentioned.

Printed in the United States of America

First Edition, 1983

Library of Congress Cataloging-in-Publication Data

Clinical problems, injuries, and complications of
   gynecologic surgery.

   Includes bibliographies and index.
   1. Gynecology, Operative—Complications and
sequelae. I. Nichols, David H., 1925–
II. Anderson, George W. (George Woodrow), 1913–
[DNLM: 1. Breast Neoplasms—surgery. 2. Genitalia,
Female—surgery. 3. Pelvic Neoplasms—surgery.
4. Postoperative Complications. WP 660 C641]
RG104.C48 1988   618.1′059   87-6151
ISBN 0-683-06496-7

5 6 7 8 9 10   92 93

To
Lorraine, Laurie,
Nancie, Julie,
Julianne, and Amanda

Foreword

In my foreword to the first edition of this book, I commented that it represented an experiment in format and style. Clearly the experiment has succeeded and now, just four years later, the second edition is ready for the printer.

This is no mere rewrite. Dr. Nichols has dismembered and restructured the text in accordance with suggestions solicited from his authors and other consultants. Sections have been rearranged and their contents reordered, eliminating a few redundancies but increasing overall by 38 chapters and 25 additional authors.

Most striking is an entire new section on Pelvic Cancer Surgery and useful additions to the sections on Laparotomy and Vaginal Surgery.

The style and content make for interesting reading of a random sort, but the volume will fulfill its true purpose when consulted with a specific situation under consideration, and for this usage, one needs contents pages with chapter titles that clearly indicate the subject matter and a properly composed index. Happily, both these have been achieved in this edition as was the case with the first.

Howard Ulfelder, M.D.
Joe Vincent Meigs Emeritus Professor of
   Gynecology
Harvard Medical School and
     Massachusetts General Hospital
Boston, Massachusetts
March 1987

Preface

This second edition of *Clinical Problems, Injuries, and Complications of Gynecologic Surgery* is intended not only to satisfy that surgical curiosity which is so intrinsic to the specialty, but to stimulate creative surgical thinking as well. To this latter end, we hope that the reader will study the case abstracts at the beginning of each chapter. The problems presented should be recognized as examples of those which might present themselves (usually without warning) to the surgeon. A decision is required. What are the various treatment options? Which should be chosen, and for what reasons? Could this problem have been avoided, and if so, how?

The problems, while uncommon, are of major importance to both house officers and surgeons in practice. They are representative of the unexpected developments that can arise in almost any gynecologic surgical operation, and that require timely and definitive responses.

After studying the case, the reader is encouraged to analyze the problem, consider the possible alternative treatments, and select an approach. Then turn to the discussion following the case—authored by contributors selected for their relevant interest, experience, and expertise—for an authoritative analysis, a response to the possible alternative treatments, and most importantly, a rigorous method of decision-making.

Recognizing that for each problem there may be a number of appropriate solutions, we present these studies not as the final word but as the best thoughts of well-known specialists on organizing one's thinking, skills, and resources to solve a surgical problem. Conveying the thought process of arriving at an effective solution is the major goal of this work, that by learning to use the process regularly one may employ it effectively in one's practice to other unexpected surgical problems beyond those treated herein.

Competence in gynecologic surgery requires that the surgeon not only accept responsibility for any intentional, accidental, or incidental damage produced in the course of an operation, but also be comfortable with the techniques to repair that damage. Refining the means of arriving at a particular surgical solution to such problems is the purpose of this book, and the reader is invited, indeed urged, to participate in this process.

D.H.N.
G.W.A.

Preface to the First Edition

As the title of the book indicates, this effort is directed at the factors involved and solutions to the complications of gynecologic surgery. During the last few years, we have participated in the development of problem-oriented cases in gynecologic surgery as part of various postgraduate programs in continuing medical education. These emphasize practical problems that can intrude unexpectedly in the day-to-day activities of anyone who practices gynecologic surgery and are of serious consequence if not handled correctly. Most of the problems, even if uncommon, are of major importance to both house officers and surgeons in practice. One of the main reasons for this book is directed to possible deficiencies of present-day education of residents in obstetrics and gynecology. In a 3- to 4-year program, the time devoted to surgical competence in gynecology must be competitive with maternal and fetal medicine, family planning, reproductive endocrinology, gynecologic oncology, and the psychologic and social aspects of understanding the proper delivery of health care to women. The current incidences of injury to the urinary tract or intestine vary from one in 500 to one in 1,000 to 2,000 cases. Very few residencies have this volume of patients compressed into the 2 surgical years of an individual resident's experience. It is possible that many residents have only had the primary responsibility for management of one or two of the complications listed in this book during their training.

The emphasis in the clinical cases in this volume has been on practicality to help the practitioner appropriately organize his thinking, skills, and resources concerning clinical dilemmas, rather than on demonstrating the clinical dexterity of the consultant. The cases chosen for this book represent important and usually unexpected problems in surgical management and decision-making that can develop in almost any gynecologic surgical operation and practice and that require timely, definitive, and surgically appropriate solutions. Fully recognizing that in most situations there can be contrasting and effective alternate points of view, the solutions presented are neither intended nor presumed to be the final words, but do represent those which in the views of the authors are likely to be appropriate. Contributors have been selected on the basis of a special expertise for which they, as individuals, are well known and represent important and sometimes sophisticated studies in anatomic relationships, skills, and techniques, based on established surgical principles and embodying information not necessarily available in the standard texts.

The format for each case presentation includes a short clinical abstract identifying the problem or complication of the surgery. The consultant makes his own analysis, responds to the possible alternate treatments with his method of decision-making, and arrives at an appropriate solution. Selected references and illustrations augment each presentation.

The patient's symptoms are not always proportionate to the findings upon physical examination. Patient disability has wide individual variation, for that which may be acceptable to one person is not to another, and the niceties of judgment require a knowledge of each patient as a person and some insight as to how she perceives her pathology and the results to be expected from surgery. Modern techniques of surgery, anesthesia, and nursing care have now made possible a safe approach to surgery for the significantly older patient, although preferably in the larger hospitals where round-the-clock professional skills are available should they be needed.

We subscribe to the view of many that not only is a surgeon responsible for any intentional, accidental, or incidental damage that he produces in the course of an operation, but he should be comfortable with the techniques to repair that damage. These skills, once learned, are not easily forgotten. The primary goal of any continuing medical education program is to provide an environment that leads to the orderly growth of a physician to the level of education and skills required of a progressive physician. The learning process is an ongoing lifetime experience. In the case of surgeons, this laboratory of learning is in the operating room. In the future, well-controlled clinical trials will be the crucial test for adoption of new therapies. Greater communication between all branches of the surgical disciplines will help solve the injuries and complications of gynecologic surgery.

D.H.N.
G.W.A.

Acknowledgments

Sincere appreciation is expressed to Jane Fallon Seleyman for her many hours of understanding help in typing the manuscript, and to Carol-Lynn Brown, Editor and to Vicki Vaughn, Associate Editor from Williams & Wilkins Company, for their faith, patience, and understanding.

Contributors

Anderson, Barrie, M.D., Associate Professor, Division of Gynecologic Oncology, University of Iowa Hospital, Iowa City, Iowa.

Anderson, George W., M.D., Lecturer, Department of Obstetrics and Gynecology, Brown University, Providence, Rhode Island, Associate Professor of Obstetrics and Gynecology, Tufts University School of Medicine, Boston, Massachusetts.

Azziz, Ricardo, M.D., Instructor, Department of Obstetrics and Gynecology, Division of Reproductive Endocrinology, The Johns Hopkins Hospital, Baltimore, Maryland.

Barber, Hugh R. K., M.D., Director, Department of Obstetrics and Gynecology, Lenox Hill Hospital, New York, New York.

Beecham, Clayton T., M.D., Emeritus Director of Gynecology and Obstetrics, Geisinger Medical Center, Danville, Pennsylvania.

Belinson, Jerome L., M.D., Associate Professor, Director of Oncology, Medical Center Hospital of Vermont, Burlington, Vermont.

Breen, James L., M.D., F.A.C.O.G., F.A.C.S., Chairman, Department of Obstetrics and Gynecology, Saint Barnabas Medical Center, Livingston, New Jersey; Clinical Professor, Obstetrics and Gynecology, Jefferson Medical College, Philadelphia, Pennsylvania.

Burchell, R. Clay, M.D., Professor of Obstetrics and Gynecology, University of Connecticut Health Center; Chief of Obstetrics and Gynecology, The Lovelace Clinic, Albuquerque, New Mexico.

Caldwell, Burton, V., M.D., Ph.D., Associate Professor of Clinical Medicine, Yale University School of Medicine, New Haven, Connecticut.

Cavanagh, Denis, M.D., Ch.B. (Glas.), F.A.C.O.G., F.A.C.S., F.R.C.O.G., American Cancer Society Ed. C. Wright Professor of Clinical Oncology, Director of Gynecologic Oncology, University of South Florida College of Medicine, Tampa, Florida.

Creasman, William T., M.D., Sims Hester Professor and Chairman, Department of Obstetrics and Gynecology, Medical University of South Carolina, Charleston, South Carolina.

Crisp, William E., M.D., Clinical Associate Professor, University of Arizona College of Medicine; Director of Gynecologic Oncology, Maricopa County Hospital, Phoenix, Arizona.

Curry, Stephen L., M.D., Louis E. Phaneuf Professor and Chairman, Department of Obstetrics and Gynecology, Tufts University School of Medicine, Boston, Massachusetts.

DeCherney, Alan H., M.D., The John Slade Ely Professor of Obstetrics and Gynecology, Yale University School of Medicine, New Haven, Connecticut.

DeLia, Julian E., M.D., F.A.C.O.G., Assistant Professor, Department of Obstetrics and Gynecology, University of Utah School of Medicine, Salt Lake City, Utah.

DiSaia, Philip J., M.D., Professor and Chairman, Department of Obstetrics and Gynecology, University of California Irvine Medical Center, Orange, California.

Drukker, Bruce H., M.D., Professor and Chairman, Department of Obstetrics, Gynecology and Reproductive Biology, Michigan State University, East Lansing, Michigan.

Ebner, Herbert, M.D., Clinical Associate Professor of Obstetrics and Gynecology, Brown University-Division of Biology and Medicine; formerly Chief of Anesthesiology, Women & Infants Hospital, Providence, Rhode Island.

Evans, Tommy N., M.D., Professor and Vice-Chairman, Chief of Gynecology, Department of Obstetrics and Gynecology, University of Colorado Health Sciences Center, Denver, Colorado.

Evrard, John R., M.D., M.P.H., Professor of Obstetrics and Gynecology, Brown University Program in Medicine, Providence, Rhode Island.

Flowers, Charles E., Jr., M.D., Professor and Chairman Emeritus, Department of Obstetrics and Gynecology, University of Alabama, Birmingham, Alabama.

Fuller, Arlan F., Jr., M.D., Assistant Professor of Obstetrics and Gynecology, Harvard Medical School; Director, Gynecologic Oncology Service, Department of Gynecology, Massachusetts General Hospital, Boston, Massachusetts.

Galle, Phillip C., M.D., Fellow in Reproductive Endocrinology and Infertility, Hospital of the University of Pennsylvania, Philadelphia, Pennsylvania.

Garcia, Celso-Ramon, M.D., F.A.C.S., F.A.C.O.G., The William Shippen, Jr. Professor of Human Reproduction, School of Medicine and Hospital, the University of Pennsylvania, Philadelphia, Pennsylvania.

Gusberg, Saul B., M.D., D.Sc., Distinguished Service Professor, The Mount Sinai School of Medicine, New York, New York.

Haning, Ray V., Jr., M.D., Associate Professor of Obstetrics and Gynecology, Brown University Program in Medicine; Director, Gynecologic Endocrinology, Women & Infants Hospital, Providence, Rhode Island.

Hoskins, William J., M.D., Capt., MC, USN, Associate Chief, Gynecology Service; Associate Member, Memorial Sloan-Kettering Cancer Center, New York, New York.

Hurt, W. Glenn, M.D., Professor, Department of Obstetrics and Gynecology, Medical College of Virginia, Virginia Commonwealth University, Richmond, Virginia.

Isaacs, John H., M.D., Professor and Chairman of Obstetrics and Gynecology, Loy-

ola University of Chicago, Stritch School Medicine, Maywood, Illinois.

Jones, Howard W., Jr., M.D., D.Sc. (Honoris Causis), Professor of Obstetrics and Gynecology, Eastern Virginia Medical School Norfolk, Virginia; Professor Emeritus, Gynecology and Obstetrics, Johns Hopkins University Medical School, Baltimore, Maryland.

Lackritz, Richard M., M.D., Associate Clinical Professor of Obstetrics and Gynecology, The University of Texas Health Science Center at San Antonio, San Antonio, Texas.

Lathrop, John C., M.D., Clinical Associate Professor of Obstetrics and Gynecology, Brown University Program in Medicine, Providence, Rhode Island.

Lee, Raymond A., M.D., Professor and Chairman, Division of Gynecology and Gynecologic Surgery, Mayo Medical School, Mayo Clinic, Rochester, Minnesota.

Lewis, John L., Jr., M.D., Chief, Gynecology Service, Memorial Sloan-Kettering Cancer Center; Professor of Obstetrics and Gynecology, Cornell University Medical Center, New York, New York.

Malinak, L. Russell, M.D., Professor, Department of Obstetrics and Gynecology, Baylor College of Medicine, Houston, Texas.

Marchant, Douglas, J., M.D., Professor of Obstetrics and Gynecology and Professor of Surgery, Tufts University School of Medicine; Director, Cancer Institute, Tufts—New England Medical Center, Boston, Massachusetts.

Marsden, Donald E., M.D., M.R.C.O.G., F.R.A.C.O.G., Senior Lecturer, Department of Obstetrics and Gynecology, University of Tasmania, Hobart Tasmania 7000, Australia.

Massey, Fred M., M.D., Associate Clinical Professor, The University of Texas Health Science Center at San Antonio, San Antonio, Texas.

Masterson, Byron J., M.D., F.A.C.S., F.A.C.O.G., Professor and Chairman, Department of Obstetrics and Gynecology, University of Louisville School of Medicine, Louisville, Kentucky.

*Mattingly, Richard F., M.D., Professor and Chairman, Department of Obstetrics and Gynecology, The Medical College of Wisconsin, Milwaukee, Wisconsin.

McDuff, Henry C., Jr., M.D., F.A.C.S., F.A.C.O.G., Clinical Professor of Obstetrics and Gynecology, Brown University Program in Medicine, Providence, Rhode Island; Clinical Associate Professor of Gynecology, Tufts University School of Medicine, Boston, Massachusetts.

Mickal, Abe, M.D., F.A.C.O.G., F.A.C.S., Professor and Emeritus Chairman of Obstetrics and Gynecology, Louisiana State University Medical Center, New Orleans, Louisiana.

Mikuta, John J., M.D. Professor, Obstetrics and Gynecology, Director Gynecologic Oncology, Hospital of the University of Pennsylvania, Philadelphia, Pennsylvania.

Mitchell, George W., Jr., M.D., Professor, Obstetrics and Gynecology, The University of Texas Health Science Center at San Antonio, San Antonio, Texas.

Moore, J. George, M.D., Professor, Department of Obstetrics and Gynecology, UCLA School of Medicine, Center for the Health Sciences, Los Angeles, California.

Morley, George W., M.S., M.D., Professor, Obstetrics and Gynecology, University of Michigan Medical Center, Ann Arbor, Michigan.

Morris, John McLean, M.D., Professor of Gynecology, Yale University School of Medicine, New Haven, Connecticut.

Nichols, David H., M.D., Professor and Chairman, Department of Obstetrics and Gynecology, Brown University; Obstetrician and Gynecologist-in-Chief, Women & Infants

*Deceased, 1986.

Hospital of Rhode Island; Surgeon-in-Chief, Department of Gynecology and Obstetrics, Rhode Island Hospital, Providence, Rhode Island. Lecturer in Obstetrics and Gynecology, Tufts University School of Medicine, Boston, Massachusetts.

Nichols, David Landel, Esq., B.A., M.A., J.D., County and District Attorney 76th and 276th Judicial Districts, Morris County Courthouse, Daingerfield, Texas.

Porges, Robert F., M.D., Professor of Obstetrics and Gynecology, New York University Medical Center, New York, New York.

Pratt, Joseph H., M.D., Emeritus Professor of Surgery, Mayo Medical School, Mayo Clinic, Rochester, Minnesota.

Randall, Clyde L., M.D., Emeritus Professor and Chairman of Gynecology and Obstetrics, State University of New York at Buffalo, Buffalo, New York.

Rock, John A., M.D., Associate Professor of Obstetrics and Gynecology; Director, Division of Reproductive Endocrinology, The Johns Hopkins University School of Medicine, Baltimore, Maryland.

Rogers, Robert E., M.D., Professor of Obstetrics and Gynecology, Indiana University School of Medicine, Indianapolis, Indiana.

Schwarz, Richard H., M.D., Professor and Chairman, Department of Obstetrics and Gynecology; Dean and Vice President for Academic Affairs, State University of New York Downstate Medical Center, Brooklyn, New York.

Simolke, Greg, B.S., Department of Obstetrics and Gynecology, Baylor College of Medicine, Houston, Texas.

Slaby, Andrew E., M.D., Ph.D., M.P.H., Medical Director, Fair Oaks Hospital, Summit, New Jersey; Adjunct Professor of Psychiatry and Human Behavior, Brown University Program in Medicine, Providence, Rhode Island.

Symmonds, Richard E., M.D., Emeritus Professor and Chairman, Division of Gynecologic Surgery, Mayo Clinic, Rochester, Minnesota.

Thompson, John D., M.D., Professor, Department of Gynecology and Obstetrics, Emory University of Medicine, Atlanta, Georgia.

Wheeler, James M., M.D., Fellow, Robert Wood Johnson Clinical Scholars Program, Department of Medicine/Department of Obstetrics and Gynecology, Yale University School of Medicine, New Haven, Connecticut.

Wheeless, Clifford R., Jr., M.D., Chief, Obstetrics and Gynecology, Union Memorial Hospital; Assistant Professor of Gynecology and Obstetrics, Johns Hopkins University School of Medicine; Associate Professor of Obstetrics and Gynecology, University of Maryland School of Medicine, Baltimore, Maryland.

Wiser, Winfred L., M.D., Professor and Chairman of Obstetrics and Gynecology, The University of Mississippi Medical Center, Jackson, Mississippi.

Contents

3. Fertility Surgery

4. Vaginal Surgery

5. Urinary Tract Problems and Injuries

6. Intestinal Problems and Injuries

7. Pelvic Cancer Surgery

8. Problems of Minor Gynecologic Surgery

9. Breast Surgery

10. Medical, Endocrine and Miscellaneous Problems

CHAPTER 1

Postoperative Necrotizing Fasciitis

RAYMOND A. LEE, M.D.

CASE ABSTRACT

A 65-year-old diabetic patient with a 3-cm grossly malignant appearing lesion on the left labia majora underwent confirmatory biopsy, radical vulvectomy, bilateral lymphadenectomy, and sartorius transplant. The following is a copy of the pathology report: "Grade 2 invasive squamous cell carcinoma, 3.5 × 3.1 cm, with 14 negative nodes."

Twenty-four hours after surgery, her temperature was 39.4 degrees C and there was evidence of necrosis of the skin edges with purulent discharge between the suture line. A culture was obtained, and she was placed on triple antibiotics Her temperature elevation continued 3 days later.

DISCUSSION

Necrotizing fasciitis is a severe, synergistic bacterial infection that results in necrosis of the superficial and deep fasciae. The patient has an unusually high fever and necrosis of the wound edges very early after operation, alerting the physician that the wound infection may be more than trivial.

Predisposing Factors

Predisposing factors include advancing age, atherosclerosis, obesity, malnutrition, diabetes mellitus, and previous radiation and operative trauma. The condition is most commonly found in the lower extremities, perineum, groin, back, or buttocks. Perineal and vulvar involvement is frequently seen in the obese diabetic patient. Minor infections may trigger the event in the compromised patient. The disease may smoulder initially and then progress rapidly, with subcutaneous necrosis of fat and fascia secondary to bacterial toxins and with thrombosis of vessels leading to gangrene and bullae in the skin. The mortality rate is from 30% to 60%. Necrotizing fasciitis is a synergistic infection usually combined with Gram-positive cocci and Gram-negative rods. Often, the offending anaerobic bacteria are *Peptococcus, Peptostreptococcus,* or *Bacteroides* species. Beta-hemolytic streptococci may be cultured in about 50% of the cases, with many other organisms probably acting as secondary contaminants.

Clinical Presentation

Necrotizing fasciitis may be fulminant or slowly progressive. The patient usually has a fever and may experience prostration due to rapid changes in fluids and electrolytes. Toxicity and leukocytosis can be striking and out of proportion to the apparent extent of the condition. Given sufficient time, the infection travels in a centrifugal direction, and the skin becomes tense and brawny and may have a purple discoloration, with vesicular formation progressing to gangrene (Fig. 1.1). The skin becomes anesthetic because the subcutaneous nerves die as a result of thrombosis of the underlying nutrient vessels within the necrotic and string fascia. The clinical clues are: (1) cellulitis that fails to respond promptly to antibiotic treatment; (2) development of blisters over an area of cellulitis; (3) development of ecchymosis over an area of cellulitis; and (4) presence

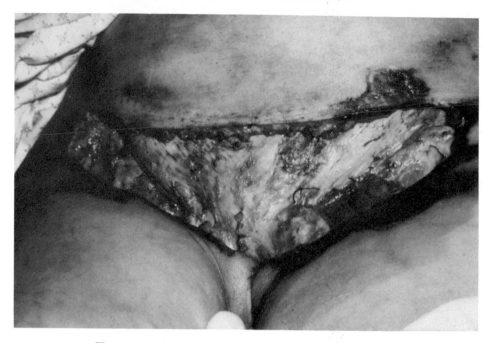

Figure 1.1.   Necrosis of operative site of radical vulvectomy.

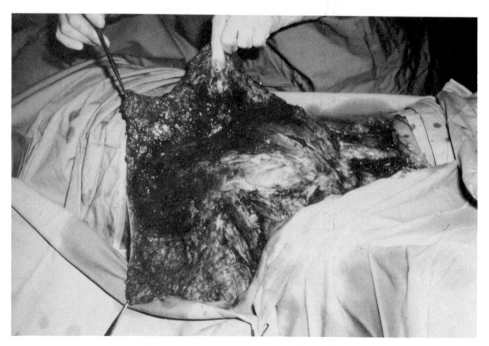

Figure 1.2.   Initial radical debridement.

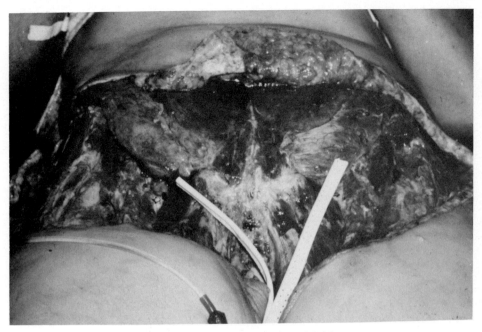

Figure 1.3.   Surgical site after fourth debridement.

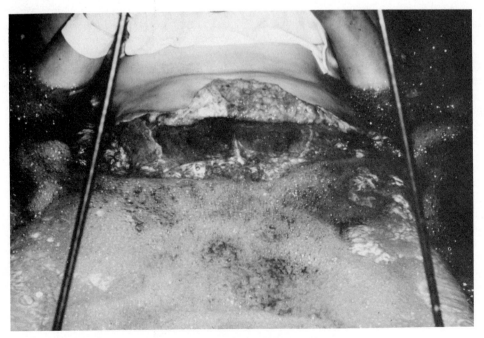

Figure 1.4.   Patient in whirlpool bath.

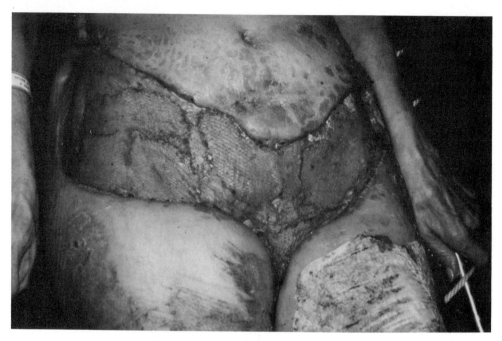

Figure 1.5.   Three days after skin graft.

of gas in the incision, as detected by palpation.

Treatment. Survival depends on early recognition and immediate surgical debridement to healthy tissue margins (Fig. 1.2). All indurated, edematous tissue that is crepitant or does not bleed easily when incised should be removed. After the initial debridement, persistent or progressive necrotizing fasciitis is suggested by the presence of continued leukocytosis, fever, or seropurulent discharge from the wound margins. Multiple debridements may be necessary (Fig. 1.3). Cleansing the wound is facilitated by whirlpool baths and frequent changes of wound dressings (Fig. 1.4). The wound should be dressed open while the patient is in strict isolation, with plans for a split-thickness skin graft later to cover the wound areas (Fig. 1.5). Broad-spectrum antibiotics are useful adjuncts to assist in the control of infection after the operation and may shorten the hospital stay, but they remain secondary to definitive operative intervention. Initial treatment consists of penicillin, clindamycin, an aminoglycoside, intravenously administered fluids, and blood transfusion as necessary, with supplemental calcium and general patient support. Death from necrotizing fasciitis is most commonly due to overwhelming sepsis or a combination of diabetes and vascular insufficiency. Early recognition and immediate surgical debridement are the hallmarks of successful management.

Selected Readings

Addison WA, Livengood CH III, Hill GB, et al: Necrotizing fasciitis of vulvar origin in diabetic patients. *Obstet Gynecol* 63:473-479, 1984.

Defore WW Jr, Mattox KL, Dang MH, et al: Necrotizing fasciitis: A persistent surgical problem. *JACEP* 6:62-65, 1977.

Roberts DB, Hester LL Jr: Progressive synergistic bacterial gangrene arising from abscesses of the vulva and Bartholin's gland duct. *Am J Obstet Gynecol* 114:285-289, 1972.

Stone HH, Martin JD Jr: Synergistic necrotizing cellulitis. *Ann Surg* 175:702-710, 1972.

CHAPTER 2

Ruptured Tubo-ovarian Abscess

RICHARD H. SCHWARZ, M.D.

CASE ABSTRACT

A ruptured right tubo-ovarian abscess was discovered at laparotomy for suspected appendicitis in a 30-year-old infertility patient. The abscess was on the patient's right side, but the appendix was not involved in the process. The tube and ovary of the left side of the pelvis were grossly normal, although now bathed in the purulent exudate from the ruptured right tubo-ovarian abscess. A 4-cm leiomyoma was palpable in the uterine fundus.

DISCUSSION

The critical problem presented by this case is to strike a balance between a desire to preserve the potential of childbearing in this relatively young infertile woman and the risk that surgical conservatism may not resolve the life-threatening problem. This decision would be far less difficult if the patient were multiparous, perimenopausal, or even if the opposite tube and ovary were grossly diseased, suggesting a poor prognosis for any future reconstructive surgery. In such circumstances, total abdominal hysterectomy with bilateral salpingo-oophorectomy would be the approach of choice and offer the most certain chance of cure. Unilateral adnexal removal, however, is the better option for this patient.

Although it is not common to have totally unilateral involvement with pelvic inflammatory disease, it is certainly more common than previously thought, or taught, to have markedly disparate involvement of the two sides. Up to 40% of tubo-ovarian abscesses are unilateral, a finding first brought to the attention of clinicians in dealing with infections associated with intrauterine contraceptive devices. This information does permit the surgeon to consider a conservative approach. The worst case outcome for the patient, if this approach is used, would be the need for a second operation. This might arise if the less obvious disease in the residual tube progressed despite perioperative antibiotics or a secondary pelvic operative site

(pelvic) abscess formed. The latter could, of course, occur even if hysterectomy and bilateral salpingo-oophorectomy were done.

The surgical procedure in this patient should be a simple salpingo-oophorectomy on the side of the abscess. The myoma described should not be removed since an incision into the uterus would provide a focus for secondary infection. Surgical steps should include: obtaining aerobic and anaerobic cultures (best done from the pus in the abscess or even a piece of the abscess wall); exploration of the abdomen to locate and break up any loculations of pus; and thorough lavage with copious amounts of warm saline solution. Although some would suggest irrigation with antibiotic solutions, I believe there is some risk of absorption of excess quantities of antibiotics from inflamed serosal surfaces. In general, I believe antibiotics are most effectively delivered in such patients by the intravenous route.

There are always questions concerning surgical drainage in these cases. Should there be drainage? Of what area? Through what portal? I believe this patient should have drainage and there are two reasonable options for the route. If the cul-de-sac is free, a drain can be placed through that area into the vagina. A T-tube or a mushroom catheter is appropriate, and placement can be facilitated by an assistant exerting upward pressure with an open-ring forceps or long hemostat placed in the posterior vaginal fornix. This same instrument can then be used to pull the drain down into the vagina after a stab wound in the cul-de-sac has been made. This route has the advantage of gravity. An alternate is placement of a drain through a lateral stab wound (drains should not be brought out through the primary incision). The tip of the drain may be placed in the cul-de-sac or at the site of the abscess. Finally, in such a patient, the wound should be dealt with by delayed primary closure of the subcutaneous tissue and skin.

Selected Readings

Brown SE, Allen HH, Robins RN: The use of delayed primary wound closure in preventing wound infection. *Am J Obstet Gynecol* 127:713, 1977.

Dawood MY, Birnbaum SJ: Unilateral tubo-ovarian abscess and intrauterine contraceptive device. *Obstet Gynecol* 46:429, 1975.

Franklin EW, Hevron JE, Thompson JD: Management of pelvic abscess. *Clin Obstet Gynecol* 16:66, 1973.

Mead PB, Beecham JB, Maeck S Jr: Incidence of infections associated with the intrauterine contraceptive device in an isolated community. *Am J Obstet Gynecol* 125:79, 1976.

Taylor ES, McMillan JH, Green BE, et al: The intrauterine contraception device and tubo-ovarian abscess. *Am J Obstet Gynecol* 123:338, 1975.

CHAPTER 3

Appendiceal Abscess with Drain

RAYMOND A. LEE, M.D.

CASE ABSTRACT

A 26-year-old patient, thought to have an ovarian abscess, was explored surgically when the abscess showed no sign of resolution. The patient had remained clinically infected and exhibited tachycardia and temperature spiking. When the abdomen was opened it was found that the right lower quadrant was filled with matted bowel, densely adherent to the side walls of the pelvis, and to the free surfaces of both large and small intestine. The tubes and ovaries, although covered with light filmy adhesions, were not involved. Probing of this ligneous mass in the right lower quadrant brought forth a free flow of thick, greenish yellow exudate, and a diagnosis of appendiceal abscess was made. The appendix itself, however, was not identified. A Penrose drain was placed into the center of this abscess through a separate stab wound in the abdomen, and the original incision was closed.

DISCUSSION

The rationale of surgical drainage of an appendiceal abscess has been accepted during the past hundred years. While the frequency of abscess formation appears to be declining (possibly as a result of patient and surgeon education) and the availability of emergency services has increased, further improvement can be expected. Almost always, the appendix can be identified and resected, and the appendiceal stump can be tied and inverted. Occasionally, the induration of the stump of the appendix and cecum is such that inversion is not possible and simple ligation with an adequate absorbable suture must suffice. Rarely, a right hemicolectomy is done because the ligneous reaction may make it difficult to differentiate the process from that of a malignancy involving the cecum. In the uncommon event that the appendix is impossible to identify, usually because of adhesive inflammatory reaction, the abscess cavity can simply be drained and irrigated, and an appendectomy can be performed 8 to 12 weeks later.

Vigorous irrigation with warm saline to remove particulate debris is beneficial, but little effort is made to dissect or tease off the fibrinous exudate from the surrounding bowel.

Currently, my colleagues and I do not use antibiotic solution for irrigation. We have changed from the use of soft Penrose drains to the use of a soft, closed-suction catheter of the Jackson-Pratt variety; we do not use firm catheters for fear that bowel erosion may result. Drainage through a separate incision has been generally accepted as the proper management of the abscess itself.

The management of the wound must be individualized; in general, the abscess is drained through a separate incision and the operative incision is closed primarily with polyglycolic acid sutures. The operative incision is also drained, but this is done separately. A small (1/8-inch) wound catheter is placed on top of the fascia, over which the skin is closed. Five to 10 ml of a solution consisting of gentamicin (80 mg), neomycin (0.5 g), polymyxin (0.10 g), and saline (1000 ml) are instilled through the wound catheter every 8 hours. Between 5 and 10 ml of this solution are permitted to remain in place for 30 minutes; otherwise, the suction catheter is on continuous suction. The wound catheter is removed on the third or fourth postoperative day; the abscess drain remains in place, depending on the clinical response and drain production. Infrequently, the incision is closed through the fascial layer, and the rest of the wound is packed with plain gauze, which is changed three times a day, thus permitting granulation of the wound, which is later closed with paper tapes.

The condition would be managed the same way if the patient was pregnant—recognizing that the greater the inflammatory reaction and the nearer the condition to the uterus, the greater likelihood that premature labor may be precipitated. Management should be dictated by the pregnancy and not by the condition of the appendix.

The risk of closed appendiceal sepsis is related to the degree of appendicitis. Usually, the patient is given cephalosporin immediately before operation. When a ruptured appendix or an appendiceal abscess is encountered, therapy is immediately changed to broad-spectrum antibiotics that is effective against gut flora intraoperatively. The place of postoperative antibiotics is less clear and continues to be debated. The use of antibiotics can be continued postoperatively until the temperature is normal for 48 hours and the leukocyte and differential counts return to normal.

Managing the interval (elective) appendectomy has been a source of controversy. In general, if the patients are left untreated, 80% to 90% will not have recurrent appendicitis. Using barium enema to identify the patients likely to have appendicitis (obliteration of the appendix) has been unrewarding. However, my colleagues and I withhold interval appendectomy only in poor-risk patients whose 10% to 20% rate of recurrent appendicitis seems to be the smaller risk.

CHAPTER 4

Postoperative Fever Following Hysterectomy

RICHARD H. SCHWARZ, M.D.

CASE ABSTRACT

At 3 a.m. on the second postoperative day following total abdominal hysterctomy, a floor nurse called the attending physician to report a temperature elevation to 102 degrees F in a patient who was otherwise asymptomatic and had not been taking antibiotics. The attending ordered a vaginal smear and culture, urinalysis and 500 mg of ampicillin to be given four times per day. The patient remained relatively asymptomatic, but a temperature elevation to 101.8 degrees F was noted at 8 p.m., this time accompanied by tachycardia.

DISCUSSION

The scenario presented by this case is unfortunately a very common one. Therapy was begun without a direct evaluation of the patient, with one appropriate and one inappropriate microbiology study and without a logical thought process leading to the selection of an antimicrobial agent.

The differential diagnosis must include infection at the operative site (wound or pelvis), urinary tract infection (a catheter was probably used at the time of surgery) and atelectasis (regardless of the anesthetic technique used). Low grade fever can occur postoperatively in the absence of infection although 102 degrees F is a bit high for that circumstance. With a single, early, low grade elevation, it is appropriate to withhold treatment if the immediate evaluation does not reveal a source of the problem. Occasionally this approach will be rewarded with no further elevations. The most likely diagnosis in the case presented, however, is operative site infection.

The initial evaluation should include a brief but focused history and physical examination. Special attention should be paid to the wound, the lung bases, the kidney areas, and the calves. There is often reluctance to perform a pelvic examination in the early postoperative period because of patient discomfort and difficulty in interpreting findings. This is an ill-founded concern and could lead to missing a pelvic collection. In addition, a culture from the vaginal cuff can only be obtained with a speculum in place. Initial microbiologic studies should include blood and urine cultures. A blind vaginal culture has little or no value unless one is looking for a specific exogenous organism, such as Group A streptococcus or *Neisseria gonorrhea*. Microscopic examination of a urine sample is very helpful if the specimen is properly obtained (clean catch or catheter). A chest x-ray would be in order only if there are suggestive physical findings. The white count will be moderately elevated as a result of the surgery and is, therefore, of limited value. A hemoglobin or hematocrit might be helpful, especially if there is concern about a collection at the operative site.

The selection of an antibiotic(s) for this patient must be based upon several considerations. The first is the most likely site of the infection. If the site is the urinary tract, there is probably a single pathogen, *E. coli*, and if it resulted from a hospital-inserted catheter there is a significant chance (30% to 40%) that it will be resistant to ampicillin. If the infection is at the operative site, in the pelvis, it is likely polymicrobial and will involve both aerobes and anaerobes from the patient's vaginal flora. Although these are not hospital acquired organisms, there are likely to be significant resistance problems, particularly with the anaerobes, and especially *Bacteroides* species. If the site is the abdominal wound, endogenous organisms are likely but the possibility of a resistant Staphylococcus must be kept in mind.

Another consideration is the clinical status of the patient. If, for example, there is a superficial wound infection in an otherwise healthy patient, antibiotics are almost secondary and the problem may be solved with drainage. If a patient is seriously ill with the threat of septic shock, however, then one must use maximal antibiotic coverage.

It is often suggested that a single bactericidal agent is superior to combinations and static antibiotics. Combinations, however, are often needed to cover the multiple organisms and cidal agents are not critical in most instances. Toxicity is a major consideration and one should always select the least toxic agent or combination that will provide the coverage needed. The beta-lactam antibiotics, penicillins, and cephalosporins, are generally less toxic agents because of their mode of action. They inhibit cell wall synthesis and human cells lack cell walls. In this day of cost containment, that is also a consideration if efficacy is equivalent.

For this patient, if my suspicion was of an operative site infection, I would probably not have selected ampicillin alone. This is a choice which might prove effective, especially if a cuff collection were drained; however, if the infection proved to be serious, it is likely that both an aminoglycoside and an agent to cover *Bacteroides* (clindamycin or metronidazole) would ultimately need to be added. If the patient appeared clinically ill at the start one might select a combination of clindamycin and gentamicin or alternatively as a single agent, cefoxitin. My preference is to treat parenterally until the patient has become afebrile and remains so for 24 to 48 hours. I would then discontinue the antibiotics and observe for an additional 24 hours and discharge without antibiotics.

The use of perioperative antibiotic prophylaxis in abdominal hysterectomy is still somewhat controversial. It is probably best decided based upon the postoperative infection rate in a gynecologist's practice. If the rate is low (less than 10%), the use of prophylaxis is probably not justified. If higher, the approach will likely reduce the rate of morbidity and shorten hospital stay. My preference for prophylaxis is to use a short (3-dose) periopeative course of a first generation cephalosporin, such as cefazolin.

The subject of an open or closed vaginal cuff is one of almost religious commitment by gynecologists. I am a fence-sitter in this area and close the cuff in "dry" uncomplicated cases with the intention of achieving faster and cleaner healing of the cuff. In patients with infection or less than a "dry" operative field, I leave the cuff open. I have no good supporting data to indicate whether the management of the cuff influences the risk of postoperative infection.

A final consideration should be failure of response. When this occurs the surgeon should first consider the antibiotic coverage. Is it complete? The areas of special concern would be resistant anaerobes especially *Bacteroides* species and *Enterococcus* which is not covered by cephalosporins or combinations without penicillin or ampicillin. If this does not seem to be the cause then the most likely explanation of failed response is an undrained collection (hematoma or abscess). Septic pelvic thrombophlebitis and drug fever are considerations as well but far less likely.

Selected Readings

Gorbach SI, Bartlett JG: Anaerobic infections. *N Engl J Med* 290:1177, 1974.

Ledger WJ, Child MA: The hospital care of patients undergoing hysterectomy: an analysis of 12,026 patients from the professional activity study. *Am J Obstet Gynecol* 117:423, 1973.

Ledger WH, Norman M, Gee C, et al: Bacteremia on an active obstetric-gynecologic service. *Am J Obstet Gynecol* 121:205, 1975.

Mead PB, Gump DW: Antibiotic therapy in obstetrics and gynecology. *Clin Obstet Gynecol* 19:109, 1976.

Schulman H, Zatuchini G: Pelvic thrombophlebitis in the puerperal and postoperative patient. *Am J Obstet Gynecol* 90:293, 1969.

CHAPTER 5

Postoperative Septic Pelvic Thrombophlebitis

JAMES L. BREEN, M.D., F.A.C.O.G., F.A.C.S.
JULIAN E. DeLIA, M.D., F.A.C.O.G.

CASE ABSTRACT

A 36-year-old multipara had undergone total abdominal hysterectomy and bilateral salpingo-oophorectomy because of chronic, recurrent pyosalpinx. She had four episodes of clinical flare-up with chills, fever, pain, and menorrhagia during the year preceding surgery. These episodes had become more frequent, with the most recent one 7 weeks prior to the surgery.

Surgery was complicated by many old and new pelvic adhesions. A right tubo-ovarian abscess spilled into the abdominal wound during the course of surgery. The pelvis was irrigated with 2 quarts of sterile saline and the vaginal vault closed.

There was considerable postoperative pain and a sustained fever varying between 102 and 104 F degrees beginning the first postoperative day. Intravenous penicillin and chloramphenicol were administered. By the third postoperative day the fever had become spiking in character, with a tachycardia sustained even when the temperature was at its lowest. Temperature spikes up to 104 degrees F were preceded by a shaking chill followed by profuse sweating. Examination at this time revealed minimum pelvic tenderness with no masses palpable.

DISCUSSION

The patient described in the case presentation fulfills the classic description of the "pelvic cripple." Despite treatment of the initial episode the patient continues to have flare-ups with fever, pain, menorrhagia, and pelvic masses. The initial episode may have been a postpartum or postabortal infection, pelvic inflammatory disease from a sexually transmitted pathogen, or as a complication of previous pelvic surgery. In most instances, regardless of age, resolution of the problem is by surgical intervention with the expectation of performing a total abdominal hysterectomy and bilateral salpingo-oophorectomy.

Based on the history, findings at surgery, the amount of surgical dissection necessary, and the rupture and "leak" of the abscess, this patient would be anticipated to have a stormy postoperative course. In light of this, several preoperative, intraoperative, and postoperative prophylactic measures could have been taken. Now, 3 days after surgery, the clinician is faced with a patient who is febrile, very ill, and unresponsive to the usual therapeutic measures.

In order to manage a gynecologic patient with postoperative febrile morbidity, it is important that the clinician understand the microorganisms involved and the techniques to identify them, the spectrum of activity and toxicity of available antibiotics, and the role of additional surgery to drain collections of pus, if necessary. We are handicapped at present by the fact that no uniformly satisfactory methods exist to culture specimens from deep-seated infections, i.e., parametritis, pelvic cellulitis, and septic pelvic thrombophlebitis. We can overcome this handicap, however, by understanding those organisms that are most likely to cause pelvic in-

Table 5.1
Organisms Recovered from Pelvic Infections

Aerobic bacteria	
Gram-positive	*Streptococcus*
	Staphylococcus
Gram-positive rods	*Diphtheroids*
	Listeria monocytogenes
Gram-negative rods	*Escherichia coli*
	Klebsiella
	Pseudomonas
	Proteus
	Enterobacter
	Serratia
Anaerobic bacteria	
Gram-positive cocci	*Peptostreptococcus*
	Peptococcus
Gram-positive rods	*Clostridium* species
Gram-negative rods	*Bacteroides* species
	Fusobacterium species

Table 5.2
Differential Diagnosis in Septic Postoperative Patients

Atelectasis and pneumonia
Urinary tract damage or infection
Infected pelvic hematoma
Wound infection (clostridial or necrotizing fasciitis)
Bacterial resistance to appropriate or inappropriate antibiotic therapy
Generalized peritonitis
Endotoxic shock
Pelvic cellulitis
Pelvic or intra-abdominal abscess
Septic pelvic thrombophlebitis

fections. Curiously, the majority of postoperative pelvic infections are caused by endogenous organisms normally found in the vaginal flora. These organisms become opportunistic pathogens in tissues damaged by trauma or exogenous pathogens; i.e., *Neisseria gonorrhoeae*. The organisms most often involved in postoperative infections in pelvic surgery are given in Table 5.1. Current investigations have demonstrated the mixed nature (aerobic and anaerobic) of pelvic and intra-abdominal infections. Of special note is the emergence of the role of anaerobic bacteria, now isolated from 70% to 100% of pelvic infections (4).

Before the cause of the postoperative fever is assigned to a vaginal cuff infection or pelvic cellulitis in this patient, it is essential to conduct a complete physical examination to rule out other causes.

Differential Diagnosis

The differential diagnosis of conditions potentially responsible for this patient's fever is outlined in Table 5.2. Pelvic surgery in the face of chronic pelvic inflammatory disease will place the patient at an increased risk for all of the complications listed. Conversely, descriptions of these conditions in texts generally list chronic pelvic inflammatory disease as a risk factor in their etiology. All must be considered in this patient, while the site of infection and organisms involved are sought. The immediate threat

to life would come from Gram-negative sepsis with endotoxic shock, clostridial sepsis, necrotizing fasciitis, and septic pelvic thrombophlebitis with widespread dissemination of septic emboli.

A common cause of early postoperative fever and tachycardia is pulmonary atelectasis which, if unrelieved, leads to pneumonitis. The patient had a prolonged operation followed by considerable pain and probable abdominal distention, all of which are contributing factors. Usually, basilar rales are heard on auscultation of the chest, and roentgenographic examination may detect more extensive involvement.

Extravasation of urine into the peritoneal cavity or retroperitoneum from bladder or ureteral injury can result in high spiking fevers and chills in the early postoperative period. Pyuria and flank pain may be present, and abdominal distention or leakage of urine from wounds will eventually appear. An intravenous pyelogram will clarify the site of injury when clinical findings suggest this possibility.

Hematoma formation or intra-abdominal bleeding in the face of active infection can also cause fever. A falling hematocrit or an expanding mass on examination would suggest this possibility, and immediate reoperation may be necessary. Eventually, this would lead to pelvic or abdominal abscess formation. Ultrasound scanning is useful to identify this and other possible complications.

Wound infections are frequent with surgery, in the presence of active pelvic infections. The quantity of bacterial contamination, blood and foreign material left in the wound, and the appropriate use of drains, delayed closure, and antibiotics will determine whether a wound infection develops. Although wound infections develop to the stage of clinical recognition 5 to 6 days after surgery, there are two exceptions, i.e., clostridial infections and necrotizing fasciitis. In necrotizing fasciitis the wound is excruciatingly painful and is characterized by dark vesicles, dusky discoloration, and widespread ecchymosis on the surrounding skin. Later, there is anesthesia of the affected area with subcutaneous and facial necrosis which results in extensive undermining of the skin. Hemolytic *Streptococcus* and hemolytic *Staphylococcus*, as well as a variety of virulent Gram-negative bacteria, are responsible. The wound and its cutaneous manifestations, along with the initial systemic signs of clostridial infections, resemble necrotizing fasciitis. Tachycardia out of proportion to the degree of fever is a constant finding. The early differential diagnosis of the two conditions can be made on a Gram's stain of the wound exudate.

The choice of an initial antibiotic regimen is not inordinately difficult when one considers the potential pathogenic organisms and their antimicrobial susceptibility. The combination of penicillin and chloramphenicol in appropriate doses provides excellent coverage of most potential pelvic pathogens. This regimen may, however, be considered obsolete in contemporary practice. Most Gràm-negative aerobes, enterococci, unusual Clostridia, and some *Bacteroides* may not be covered. Other recently recommended regimens that are more appropriate for this patient are an aminoglycoside/clindamycin or aminoglycoside/metronidazole combination (5).

Penicillin is the drug of choice for all anaerobes except *Bacteroides fragilis*. Lately, there has been an increasing awareness of the role of Bacteroides in septic conditions originating below the diaphragms. Although in vitro activity of chloramphenicol has been excellent against this organism, multiple reports have appeared of patients who have failed to respond clinically to chloramphenicol (6).

One final concern in antibiotic failure is the observation that the antibiotic susceptibility patterns of bacteria, especially the Gram-negative enteric bacilli, vary from hospital to hospital. Clinicians should be familiar with updated results of sensitivity patterns of clinical isolates from their microbiology laboratories to aid in directing antibiotic therapy.

Generalized peritonitis and endotoxic shock are common complications of spontaneous rupture of a tubo-ovarian abscess. Although a tubo-ovarian abscess was ruptured during surgery, appropriate measures were taken. It is the delayed operation in the face of rupture that causes the high mortality associated with this condition. With the signs and symptoms of septicemia manifested by this patient, careful observation for signs of shock are indicated. It is important to note that, although Gram-negative aerobes, the organisms most often associated with endotoxic shock, are generally sensitive to chloramphenicol, it is not considered the drug of choice. The greatest number of these organisms will respond to an aminoglycoside. Aminoglycosides are bactericidal, while chloramphenicol is bacteriostatic. The addition of an aminoglycoside without discontinuing the penicillin, chloramphenicol, or clindamycin will provide coverage of most pathogens in septic gynecologic patients.

Infections at the operative site are the most common cause of fever following hysterectomy. There is an expected febrile morbidity of 20% to 30% for abdominal hysterectomy and 30% to 40% for vaginal hysterectomy. These infections range from minimal pelvic cellulitis to pelvic abscess formation or septic pelvic thrombophlebitis. Serious infection manifested by early-onset sepsis or late-onset abscess formation can occur after surgery, especially if the operative field was contaminated. Prolonged operating time, raw surfaces, and poor hemostasis also enhance growth of bacteria.

These infections, although classified separately, are essentially a single infection caused by a mixed aerobic and anaerobic bacteria found in the flora of the lower genital tract and bowel. The infection, as recently demonstrated in the animal model, occurs in two phases (9). The first phase, manifested by peritonitis and sepsis, was due to Gram-negative facultative aerobic bacteria, especially *Escherichia coli*. The second phase, characterized by the formation of abscesses, was associated with anaerobic bacteria, in particular, *B. fragilis*. The biphasic disease process occurs in those pelvic infections that the obstetrician-gynecologist encounters, i.e., postpartum infections.

The diagnosis of pelvic cellulitis is suggested by fever (<102 degrees F) appearing 2 to 4 days after surgery, with minimal pelvic pain and tenderness. Although some induration may be noted, no masses are palpable on bimanual examination, and no drainage occurs on probing the vaginal cuff.

A vaginal cuff abscess typically presents 3 to 6 days after surgery and is accompanied by fever (<102 degrees F), pelvic pain or rectal pressure, and a palpable fullness at the apex of the vault. Drainage is generally seen on probing. An ultrasound scan aids in locating intra-abdominal abscesses and demonstrates their regression or progression. The signs and symptoms of sepsis will persist in the presence of an abscess despite adequate antibiotics until drainage is established, either spontaneously or surgically.

Septic pelvic thrombophlebitis has been described as "enigmatic fever," that is, persistent in spite of proper antibiotic therapy. High spiking fevers (>102 degrees F) with disparate tachycardia, chills, and minimal pelvic findings are the rule. With the absence of pelvic findings, it can be tentatively diagnosed in this patient. The use of heparin at this point would be both therapeutic and diagnostic. The response to heparin is usually dramatic in septic pelvic thrombophlebitis. Consequently, it would be reasonable to allow 24 to 48 hours for a therapeutic trial with heparin before going to the next step, which would likely be a laparotomy. Heparin will not mask other types of infection. Anaerobic bacteria have a propensity for causing phlebitis and *Bacteroides fragilis* produces a heparinase that facilitates septic phlebitis. It is unknown, at this time, why the appropriate antibiotics alone do not resolve the condition without the addition of heparin. If a response is noted, the diagnosis is assured, and therapy should be continued for 10 days. We prefer the intravenous route, by continuous infusion, with a goal of maintaining appropriate clotting tests two to two and one-half times the control value. The antibiotics should also be continued.

Prophylactic Measures

When performing surgery for residual pelvic inflammatory disease, postoperative morbidity should be anticipated and prophylactic measures taken. These measures may include: (a) proper timing of surgery, (b) preoperative antibiotics, (c) careful dissection and hemostasis, and (d) proper use of drainage.

The optimal time to perform surgery for chronic pelvic inflammatory disease is between flare-ups rather than when the patient is acutely ill. At least 4 to 6 weeks from the last attack would be ideal. However, an acute inflammation not responding to medical therapy is also an indication for operative intervention. In series where more aggressive approaches were taken during the active phases, significant intraoperative and postoperative complications occurred (2).

The use of prophylactic antibiotics for routine surgery is somewhat controversial. However, in high-risk cases where pelvic infection is the indication for surgery, their use is recommended to decrease their inoculum size. Guidelines for their use have been outlined (7). Many regimens have been proposed with equally successful results; therefore, it would be hard to be dogmatic about specific drug use. We utilize a single drug of low cost and toxicity (ampicillin, a first generation cephalosporin, or a tetracycline), saving more potent antibiotics to combat resistant infections. The antibiotic should be given immediately preoperatively to afford delivery to the operative site and be continued for only two to three doses postoperatively. Thereafter, the antibiotic used for prophylaxis should not be used for therapy if a clinical infection develops.

Failure to adhere to good surgical principles often results in postoperative complications. Gentle handling of tissues, meticulous hemostasis, eliminating dead space, avoiding bowel and urinary tract damage, and avoiding the spread of purulent material with liberal use of lavage are of utmost importance in these cases.

The final consideration in this case is drainage. We see three areas where drainage may have been indicated. In light of the bacterial contamination of the wound, a subcutaneous drain (Penrose), brought out lateral to the skin incision, is indicated. In severe infections, however, it is sometimes better to leave the wound open and afford secondary closure at a later date (1). The use of intra-abdominal drainage will depend on factors such as the extent of raw surfaces and the inability to excise the abscess cavity completely. We would bring this drain (Penrose) out through the vaginal vault. It has been shown that even in an uncomplicated hysterectomy a considerable amount of serosanguineous fluid collects in the retroperitoneal space (3). Postoperative morbidity is reduced if this fluid is evacuated. Alternatively, a closed suction sump drain may be placed retroperitoneally and brought out through the flank if the vaginal vault is closed. Lastly, we would employ nasogastric suction to avoid an ileus that is almost certain to occur if significant bowel manipulation and contamination occur. Two of the most commonly associated findings in wound dehiscences are bacterial contamination of the wound and mechanical factors such as abdominal distention. In addition, if a midline incision would be preferred, a Smead-Jones wound closure may be used (8). With a mortality of 10% to 20%, dehiscence is a complication to be avoided.

References

1. Brown SE, Allen HH, Robins, RH: The use of delayed primary wound infections. *Am J Obstet Gynecol* 127:713, 1977.
2. Kaplan AL, Jacobs, WM, Ehresman, JR: Aggressive management of pelvic abscess. *Am J Obstet Gynecol* 98:982, 1975.
3. Swartz WH, Tanaree P: Suction drainage as an alternative to prophylactic antibiotics for hysterectomy. *Obstet Gynecol* 45:305, 1975.
4. Sweet RL: Anaerobic infections in the female genital tract. *Am J Obstet Gynecol* 122:891, 1975.
5. Sweet RL, Yonkura ML, Hill G, et al: Appropriate use of antibiotics in serious obstetric and gynecologic infections. *Am J Obstet Gynecol* 146:719, 1983.
6. Thadepalli H, Gorback SL, Bartlett JG: Apparent failure of chloramphenicol in the treatment of anaerobic infections. *Curr Ther Res* 22:421, 1977.
7. The Medical Letter 27(703):105, 1985.
8. Wallace D, Hernandez W, Schlaerth JB, et al: Prevention of abdominal wound disruption utilizing the Smead-Jones closure technique. *Obstet Gynecol* 56:226, 1980.
9. Weinstein WM, Onderdonk AB, Bartlett JG, et al: Experimental intraabdominal abscesses in rats: Development of an experimental model. *Infect Immunol* 10:1250, 1974.

CHAPTER 6

Ovarian Remnant Syndrome

RAYMOND A. LEE, M.D.

CASE ABSTRACT 1

A 38-year-old gravida 1, para 1 underwent total abdominal hysterectomy and bilateral salpingo-oophorectomy for symptomatic pelvic endometriosis. The postoperative course was uneventful. During routine bimanual pelvic examination 2 years later, a 4-cm, slightly tender and mobile left-sided pelvic mass was found above the vagina. No supplemental estrogens had been prescribed postoperatively, there was no history of "hot flashes," and the vaginal skin did not appear to be atrophic. She was examined every 6 weeks and the size of the mass essentially unchanged over the year. A sonogram reported a 5-cm left "adnexal mass" containing a solid rim posteriorly and a 3-cm cystic area anteriorly. Despite the history of left oophorectomy, this mass had the appearance of an enlarged left ovary containing a cyst.

CASE ABSTRACT 2

Total abdominal hysterectomy and bilateral salpingo-oohorectomy because of severe and chronic pelvic inflammatory disease had been performed 10 years ago on a now 34-four-year-old nullipara. The patient presently has a three month history of progressively disabling left iliac pain with some radiation to the lower back, but not down the leg. Pelvic tenderness without the discrete mass was noted on pelvic exmaination, and sonography identified a 3 X 4 cm cystic mass on the left side of the pelvis, apparently retroperitoneal. An intravenous pyelogram showed extrinsic compression of the lower third of the left ureter by this mass. A review of the previous operative record described considerable difficulty encountered in mobilizing and removing a left tubo-ovarian mass, which had been adherent to the pelvic side wall.

DISCUSSION

Typically, the patient with the ovarian remnant syndrome has pelvic pain (with or without a mass) or has a palpable pelvic cystic mass (without symptoms) after undergoing bilateral salpingo-oophorectomy, and residual ovarian tissue is found at reoperation.

Predisposing Factors

Conditions associated with dense adhesions, diffuse inflammatory reaction, or distortion of pelvic anatomy leading to a difficult dissection may result in the inadvertent retention of a fragment of ovarian tissue. The most frequent predisposing conditions are endometriosis, pelvic inflammatory disease, diverticulitis, and a previous operation with resultant adhesions. The operative procedures are usually appendectomy or a conservative gynecologic procedure. This syndrome can be prevented by the excision of the peritoneum of the pelvic sidewall and cul-de-sac when the ovary is solidly adherent to these areas as a result of an inflammatory process.

Symptoms. Usually, the syndrome occurs within 5 years after bilateral salpingo-oophorectomy. The most frequent presenting symptom or sign is pelvic pain with a mass. Occasionally, the patient may have pelvic pain without a discernible mass or may have an asymptomatic mass. The pain may vary from a sensation of pelvic pressure to a dull ache to a sharp stabbing pain. Occasionally, there may be dyspareunia, and gastrointestinal and gastrourinary symptoms may be part of the clinical pattern. The patient may experience temporary hot flushes immediately after operation, only to have them spontaneously disappear, suggesting the resurgence of estrogen production.

Diagnosis.   The diagnosis is usually suggested by the history and physical findings. Because of the frequent extraperitoneal location or presence of extensive adhesions, laparoscopic examination is rarely beneficial or necessary. Ultrasound examination and computed tomographic scans are helpful in further delineating the size and location of the mass. A preoperative intravenous pyelogram or retrograde studies may show obstruction (Fig. 6.1); however, the absence of apparent involvement should not misguide the surgeon. The surgeon should be prepared to dissect the ureter throughout its pelvic course because it always will have some involvement.

Treatment.   It has been suggested that pelvic radiation be may used in the management of this syndrome, yet one hesitates to advocate

radiation for a benign condition. My colleagues and I have seen several patients with persistent symptoms despite various hormonal therapies or pelvic radiation (or both). We prefer an operative approach without preoperative placement of ureteral catheters regardless of the preoperative intravenous or retrograde pyelography findings. Prevention of ureteral injury requires that the peritoneum be opened laterally, well above the pathological process. The ureter is then followed inferiorly, and sharp dissection is used to ensure minimal trauma to its sheath. If during this dissection a ureteral catheter is to be placed, the bladder is opened in an extraperitoneal location and a no. 5 ureteral catheter is passed in a retrograde fashion. Usually, a ureteral catheter is unnecessary and is not routinely placed because its unyielding nature may add to the potential of ureteral injury. Excellent exposure with appropriate traction and countertraction and good hemostasis will facilitate the dissection of contiguous structures (bowel, bladder, vessels, and nerve roots) to ensure safe, complete removal of the ovarian remnant (Fig. 6.2). Usually, the entire

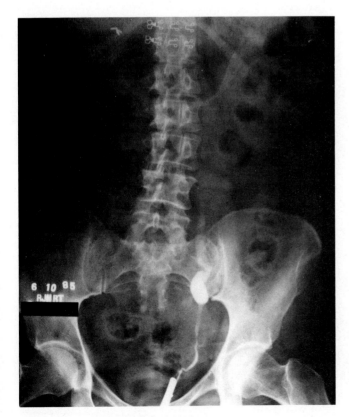

Figure 6.1. Preoperative retrograde pyelogram demonstrating narrowing of lower ureteral segment, with dilated ureter proximal to ovarian remnant mass.

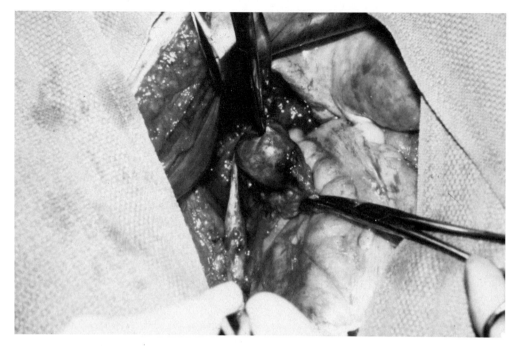

Figure 6.2.   Early dissection showing ureter dissected at pelvic brim with ovarian remnant intact and medial to ureter.

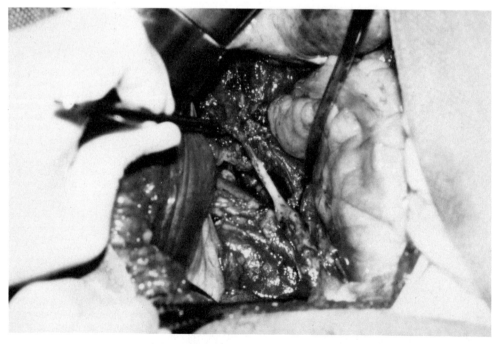

Figure 6.3.   Ureter dissected throughout its pelvic course from pelvic brim to entrance into bladder.

pelvic course of the ureter is dissected before the ovarian remnant is safely removed (Fig. 6.3).

Selected Readings

Berek JS, Darney PD, Lopkin C, et al: Avoiding ureteral damage in pelvic surgery for ovarian remnant syndrome. *Am J Obstet Gynecol* 133:221-222, 1979.

Christ JE, Lotze EC: The residual ovary syndrome. *Obstet Gynecol* 46:551-556, 1975.

Lee RA, Silverman LF, Pratt JH: Sigmoidal complications of left ovarian enlargement. *Minn Med* 55:565-567, 1972.

Symmonds RE, Pettit PDM: Ovarian remnant syndrome. *Obstet Gynecol* 54:174-177, 1979.

CHAPTER 7

Pending Evisceration Post-Laparotomy

CHARLES E. FLOWERS, JR., M.D.

CASE ABSTRACT

Because of symptomatic leiomyomata, a total abdominal hysterectomy had been performed in an 40-year-old diabetic. On the morning of the sixth postoperative day, there was a serosanguinous discharge from the wound, the dressing was changed, and the floor nurse called the attending surgeon. Four hours later, it was observed that the recently changed dressing was now soaked with a serosanguinous fluid. The surgeon probed the wound with the tip of a Kelly hemostatic forceps, for what seemed to the full depth of the wound. The patient was afebrile, and there was no purulent discharge. A superficial Penrose drain was placed in the site that had been probed, and a tight strapping of the edges of the wound was performed. Over the next 36 hours the amount of serosanguinous drainage progressively increased, although the patient remained asymptomatic.

DISCUSSION

When an abdominal wound exudes serosanguinous fluid, a total wound breakdown with evisceration is the diagnosis which must be excluded. It is essential to investigate the wound until the proper diagnosis is made. The condition is due to a myriad of cellular responses related to healing that did interdigitate. Some of the factors that interfere with this process are age, malignancy, radiation, poor nutrition, blood supply, protein, caloric and vitamin intake, infection, and poor surgical technique.

The differential diagnosis in this patient is impending evisceration versus fat necrosis, a seroma, or a small peritoneal fistula that will not require surgical repair.

The diagnosis is made by probing the wound in an effort to determine the integrity of the fascia. If a portion of the skin incision must be broken down to make the diagnosis, then break it down! If is necessary to take the patient back to the operating room and investigate the wound; do so! One must not be falsely assured if there appears to be only a very small area of dehiscence. If the process of healing is absent in a small portion of the wound, the integrity of the entire wound must be suspect. X-ray or ultrasound studies of the wound are not rewarding.

This case history indicates there is dehiscence. The continued exuding of serosanguinous fluid for 4 hours after the wound has been probed would indicate that the patient should be taken to the operating room. Nothing was gained with the 36-hour delay: a great deal could be lost in terms of fluid, electrolytes, and protein, and the development of generalized infection.

It is appropriate to consider how this surgical complication could be prevented. The patient is obese, 40 years old, and a diabetic. This places her in an extremely high-risk category for wound dehiscence. The preferable closure of the fascia would have been with polydioxanone (PDS) or polypropylene suture run continuously with each suture being at least 2 1/2 to 4 cm from the midline and advanced only 1 1/2 cm with each stitch.

An interrrupted Smead-Jones stitch with a PDS suture would be an excellent choice. It is felt that catgut, or polyglycolic acid suture should not be used in such a high-risk patient.

Appropriate preoperative preparation of this patient is mandatory prior to the reoperation, i.e., fluid electrolyte replacement, regulation of glucose metabolism, initiation of broad spectrum antibiotic coverage, and blood transfusion if the patient has a hematocrit below 25.

Whether general anesthesia with muscle relaxants, spinal anesthesia, or epidural anesthesia is used is not nearly as important as the skill of the anesthesiologist.

Since this patient has had dehiscence of the wound for a considerable period of time, it is likely that the bowel is adherent to an underportion of the incision and if great care is not taken, bowel mucosa can be denuded over a large area or the bowel can be perforated. It is, therefore, important that the incision be carefully opened and the bowel be handled gently. If an area of dense adhesions is present, it is preferable to use a very sharp knife and leave a portion of the fascia on the bowel. The incision should be thoroughly irrigated with normal saline and the borders of the incision carefully inspected to determine if any areas of necrosis should be removed.

The principle of the repair of a dehiscence is to use through- and-through sutures which will maintain the integrity of the wound for 14 to 21 days. The separate suturing of the fascia is preferable but not absolutely mandatory. The peritoneum does not need to be closed.

The preferable repair is with a continuous suture of polypropylene or polydioxanone (PDS or polyglyconate (Maxon) placed 2 1/2 to 4 cm from the midline on each side with the abdominal wall being closed with through-and-through sutures of nylon or Dermalon. Before the nylon sutures are tied, one must be certain that there is no bowel insinuated between the fascial closure and the sutures.

An ideal through-and-through suture is silver wire but this is rarely readily available. Nylon is an acceptable substitute. The subcutaneous fat should not be closed in any operation and certainly not following the dehiscence of a wound. If there is fat necrosis or considerable exudate coming from the fat, a closed catheter drainage should be placed. There is no contraindication to closing the skin incision with skin clips.

CHAPTER 8
Intraoperative Hemorrhage

BYRON J. MASTERSON, M.D., F.A.C.S., F.A.C.O.G.

CASE ABSTRACT 1: INSECURELY TIED INFUNDIBULOPELVIC LIGAMENT

During a total abdominal hysterectomy and bilateral salpingo-oophorectomy performed through a Pfannenstiel incision to relieve a 35-year-old patient of a symptomatic fibroid uterus, it was evident that there was some unexpected ovarian endometriosis present. As an initial step in the operation, it was decided to perform a simultaneous bilateral salpingo-oophorectomy. The infundibulopelvic ligament on each side was clamped and ligated, and the hysterectomy was commenced. Exposure was a problem, and several packs were inserted to push the bowel away from the operative field. When the removal of the uterus had been completed, pelvic peritonealization considered, and the lower packs removed, it was evident that the tie holding the right infundibulopelvic ligament had partially slipped. A 5 × 7 cm hematoma was already evident in the stump of the right infundibulopelvic ligament. The tie was removed and dissection initiated to find the source of bleeding. The hematoma rapidly increased in size and bleeding increased, but the specific source of bleeding became more elusive.

DISCUSSION
Identification of the Problem

The patient has had an ovarian artery or vein retract from the original tie and is now bleeding into the retroperitoneal space. The operator should always aggressively identify this type of bleeder at the time of surgery. Retroperitoneal accumulation of blood, with associated protracted ileus, abdominal discomfort, and on occasion retroperitoneal abscess formation, can produce significant morbidity.

Prevention of the Problem

The term "infundibulopelvic ligament ligation" should be abandoned, as the process involved is really the ligation of the ovarian artery and veins. The use of large crushing clamps across the venous plexus is hazardous. The most secure method is to pass a suture around the vessels after they have been dissected free and the ureters have been identified. This should be followed with a suture ligature placed distally with the needle placed to the central portion of the venous plexus and tied in front and behind. Ovarian vein hematomas will almost never be seen if the veins are handled this way. If, however, the crushing clamps are placed, particularly if the less desirable double clamp technique is used, hematomas are not uncommon.

Management of This Problem

The operator is now faced with the difficulty of identifying a vessel in a somewhat edematous and engorged space. The operator should grasp the lower end of the veins with a small clamp, identify the ureter, and dissect sharply upward in the retroperitoneal space, constantly observing the ureter. Additional exposure can be attained by incising up either gutter and reflecting the colon, or medially and reflecting the peritoneum.

As soon as one has reached the top of the hematoma as identified by resumption of the veins into a more normal caliber, place a right angled clamp about them. Pass a tie around the veins at this point, again carefully identifying the ureter. One may perform either suture ligature, noted above, or occasionally a large clip may be placed below the vein. The hematoma, thus isolated, should be removed. Any small venous contributors to this hematoma should be clipped with small clips, or the electrocautery may be used. The distal end of the veins near the hysterectomy site should again be inspected to make sure that they are not contributing to the hematoma formation. A dry pack should be placed with some pressure over the site where the hematoma had been removed. One rarely will encounter difficulty in controlling such bleeding where sharp dissection and precise vessel ligation are performed. The operator should avoid the tendency to place large clamps and sutures in and around this hematoma as he will only injure adjacent structures and almost never accomplish the desired results of precise ligation of the contributing vessels and removal of the trapped hematoma. If necessary, the ovarian artery of either side may be ligated near its origin from the aorta just below that of the renal arteries, proximal to the hematoma.

CASE ABSTRACT 2: DAMAGE TO INTERNAL ILIAC VEIN

During ligation of the left internal iliac artery for control of persistent angle bleeding following hysterectomy, the wall of the internal iliac vein was lacerated. Hemorrhage was temporarily controlled by direct pressure to the vein. A call for a vascular surgeon was fruitless.

DISCUSSION

Injury to adjacent structures in pelvic surgery almost always is due to poor exposure. Exposure may be limited by too small an incision, inadequate assistance, poor instruments, pelvic masses such as cervical fibroid obscuring the area, blood obscuring the visualization, inappropriate anesthesia, or poor operative lights. The injury has occurred in this particular case at the time of ligation of the internal iliac artery for control of bleeding at the vaginal angle. The author would disagree with the surgeon that unilateral ligation of an internal iliac artery is of much value in the control of pelvic bleeding from the vaginal angle. One need only look at the intense arterial anastomosis around the vaginal tube to realize such a maneuver offers little chance of producing hemostasis. A much more appropriate maneuver would be to isolate the artery in question with appropriate exposure and to ligate it at its source. Secondly, bleeding as described in this case, at the vaginal angle, is often venous in origin and not influenced by isolating and ligating the internal iliac artery. One can demonstrate this by ligating the internal iliac artery during the course of a radical hysterectomy and then producing an operative injury in an area which will subsequently be excised. Bleeding will be brisk and not affected by unilateral internal iliac artery ligation. If the reader is still unimpressed, place a vascular clamp across the entire arterial tree and divide an artery or vein below the site of ligation. One will be unable to detect the difference in bleeding volume whether the vessel is clamped or not, due to the intense pelvic anastomosis so well demonstrated with pelvic arteriography. In managing the defect produced, the operator is faced with the control of bleeding in a structure which frequently cannot be mobilized. The exiting branches of the internal iliac vein are fixed, fragile, and may produce almost uncontrollable hemorrhage if injured. Great care must be exercised in manipulating this venous tree. The initial response to such bleeding should be prompt pressure directly applied upon the defect against the pelvic wall. The surgeon should then advise the anesthesiologist to secure an additional 4 units of blood for transfusion, immediately secure additional lighting, both overhead and the flexible intraoperative type, and get an additional suction and any additional assistance needed. Delicate thumb forceps, needle holders, bulldog clamps, and other vascular instruments should be brought to the operative site, and hopefully such instruments are in the operator's usual instrument set. Kocher and Heaney clamps and other nonvascular instruments are hazardous in the extreme in handling delicate branches of the internal iliac vein. Delicate swedged-on vascular suture of 5-0 size, monofilament type is most useful, and hemostatic clips of both small and large size with long appliers should be immediately at hand.

Direct an assistant to maintain pressure on the vein by pressing it gently against the pelvic wall. Proceed to expose the vein by lifting the left round ligament strongly upward. Place a medium Deaver retractor above the femoral artery and dissect upward to the bifurcation of the common iliac artery. Identify the ureter and direct the scissor downward along its medial leaf. Enter the pararectal and paravesical spaces and identify the obliterated hypogastric artery and the obturator nerve. Be reassured as the entire internal iliac venous tree may be ligated with impunity, as may any of its branches, so that one need not preserve the integrity of this vein to continue vascular function of the pelvis. Place two suction tips in the wound, place a flexible fibroptic light source over the pelvic wall, and gently remove the sponge stick pressed against the venous defect. The operator may be delighted to find that the bleeding has ceased. Less fortunately, he may be amazed by the volume of blood escaping from a relatively small defect in the vein. Do not attempt to operate on this venous defect with Kocher, Heaney, or other large crushing toothed clamps. One may convert a small defect, which can be easily managed with a single clip, to a laceration involving two or three venous trunks, which may only be controlled by a complex procedure requiring numerous blood transfusions.

As soon as the operator has clearly identified the defect and its size, replace the sponge stick. Put a sucker directly near the defect. If the defect is small, a small clip or two will quickly close the hole in the vein and control bleeding. The presence of a clip on the defect makes its suture infinitely more difficult, as the clip will be incorporated in the suture and the defect will not close. Therefore, avoid using clips with large lacerations when suture is contemplated. If the defect is large, one may divide the vein by placing large clips on each of the defect. Remember the vein in this area is not a simple tube but a branching system which may have veins entering its lateral surface which cannot be seen by the operator. In this case, one may place a running vascular suture in the vein and control bleeding. If, however, the laceration is large, and several venous trees have been torn where several perforators enter, a truly hazard-

ous circumstance exists. Where concerted effort does not produce control of the bleeding, and hemorrhage is life threatening, two maneuvers remain: (a) sew over the entire area with a 0 chromic suture in a continuous fashion; (b) realize that some of the pelvic plexus of nerves may sustain some injury during this maneuver, and inform the family at the conclusion of the procedure.

As a last resort, tightly pack the pelvis with a large breast roll gauze and layer the gauze into the pelvis in such a way that its removal will not produce knots, causing difficulty in its extraction from the wound. Before placement, soak the upper portion of the roll with Betadine and bring it out the edge of the abdominal wound. Close the wound with retention sutures and leave a 4- to 5-cm defect for pack removal untied. Send the patient to the intensive care unit and observe her carefully. If bleeding is controlled bring the patient back to the operating room in 48 hours. Administer a light anesthetic, remove the pack, and irrigate the wound gently to remove any superficial hematoma. Tie the retention sutures, do not manipulate the area of the old venous injury, and do not use any sutures in the skin. While hernias are increased when packs are used through the incision, little other morbidity is usually noted. Other methods to be considered are arterial catherization and selective Gelfoam embolization. Pitressin infusion may also be useful.

Avoid injury to the internal iliac venous system by carefully exposing the area before any manipulations are performed, and avoid the double clamp system of pelvic surgery. One will rarely be faced with a lacerated internal iliac vein if this advice is followed.

Selected Readings

Bergan JJ, Dean RH, Yao JT: Vascular injuries in pelvic cancer surgery. *Am J Obstet Gynecol* 124:562, 1976.

Magrina JF, Moffat RE, Masterson BJ, et al: Selective arterial infusion of Pitressin for the control of puerperal hemorrhage after hypogastric artery ligation. *Obstet Gynecol* 58:646, 1981.

Masterson BJ: *Manual of Gynecologic Surgery*, 2nd ed. Springer-Verlag, New York, 1986.

CHAPTER **9**

Dyspareunia after Radical Hysterectomy

ABE MICKAL, M.D., F.A.C.O.G., F.A.C.S.

CASE ABSTRACT

A Wertheim radical hysterectomy with bilateral salpingo-oophorectomy and pelvic lymphadenectomy had been performed upon a 44-year-old multipara. One year after surgery, there was no evidence of malignant disease in the pelvis, but the patient and her husband complained of the vagina now being too short for marital comfort. This observation was confirmed on pelvic examination where a depth of but 3 inches was determined. There was a thick ligneous scar occupying the vault of the vagina.

DISCUSSION

The Patient, Cancer, and Quality of Life

The main thrust of therapy for cervical cancer as well as for all gynecologic malignancies is for a high cure rate and/or a respectable survival rate. In the past, emphasis on cure took precedence over the well-being of the patient with regards to the emotional, sexual, and psychologic aspects of her life. Fortunately, these views are being constantly modified as doctors learn to better relate with and treat the cancer patient as a total being and not just focus on the disease process itself.

Vasicka and associates (11) called attention to this problem. They state that:

"although the cure of the disease is the primary objective in the therapy of cervical cancer, preservation of function of organs adjacent to the diseased area, namely the bladder, vagina, and rectum seems to be of no less importance. Each, however, has functions which are difficult to replace . . . the vagina is not functionally comparable to urinary bladder or rectum, and therefore it has been much more frequently neglected during the application of therapeutic measures for cancer of the cervix . . . Even though the mutilation, shortening, or complete occlusion of the vagina does not kill the patient, it may produce serious psychosomatic implications which may make adequate social and marital post treatment adjustment impossible."

They further state that the doctor's objective is not only to save life but to make that life worth living, and especially is this true with patients suffering from cervical carcinoma.

Seibel et al (9, 10) compared sexual enjoyment in patients with carcinoma of the cervix who had been irradiated versus those who had been surgically managed: 45% of the irradiated patients reported decreased enjoyment as compared to 25% of the surgically treated patients. Sexual enjoyment was the same or improved in 28% of the irradiated patients as compared to 70% of those managed surgically.

Abitbol and Davenport (1) similarly reported shortening of the vagina and interference with sexual functions in 22 of 28 patients irradiated for cervical cancer as compared to only 2 of 32 surgical patients. Decker and Schwartzman (3) reported similar findings.

The foregoing reports illustrate that sexual function is definitely affected in the treatment of invasive cervical cancer, with irradiation therapy being the more serious offender. One must be very careful in evaluating such subjective data as no two women have similar sexual behavior nor do they have the same degree of malignancy or anatomic configurations. The emotional and psychic impact of cancer on a particular patient, her mate, and their relationship is also difficult to assess. There are no other areas in gynecology where more individualization is required in the overall management of patients than with cervical cancer and its impact on the anatomic, psychosomatic, and sexual aspects of a patient's life.

Preservation of ovarian function at the time of surgery for cervical carcinoma results in less degenerative changes of the vagina. Sexual function is improved by making coitus less painful and more enjoyable. Other causes or factors in dyspareunia besides the postsurgical are post-traumatic, infections, lack of communication between couples, poor or incomplete knowledge of the sex act (psychosexual), as well as fear and pain.

Prevention of Complications

The patient presented for discussion was 44 years of age, and certainly removal of the ovaries was warranted. The ligneous scar at the vault was most likely caused by a postoperative infection. It is assumed that the cervical cancer has been cured to date and the problem at hand relates to a shortened, scarred vagina with dyspareunia.

One is concerned that the complaints of the couple occurred 1 year postsurgery, as this should have been the year of most frequent observation and evaluation. Much of the problem now presented may have been averted if preventive measures and counseling had been instituted earlier during this first post-therapy year.

There appears to be no contraindication to the use of estrogens in cases of carcinoma of the cervix. In younger patients with this disease process, the ovaries are left in situ with no apparent complications. The late Dr. Milton McCall (6) of Louisiana State University Gynecologic Service had a large series of patients with early malignant lesions of the cervix for whom a Schauta-Amreich vaginal hysterectomy was done with the ovaries left in situ. These patients have been followed on the service for many years, and their prognosis has not been noticeably affected nor were there any serious consequences to the ovaries being left in place. There was minimal shortening of the vagina in these patients, and the vast majority reported no serious compromise of their sexual activity.

My Approach to This Problem

The procedures used in helping this couple to regain a satisfactory sexual life would be, in my opinion, as follows:

1. Frank discussion of the problem with husband and wife. This would involve complete disclosure of their sexual attitudes, including the positive as well as the negative aspects. Encouragement to both partners, regarding free discussion with each other of the good and painful aspects of their relationship. They need to freely advise and help each other in seeking solutions to a more pleasant experience.

The attitude, concern, and compassion of the physician will do much to breach the barriers of a troublesome sex life. Many couples' frustrations are benefited by good dialogue with an understanding physician. The feeling of help on the horizon is oft times a very effective medication.

2. Oral use of low-dose estrogen, 0.3 mg Premarin or similar preparation, on a daily basis until desired results are achieved, then on a cyclic basis—3 weeks on, 1 week off or one tablet every other day indefinitely as long as results are satisfactory.

3. The use of a vaginal lubricant at times of coitus (K-Y jelly, an estrogen cream, or a short burst of a vaginal foam principally directed at the introitus). If penetration can be easily facilitated, then the rest of the performance may be enhanced.

4. Vaginal evaluation and dilation at 7- to 10-day intervals in the office after 10 to 14 days on estrogen therapy may induce elasticity of the vaginal canal. This, coupled with an active sex life at home, may reap the desired results.

5. I would not recommend surgery as long as progress is being made. If after 4 to 6 months there is no noticeable improvement, then I would contemplate the following surgical approach: (a) Multiple linear transverse incisions of the stenosed or ligneous scarred vault. The incisions must be through the total thickness of the vaginal wall. (b) Suture ligation of active bleeding areas only. (c) Tight packing of vagina after estrogen cream application to the vault for 36 to 48 hours. (d) Excision of any of the ligneous scar (8) should be limited to only the thick, dense areas. One should not sacrifice any more vaginal wall than absolutely necessary, as we are dealing with a restricted vagina.

6. If after a sufficient period of concentrated efforts, including the incision of the scarred vault, no satisfactory progress has been achieved, then one must consider additional surgical procedures. The time frame of events would be 10 to 12 months from the beginning or 6 to 8 months after the initial surgical approach to the vault. It is expected or hoped that

with estrogen therapy, dilation, and incising of the vault scar that the patient's problem is minimized. The patient had a 3-inch vagina to begin with, and hopefully these efforts increased the depth by 1/2 to 1 inch.

The two surgical procedures most often used to increase the vaginal depth are the Williams (12) and the McIndoe (7) operations. Which of these two procedures will produce the best results in this case would depend on:

1. Complete evaluation of the couple's problems as of this time and an assessment of their needs for satisfactory sexual relations. This must be done individually and collectively in order to understand their individual as well as their combined problems.

2. Explanation of surgical procedures available with the positive as well as negative aspects, including operative risk and postoperative care.

3. My choice would be a modified Williams operation as only about an inch or so is needed to achieve a 5-inch vagina, which in the majority of cases would be most satisfactory, unless we are dealing with an unusual situation. The Williams operation would be less traumatic to perform, and recovery would be more rapid than with the McIndoe procedure. We must remember that this patient had an invasive cancer of the cervix treated by a radical Wertheim hysterectomy. Fibrosis and adhesions increase the risk of bladder or rectal perforation.

Ingram (5) has used specially designed dilators in the vagina with the use of a bicycle seat to exert pressure in dilating a stenosed or constructed vagina. This rationale is logical and workable, although I have no experience with this method.

Individualization cannot be overstressed in cases of this type. The gynecologist (2, 4) must continually involve himself/herself with the whole female patient as related to her life within her environment. Good dialogue with the patient and her mate before, during, and after surgery is mandatory, especially in dealing with a cancer patient. One must not treat the disease only at the expense of the patient. Long-term survival and cures are necessary goals in the surgical management of the patient, especially those in whom invasive malignant disease is diagnosed. They also need, more than others, the concerned understanding and honest dialogue of a compassionate physician who is interested in the overall well-being of his patient. Neglect, avoidance, or indifference on the part of the physician produces dire traumatic emotional consequences within the patient. No physician should be guilty of any such accusations.

References

1. Abitbol MM, Davenport JH: Sexual dysfunction after therapy for cervical carcinoma. *Am J Obstet Gynecol* 119:181, 1974.
2. Adelusi B: Coital functions after radiotherapy for carcinoma of the cervix uteri. *Br J Obstet Gynecol* 87:821, 1980.
3. Decker WH, Schwartzman E: Sexual function following treatment for carcinoma of the cervix. *Am J Obstet Gynecol* 83:401, 1962.
4. Dennerstein L, Wood C, Burrows GD: Sexual response following hysterectomy and oophorectomy. *Obstet Gynecol* 49:92, 1977.
5. Ingram JM: The bicycle seat stool in the treatment of vaginal agenesis and stenosis: A preliminary report. *Am J Obstet Gynecol* 140:867, 1981.
6. McCall JL, Keaty EC, Thompson JD: Conservation of ovarian tissue in the treatment of carcinoma of the cervix with radical surgery. *Am J Obstet Gynecol* 75:590, 1958.
7. McIndoe A: Treatment of congenital absence and obliterative conditions of the vagina. *Br J Plast Surg* 2:254, 1950.
8. Nichols DH, Randall CL: *Vaginal Surgery*, ed. 2. Baltimore Williams & Wilkins, 1983.
9. Siebel MN, Freeman MG, Graves WL: Carcinoma of the cervix and sexual function. *Obstet Gynecol* 55:484, 1980.
10. Siebel MN, Freeman MG, Graves WL: Hysterectomy for carcinoma-in-situ and sexual function. *Gynecol Oncol* 11:195, 1981.
11. Vasicka A, Popovich NR, Brausch CC: Post-irradiation course of patients with cervical carcinoma: A clinical study of psychic, sexual and physical well-being of sixteen patients. *Obstet Gynecol* 11:403, 1958.
12. Williams EA: Congenital absence of the vagina: A simple operation for its relief. *J Obstet Gynaecol Br Commonw* 71:511, 1964.

CHAPTER 10

Panniculectomy as Incidental Procedure

JOSEPH H. PRATT, M.D.

CASE ABSTRACT

A chronically obese 42-year-old patient with a symptomatic myomatous uterus was advised to have an abdominal hysterectomy. She agreed to this recommendation and expressed the wish that her surgeon remove her abdominal panniculus at the same time.

DISCUSSION

Whalers called it flensing; in the stockyards it is called rendering; but in the average overweight American woman who is middle-aged or older, it is delicately referred to as a "tummy tuck" or panniculectomy.

Regardless of its name, it is the removal of excess fatty tissues and skin for its oil content, to make lard, to provide access to the abdomen, or to leave the female patient with an improved appearance. Unfortunately, gynecologic surgeons have almost completely overlooked this very obvious part of the total patient care of a surgical patient. The plastic surgeons, however, have most adequately filled the void, and their literature abounds in variations of techniques for the removal of excess adipose tissues and the reconstruction of the body's surface (4, 6).

The first panniculectomies were done for relatively enormous aprons and folds of skin and fat. Kelly (1) wrote in 1910 that these masses should be removed, if only for cosmetic effect to the patient. As much as a 78-lb (35.4-kg) panniculus has been reported (3) but 19 lb (18.6 kg) is the largest I have excised (5). A panniculectomy per se, utilizing large compressing stay sutures, will result in a relatively small loss of blood. A panniculectomy, as a part of a surgical procedure to aid in removal of the uterus, must be done in a manner that leaves the lower abdominal wall exposed for a laparotomy incision, and for this reason,

200 to 400 ml of blood may be lost during the panniculectomy.

There are two indications for a panniculectomy in association with an abdominal hysterectomy. Most women have some excess fat in the lower abdominal wall, and in some, the fat may be 6 to 9 cm in thickness. There also may be large hanging aprons of tissues that actually rest against the front of the thighs. The skin beneath these folds is often chronically excoriated, inflamed, thickened, and pigmented. The most effective method to sterilize such an area is to remove it in toto, along with the thickened adipose tissues. Thus, one indication for a panniculectomy is to excise chronically infected areas and facilitate the exposure of the lower abdominal wall. This method requires transverse elliptic incisions that excise a large "watermelon" section of tissues (2). The lower abdominal wall thus exposed is only 1 to 2 cm in thickness from external fectus fascia to peritoneum, and any further incisions give excellent exposure to the pelvis.

The second indication for a hysterectomy-panniculectomy is for appearances. There may not be enough adiposity to make the hysterectomy more difficult, yet, by the addition of a modified panniculectomy, the surgeon can with almost no risk remove the majority of unsightly "stretch" marks, tightened up excess flabby abdominal skin, and remove enough lower abdominal wall and fat to give the patient a more stylish figure. Of course, along with removal of such excess unsightly tissues, hernias should be repaired if they are present. A diastasis recti, or even relaxed rectus fascia, can be imbricated to aid in the reconstructed appearance of the lower abdomen. Not only is there no increased risk of a resulting ventral or umbilical hernia, but, because of attention to technique, imbrication of fascia, and removal of excess loose skin, the abdominal wall is better supported than it was preoperatively.

In the first instance, the approach to the pelvis is facilitated, and, in both instances, the patient's general appearance is improved. There are drawbacks such as ''dog ears'' at the end of large transverse incisions when a large quantity of tissue is removed. Hematomas or seromas may require drainage, and some decreased sensation is always present from the extensive undermining of skin that is often necessary.

The umbilicus poses a problem. If considerable skin must be removed, the umbilicus will be displaced downward. In such cases, the best technique is to leave the umbilicus attached by a pedicle to the fascia, excise what tissues are necessary, then bring the umbilicus out through a small circular midline incision that does not displace the umbilicus from its physical rela-

tionship to costal margins, symphysis, and iliac crests. Four to six skin sutures are all that are required to reattach the umbilicus to the skin.

For excision of a moderate or large panniculus in association with or as preparation for primary pelvic surgery, a transverse elliptic incision should be used. The fascia is widely exposed, and access to the abdomen is facilitated. The transverse diameter may be of any size, and often is betweem 30 to 70 cm. A vertical V of tissue may be excised in the midline to shorten the incision, and very often a V incision is necessary at the lateral ends to reduce the quantities of tissues there. Drainage is always necessary because of the extensive raw surfaces. Large vertical figure-of-eight sutures will help tack the skin flaps to the fascia, obliterate cavities, and hold the skin in apposition. These transverse incisions of the lower abdomen are large, suture scars also show, and the incisions are not cosmetically pleasing (Fig. 10.1).

When a panniculectomy or a ''tummy tuck'' is basically for cosmetic purposes, not as a specific aid to the pelvic procedure, then a different approach is indicated. A review of some of the articles in the plastic surgery journals is

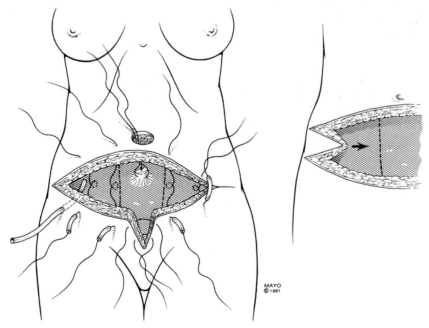

Figure 10.1. ''Watermelon'' incision with lower flap V; transplantation of umbilicus. At right is representation of incision closure to prevent ''dog ears.''

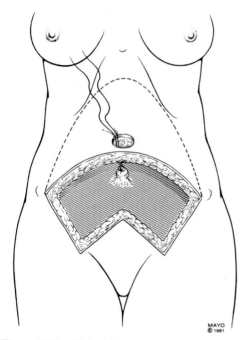

MAYO
© 1981

Figure 10.2.   W incision.

skin flap almost always is longer than the lower, some modification of a W incision in the lower skin flap is a helpful technique (Fig. 10.2).

Postoperatively, one watches for evidence of seromas or hematomas. All extensive incisions require drainage for at least 2 days. When tension on the suture line is considerable, and some tension is necessary to make the skin flap adhere to the facsia, then a modified ''jackknife'' position in bed is helpful for the first 48 hours. When snug compression dressings are utilized postoperatively to compress the skin to the fascia, the patient must be observed for evidence of respiratory difficulties.

As a general statement, the patients are very happy to have this added attention to their ''tummies,'' since this is the only part of an operation they can really see. It behooves the gynecologic surgeon to be acquainted with techniques, to be cognizant of possible complications yet ready to advise the patient first of possible improvements in appearance, and to vary his normal operative approach as seems indicated.

most helpful. These surgeons have spent much time and thought on the problem. In an effort to remove stretch marks, excise unsightly flabby skin, and so forth, undermining may be carried up to the costal margins. The lines of the incision should be marked preoperatively to be certain of symmetry. Depending on the tissue to be removed, the umbilicus may be transplanted through the upper skin flap. The final transverse skin incision should be at or below the hairline and be compatible with the wearing of a bikini bathing suit. Since the upper

References

1. Kelly HA: Excision of the fat of the abdominal wall—lipectomy. *Surg Gynecol Obstet* 10:229, 1910.
2. Masson JK: Lipectomy: The surgical removal of excess fat. *Postgrad Med* 32:481, 1962.
3. Meyerowitz BR, Gruber RP, Laub DR: Massive abdominal panniculectomy. *JAMA* 225:408, 1973.
4. Pitanguy V: Abdominal lipectomy: An approach to it through an analysis of 300 consecutive cases. *Plast Reconstr Surg* 40:384, 1967.
5. Pratt JH, Irons GB: Panniculectomy and abdominoplasty. *Am J Obstet Gynecol* 132:165, 1978.
6. Regnault P: Abdominoplasy by the W technique. *Plast Reconstr Surg* 55:265, 1975.

CHAPTER 11

A Small Transverse Pfannenstiel Incision and a Large Pelvic Tumor

WILLIAM E. CRISP, M.D.

CASE ABSTRACT

A 46-year-old patient has known for years of some fibroid tumors, but in the year preceding admission the tumors had slowly and progressively enlarged. Menses were regular, and no menopausal symptoms were evident. The uterus now extended to the patient's umbilicus. Total abdominal hysterectomy was recommended.

The abdomen was opened through a small Pfannenstiel incision and the pelvis was explored. The presence of multiple fibroids within the uterus was confirmed; the ovaries and tubes appeared grossly normal. There were so many large nodularities in the uterus that it could not be delivered "in one piece" through the incision.

DISCUSSION

The operating surgeon has a large irregular central pelvic mass thought to be multiple uterine fibroids that has enlarged dramatically over the past year.

The abdomen has been opened via a small suprapubic Pfannenstiel incision and suspected pathology confirmed, but the surgeon could not deliver the uterus through the incision. The problem is that the surgeon has compromised his proposed operation by an inappropriate incision. How could this predicament have been avoided?

The problem could have been avoided by examining the patient under anesthesia before surgery. Despite one's confidence in the office examination, we have all been surprised by pelvic findings under anesthesia. If there is still doubt about the uterus size versus possible adnexal pathology, the uterus should be sounded.

The incision then can be tailored to the findings after examination under anesthesia. If there is doubt about the findings or suspected pathology, especially adnexal pathology or malignancy, then a lower midline incision or a paramedian incision should be made so the abdomen can be adequately explored and the surgery not compromised.

Solution

The operative findings confirm the presence of a uterus irregularly enlarged with multiple fibroids. The solution to the problem is to either modify the Pfannenstiel incision to get more room or decrease the size of the uterus by myomectomy.

In this particular patient both adnexa are normal and there are multiple leiomyomata so the risk of sarcoma is minimal because a sarcoma will usually present as a single uterine enlargement. The menses have been regular and the patient is only 46 years old so the risk of an endometrial cancer is also minimal. The patient, therefore, is a good candidate for myomectomy.

The technique of myomectomy depends on the location of fibroids in the uterus. Ideally, it is best if you can ligate as much of the blood supply of the uterus as possible before removing the fibroids. If technically possible, both infundibulopelvic ligaments should be ligated and cut. The bladder flap should then be taken down so that the uterine vessels can be easily ligated. The peritoneal surface over the greater curvature of the fibroid is then incised and the fibroid can usually be bluntly dissected from its uterine base. If the uterine blood supply cannot be safely ligated, a uterine tourniquet can be placed around the uterus or the uterus can be debulked in a similar manner and bleeding controlled with figure of eight sutures. The Bonney clamp which was designed for myomectomy has not proven useful with a large uterus.

If the fibroids are intraligamentary, the broad ligament should be opened and the course of the ureter identified as well as any distortions of vascular anatomy before the fibroid is removed.

Once the size of the uterus has been decreased, it usually can be removed without difficulty in a routine manner. If it is the surgeon's choice to modify the incision, he has several options. If the Pfannenstiel incision is immediately suprapubic, it can be converted to a Cherney incision by cutting the tendinous insertion of the rectus and pyramidalis muscles and then extending the incision in a curvilinear manner toward the anterior superior spine of the ileum.

In closing the Cherney incision, it is important to identify the full thickness of the cut ends of the tendon and reattach it with permanent suture, such as O Prolene, with parallel mattress sutures which are tied all at the same time. This is because the tendon of the rectus retracts with potential hernia formation.

If the original incision was placed more cephalad over the body of the rectus muscle it could then be converted to a muscle cutting (Maylard) incision and then that incision could be extended in a curvilinear manner toward the anterior superior spine of the ileum as noted above. The rectus muscles are divided completely in a transverse fashion. The inferior epigastric vessels are always encountered and must be identified and ligated. The segmental innervation of the rectus muscle from the lateral edges of the muscle allows it to heal automatically with a new inscription, obviating the need to approximate the cut ends of the rectus.

If the patient's anatomy or the pelvic pathology would still limit the advantages of the extended transverse incision, the surgeon should not hesitate to convert the Pfannenstiel incision to a midline incision giving the patient a T-shaped scar. Cosmesis should be a secondary consideration to adequate exposure.

Selected Readings

Mattingly RF, Thompson JD: *TeLinde's Operative Gynecology,* ed. 6, Philadelphia, JB Lippincott, 1985.
Rovinsky JJ: Operations of the abdominal wall. In Sciarra JJ (ed): *Gynecology and Obstetrics,* Hagerstown, MD, Harper and Row, 1979, Chap 57.
Wheeless CR Jr: *Atlas of Pelvic Surgery.* Philadelphia, Lea & Febiger, 1981.

CHAPTER 12

Transabdominal Myomectomy— Broken Needle

L. RUSSELL MALINAK, M.D.
JAMES M. WHEELER, M.D.
GREG SIMOLKE, B.S.

CASE ABSTRACT

Myomectomy is planned for a 28-year-old nulligravida with hypermenorrhea and an enlarged, irregular uterus. Following enucleation of the fibroid tumors from the uterus, the myometrium was being closed in layers. As the deeper stitches were being placed, an audible "clack" was heard. Upon withdrawing the needleholder, it was evident that the tip of the needle had been broken. The location of the broken tip was unknown; the surgeon suspected it was retained by the myometrium.

DISCUSSION

Exposure is often a problem when operating in the depths of the female pelvis. Manipulation of instruments in restricted spaces with restricted visualization is associated occasionally with a surgical complication—a broken needle. This event invariably occurs in the deepest, most inaccessable layer of a closure, as in the myomectomy described above. A broken needle implies an imbalance of forces—either excessive resistance offered by the tissue, the use of an inappropriate needle, or the application or undue force by the surgeon.

In order to minimize the likelihood of this complication, proper needle selection is necessary. The characteristics of the specific needle are mandated by the type of tissue to be sutured. Tissue tensile strength, shear strength, weave, penetrability, density, elasticity, and thickness are mechanical factors that should be considered (8). Clinical situations may further affect these mechanical factors. For example, fibrosis in the myometrium adjacent to a myoma or lack of a discreet capsule as with an adenomyoma may complicate closure.

One basic assumption must be made in consideration of the ideal needle for a given application: the tissue being sutured should be altered as little as possible by the needle, since the only purpose of the needle is to introduce the suture into the tissue. The needle should be constructed of suitably strong material and designed so as to minimize needle damage, breakage, or alteration of its physical characteristics (8).

Breakage of surgical needles can be avoided by proper use of needle holders. There are two important considerations in grasping the needle: location and angle. The needle may be grasped near the sweged eye, so that the point protrudes after inserting the stitch, making it easier to retrieve the needle from the tissue. This maneuver is suitable for soft tissues such as subcutaneous fat. For greatest driving force in tough tissue, the needle is grasped between midpoint and tip. As the needle is advanced, the holder is repositioned nearer the midpoint, and the needle is further thrust through the tissue—the so-called "ratchet" technique. In dense tissue, the needle should not be grasped near the eye.

The angle of the needle to the needle holder may be perpendicular, obtuse, or acute. A perpendicular angle is preferred, as the needle can be driven through tissue by rotating the needle holder on its long axis. This results in more controlled delivery of the needle through tissue. In situations where perpendicular application is not practical, the least acute or obtuse angle of application is preferable.

The importance of the surgeon's grip of the needle holder is related to the strength with which needles may be thrust into tissue. The pencil grip, used in gynecologic microsurgery, is the most delicate grip, and is unlikely to provide the force necessary to break a needle. The thenar and thumb-ring finger grips are intermediate in strength to the palmed grip. The palmed grip, therefore, is most likely associated with broken needles, as surgeons adopt this grip only when they expect significant tissue resistance (1).

In the interest of saving operating time, it is common during closure after myomectomy that the surgeon will attempt to force the needle through both sides of the myometrial defect. It is usually prudent, however, to pass the needle through one side of the myometrium, bring it completely out at the deepest point, and then enter the myometrium of the other side.

Needles bend before they break. If a surgeon feels a needle bending, this is a signal that excessive force is being applied. Perhaps a thicker, more stout needle should be selected. All needles that are bent should be discarded, never to be straightened and reused. In the ideal situation, the surgeon should inspect each needle for its integrity prior to placing it into the patient.

To summarize thus far, proper selection of suture materials and use of surgical technique are of paramount importance in preventing breakage of needles in tissue. The surgeon must:

(1) Appreciate the nature of the tissue about to be sutured.
(2) Know the needle characteristics and their practical application to various tissues.
(3) Use the proper needle location and angle in grasping with the needle holder.
(4) Use a grip on the needle holder that will not transmit excessive force.
(5) Discard bent needles; it is wiser to have wasted a bent needle than to risk breakage.

In gynecologic surgery, needle breakage is most common in difficult settings where exposure is poor and the surgeon is in some way compromising good technique.

What techniques can the surgeon use to identify and remove the broken needle tip from his patient?

Perhaps the initial question is, "does the needle tip need to be removed?" Although patients live normally with a variety of foreign bodies in their tissues, there are specific reasons why broken needles should be removed (6). The needle could migrate to a position in which adjacent anatomic structures might be compromised (3). The needle can move to a surgically less accessible position (2). Long-term medical complications of retained broken needles include infection and nerve irritation (9). Psychologically, many patients will manifest anxiety regarding a retained needle in their genital tracts, including fears of damage to their sexual partner or their fetus. Medicolegally, plaintiffs with retained foreign bodies have been awarded compensation even if no demonstrable harm has occurred, simply on the principle that a surgical instrument—especially one that breaks—is ipso facto negligence.

Although in other subspecialties (e.g., neurosurgery) it may be of greater risk to attempt removal of a broken needle than to leave it behind, in most situations in gynecologic surgery attempted removal of the needle is indicated.

Immediately on hearing the telltale "clack" of a broken needle, the surgeon should not withdraw the needle holder, nor should he avert his gaze from the surgical field. All available light should be directed onto the field. Good retraction and assistance is mandatory. A radiopaque marker, such as a surgical hemostatic clip, should be placed at the entry point of the needle (5). A different sized clip can mark the expected exit site of the needle as if it had continued to arc through the tissue. Once the field is marked, the surgeon can gently probe the wound so as not to advance the broken tip any deeper into the tissue. It may be difficult to appreciate the "feel" of the needle fragment when it is small or the surrounding tissue is particularly firm. Often, a small incision made perpendicular to the expected course of the needle will reveal the retained part. Use of a sterile strong magnet has been described to retrieve metallic foreign bodies. Small hand-held electronic instruments (Roper-Hall electroacoustic metal foreign body locator) which are used in ophthalmologic surgery for localization of metallic foreign objects may be useful. If multiple attempts at probing the wound fail, then an imaging technique is indicated to help localize the retained needle (7).

The most available technique to help demonstrate a retained metallic object is radiography. An x-ray will confirm the presence of the fragment. This is the first priority if incision or probing fails to reveal the needle. A minimum of two views—AP and lateral—with the use of markers (e.g., 18 to 20 gauge needles) inserted perpendicularly to the expected path of the broken needle may aid in localization. We question the utility of this method for localization. Recent experimental attempts at radiographic localization of a broken needle in an extirpated uterus were very difficult. Intraoperative fluoroscopy via c-arm device is the preferred radiographic technique. Needles can be advanced in one or several planes under fluoroscopic control until their tips lie in close proximity to the buried metal object; an incision can then be made down the shaft of the needle to retrieve the foreign body.

Ultrasonographic localization of retained metallic fragments is is increasingly available. Modern ultrasound units found in obstetric departments often have sector scanning capability; linear array units are unlikely to have the resolution necessary to retrieve needle tips. Currently, small transducers for sector scanners are available to perform transvaginal pelvic ultrasonography. These transducers are 1 cm square and would be small enough to help in needle localization in abdominal or vaginal cases. Ideally, if probing the wound fails to retrieve the needle tip, an ultrasonographer is consulted. A 7.5 or 10 megaHertz in-line transducer is placed within a sterile probe cover (a surgical glove will do); sterile sonographic gel is placed in contact with the transducer inside the probe cover—it is not smeared on the uterus. With serial scanning and use of one or several probes, most needle fragments will be localized. When the retained needle is found, it should be grasped with a needle holder, then "backed-out" or advanced along the tract of prior anticipated passage. It should not be pulled straight-up from its imbedded site in most cases. This maneuver would be acceptable if an incision large enough to expose the entire needle has been made, an unlikely situation in myomectomy closure. A needle holder with a finer point than that in use when the needle broke may be useful.

A hand-held imaging device called a lixiscope, an acronym for Low Intensity X-ray Imaging, combines the features of fluoroscopy and real time ultrasonography in a portable unit. The lixiscope has been used in the operating room to ascertain correct setting of orthopaedic pins and in the office to identify foreign bodies in soft tissues. A safe instrument that emits so little radiation that shielding is not necessary, the lixiscope may become the ultimate tool in finding radiopaque foreing bodies intraoperatively (4).

Although computerized tomography (CT) and nuclear magnetic resonance (NMR) have superior resolution in identifying metallic objects, their bulk makes them highly unlikely to be of any use in the intraoperative location of a broken needle. These advanced instruments may have their greatest utility in carefully following migration of retained foreign bodies toward vital structures.

References

1. Anderson RM, Romfh RF: *Technique in the Use of Surgical Tools.* New York, Appleton-Century-Crofts, 1980, pp. 41-58.
2. Crouse VL: Migration of a broken anesthetic needle: Report of a case. *SC Dent J* 28:16-19, 1970.
3. Fraser-Moodie W: Rcovery of broken needles. *Br Dent J* 105:79-85, 1958.
4. Healthmate, Inc., Lixiscope (Pamphlet), 1983.
5. Leidelmeyer R: The embedded broken off needle. *JACEP* 5:362-363, 1976.
6. Orr D: The broken needle: Report of a case. *J Am Dent Assoc* 107:603, 1983.
7. Roper-Hall MJ (ed): *Stallard's Eye Surgery,* 6th Ed., Philadelphia, JB Lippincott, 1980, pp. 773-801.
8. Trier WC: Considerations in the choice of surgical needles. *Surg Gynecol Obstet* 149:84, 1979.
9. Wigand FT: Otalgia caused by a broken needle in the pterygomandibular space: Report of a case. *J Oral Surg* 18:77-78, 1960.

CHAPTER 13
The Missing Sponge

CHARLES E. FLOWERS, JR., M.D.

CASE ABSTRACT

Following completion of a vaginal hysterectomy and repair, a final sponge count was reportedly short by one. A recount was unrewarding.

DISCUSSION

It is important that the surgeon believe the sponge count: there is a missing sponge until every possiblity of error is eliminated. Today, it is rare for operating personnel to make mistakes in the sponge count. In the majority of hospitals, laparotomy pads are placed in five units in each pack, and sponges are placed in ten units of each pack. When a pack is broken on the operating table, the scrub nurse and the circulating nurse both count the sponges. If there is an error, that group of sponges is removed from the operating theater. After sponges are used they are placed back in a container, five being placed in the laparotomy sponge container and ten placed in each sponge container. At the conclusion of the procedure, it is only necessary to count the remaining sponges to be sure that all are present.

If a sponge is missing, the pathology specimen is first checked, the space around the operating table is checked: the shoe soles of the personnel in the operating theater are checked and a recount is made. If the sponge is still missing, an x-ray of the abdomen is mandatory.

The operator must assume the responsibility for every sponge he uses in a procedure. Appropriate surgical technique dictates that no free sponges be used in the abdomen and all laparotomy pads be marked with a ring or instrument. If it is necessary to place a free sponge deep within the pelvis or the recesses of an anterior or posterior repair, it is preferable to put a suture through the sponge and clamp it with an instrument so that it can be easily retrieved.

If a fairly large sponge is necessary, a laparotomy pad may be cut in half or thirds and appropriately marked.

During the time that the flat plate of the abdomen is being ordered and taken, a recheck of the count is made. However, one should not yet take down the anterior or posterior repair or open the peritoneum. One should wait until the flat plate of the abdomen is available and can be examined in the operating room. When the sponge is located, it is retrieved by the simplest method possible. Remember that a blood soaked sponge or pad more or less assumes the color of its operative environment, making it more difficult to spot.

The old adage "an ounce of prevention is worth a pound of cure" is also true in surgery. The surgeon should refrain from using free sponges, mark the sponges he does use, and work very closely with the operating room personnel.

In this litiginous society, one must be thoughtful about what is told a patient. If the sponge is found before the peritoneal cavity is closed, simple operative maneuvers can be made to retrieve the sponge: it is unnecessary to inform the patient concerning the event. However, if an x-ray of the abdomen was taken to locate a sponge it is important to indicate to the patient what was done.

An obstetrician and gynecologist can usually see the opaque string of the sponge. However, consultation with a radiologist is extremely important if there are problems of interpretation. Occasionally, it may be necessary in the obese patient to make a second film of greater intensity.

CHAPTER **14**

Trauma From Sexual Assault

JOHN R. EVRARD, M.D., M.P.H.

CASE ABSTRACT

An 11-year-old girl was brought to the emergency room in a state of shock and confusion. There had evidently been a sexual assault, and a blood-tipped broom handle was found nearby. Gentle pelvic examination revealed multiple lacerations of the wall of the vagina, and penetration of the vault of the vagina, presumably communicating with the peritoneal cavity. The patient was promptly taken to surgery where first the vaginal lacerations were repaired. It was clear that the vault of the vagina had been fractured, and this area of rupture communicated with the peritoneal cavity. A laparotomy was performed.

At surgery, it was found that damage was limited to penetration of the cul-de-sac of Douglas. There was no evidence of trauma to the gastrointestinal system or the internal genitalia.

DISCUSSION

This 11-year-old sexual assault victim has a serious, life-threatening injury and she must be handled expeditiously from a surgical standpoint as well as for evidentiary examination. Perforation of the peritoneum from the vagina presents unique problems which are enhanced by the fact that this child is prepubertal. Discussion therefore will include prepubertal factors influencing managemnt, general and evidentiary examination, and the specific surgical management of this case.

Prepubertal Factors

The physiology of the genital tract of a prepubertal child is quite different from that of a postpubertal child, and may, in fact, predispose to vaginal perforation into the peritoneal cavity. Anatomically, the prepubertal vagina is thin, red, and narrow with atrophic labium minora. The vaginal fornices are not well developed, the pH of the vagina is higher and the cervix may be a bizarre shape with transverse rugae. Because the vagina is not under the influence of estrogen, the lining epithelium is only four to five cell layers thick, compared to 30 to 35 cells after puberty, thereby making the vagina more prone to perforation. Vaginal cy-

tology, prepubertally, typically reveals parabasal cells, small oval cells with large nuclei, and a small amount of cytoplasm. As the child approaches puberty, intermediate cells are found, and finally 4 to 6 months before puberty many superficial cells, large polyhedral cells with abundant cytoplasm, and small nuclei are found.

The vaginal flora in the prepubertal child, is quite different from that of a woman in the childbearing age. Hammerschlag et al, in a study of 25 healthy girls ranging from 2 to 15 years, found that the vaginal flora commonly had both facultative anaerobes as well as obligate anaerobes colonizing the vagina. *Bacteroides fragilis*, peptococci, and peptostreptococci were commonly identified. These findings have certain implications regarding perioperative antimicrobials in this particular case.

General Principles in Management of Sexual Assault

Empathy is the key word in management of a sexual assault victim. The child should be treated as a patient rather than managed as a piece of evidence. Generally, she should be seen initially by a social worker or counselor familiar with managing sexual assault cases so as to minimize subsequent emotional sequelae. In this case, because of the life-threatening nature of the injury, the injury must be managed first. Rape crisis intervention centers all agree that it is relatively easy to manage injuries, prevent pregnancy and venereal disease, but difficult to prevent early or late emotional sequelae following sexual assault. There are three essential dicta for management of the sexual assault victim: (1) manage the patient's emotional needs; (2) manage the patient's medical needs (detect and repair injuries, prevent pregnancy and sexually transmitted disease); and (3) perform an appropriate evidentiary examination.

Permits

The following permits must be obtained before caring for the sexual assault victim:

1. Permit for history and physical
2. Permit for photography
3. Permit for gathering specimens
4. Permit for release of the above information to proper authorities.

In the case of this 11-year-old girl, her parents or guardian should sign the permits. On the other hand, if the parents are not present, and not easily available by telephone, the emergency nature of this case would justify proceeeding without parental consent.

History

Allow a parent and a social worker skilled in sexual assault management to remain with the child during the history and physical. The social worker will be skilled in helping elicit the history, frequently with the aid of sexually explicit dolls. All tests and interventions should be explained to the parents and a separate permit should be obtained for the surgical procedure. The patient should be allowed to tell her story in her own words. Following this, these questions should be asked:

What time did the assault occur? Did the patient change clothing, bathe, shower, douche, or defecate subsequent to the assault? Has the patient had any vaginal surgery or any vaginal injury prior to the current trauma? Has the patient had any emotional problems or does she have a history of mental illness or retardation?

The patient's answers are useful in the gathering and interpretations of the evidentiary examination.

Physical Examination

The general condition of the patient and her emotional state should be described and should include a description of her clothing (e.g., torn, bloody, soiled). She should be undressed over a white sheet so than any detritus adherent to her clothing may be saved. The clothing should be examined under a Woods light in a dark room for semen stains which fluoresce a bright yellow green. The clothing should be aired and placed in a sealed paper bag from the rape kit.

She should be examined completely under a good light with special attention given to the face, neck, conjunctivae, buccal mucosa of the lips and back since extragenital injuries with sexual assault are common. Injuries should be photographed with a Polaroid camera, each photograph bearing on the reverse side the time, date, and signature of the photographer.

The Woods light in a darkened room should also be used to examine the patient for suspected semen stains. If any are found they may be reconstituted with saline and the applicators placed in a vial in the rape kit marked with date, time, and location of the stain. Fingernail scrapings must also be placed in an appropriately marked vial since they may be helpful in identifying the assailant.

Other laboratory tests which should be performed beside the assays for sperm and acid phosphatase are blood typing and serologic testing for syphilis. If oral, rectal, or vaginal penetration has occurred, these cavities must be examined for traumatic injury, cultured for gonorrhea, and tested for sperm acid phosphatase. A wet smear of the vagina should also be examined immediately to detect motile sperm.

Management of the Present Case

The child was examined under anesthesia and vaginal lacerations were encountered. With the exception of the laceration perforating into the peritoneal cavity, these were repaired with O Dexon. Two applicators of the vaginal secretions were placed in vials for a determination of sperm and acid phosphatase. The child was catheterized to be certain that the urine was not bloody and the anus and rectum were examined to exclude fissures of the anus and injury to the rectum itself.

A flat plate of the abdomen was then obtained to ascertain any possible radiopaque foreign bodies in the peritoneal cavity, since vaginal examination clearly demonstrated perforation from the vagina into the peritoneal cavity. With positive evidence of vaginal penetration into the peritoneal cavity, and the knowledge that a broomstick was probably forced into the vagina, the possibility of serious injury to the bowel, mesentery, or other abdominal viscera demanded that the abdomen be thoroughly explored, preferably through a longitudinal abdominal incision. It is not possible to examine adequately the mesentery or upper viscera through a Pfannensteil or transverse incision. Similarly, there is no place for laparoscopy for the exploration of the peritoneal cavity in circumstances such as this. The abdomen was opened through a longitudinal incision from the symphysis and to the right side of the umbilicus. The small bowel and mesentery were explored from the ligament of Treitz to the cecum and found to be intact and, similarly, the colon and its mesentery were visualized and found to be undamaged. Had there been any lacerations, vascular injuries, or bleeding in the mesentery, the areas would have been repaired or the bowel resected and reanastomosed in case the area was considered nonviable.

Next, attention was given to the pelvic peritoneum and the perforation of the vagina reconfirmed.The pelvic peritoneum was then examined for any fluid which could be aspirated and placed in a vial for later assessment for sperm and acid phosphatase. The fluid was also examined immediately for motile sperm, and cultured for gonococcus, aerobes and anaerobes, as well as chlamydial infection. (Should there have been no fluid within the peritoneal cavity, a small amount of saline would have been used to wash the pelvic peritoneal cavity and this fluid collected for the above test).

At the site of the perforation, the vaginal mucosa was identified, debrided, and repaired with interrrupted O Dexon sutures. Figure-of-eight sutures were avoided since they could compromise the blood supply of the vaginal mucosa. The peritoneum was then irrigated with warm saline and aspirated. Following this, a Jackson-Pratt drain was placed through a stab wound in the abdomen. The abdominal peritoneum was closed with a running O chromic suture, the fascia closed using interrupted sutures of O Dexon, and the skin closed with staples.

Antimicrobial Therapy

Antimicrobial therapy for this 11-year-old girl should cover the following organisms: *Neisseria gonorrheae*, *Chlamydia trachomatis*, *Treponema pallidum*, Gram-positive and Gram-negative aerobes and the anaerobes. Perioperative antimicrobials are most effective when on board at the time of surgery. Preferably they are given before surgery, since deaths have occurred apparently due to an allergic reaction when a cephalosporin has been administered intravenously under anesthesia.

One recommended regimen:

Polycillen (Ampicillin) 500 mg administered intravenously preoperatively, followed by 500 mg every 6 hours for three more doses. This could be given orally if the child tolerates oral medication.

Cefoxitin sodium (Mefoxin) 300 mg/kg with the first dose given preoperatively intravenously and the other two doses 6 and 12 hours after the first.

Doxycline hyclate (Vibramycin IV) 2.2 mg/kg perioperatively and 12 hours later intravenously, succeeded by (or followed by) Vibramycin (doxycline monohydrate) 1.1 mg/kg bid orally for 7 days.

This regimen would cover most Gram-positive aerobes, many of the Gram-negative aerobes, *Gonorrhea*, *Chlamydia* and many of the anaerobes. It would prevent incubating syphilis. Perioperative treatment with Ampicillin and Mefoxin should be sufficient but the Vibramycin should be continued for 7 days. Should this child be allergic to penicillin, Vibramycin therapy would be recommended since it would cover *Chylamydia trachomatis*, *Neisseria gonorrheae*, and prevent incubating syphilis.

Emotional Support

Postoperatively, this child and her parents were followed by the social worker who saw her initially. Since these professionals are skilled in managing sexual assaults, they are useful in working out emotional problems associated with the assault. The child was followed up by the surgeon to see that all of her injuries healed and she was followed by the social worker to minimize the emotional trauma.

Selected Readings

Hammerschlag MR, Alpert S, Onderdonk AB, et al: Anaerobic microfloro of the vagina in children. *Am J Obstet Gynecol* 151:853-858, 1978.

Haney AF: Vaginal evisceration after forcing coitus with intra-abdominal ejaculation. *J Reproduc Med* 21:254-256, 1978.

Hicks DJ: Nichols D, Evrard J (eds): In *Ambulatory Gynecology*. Philadelphia, Harper & Row, 1985, pp. 473-487.

Rimsza ME, Niggeman EH: Medical evaluation of sexually abused children: A review of 311 cases. *Pediatrics* 69:8-14, 1982.

Wilson R, Swarz D: Coital injuries of the vagina. *Obstet Gynecol* 39:183-184, 1972.

Wynn JM: Injuries to the genitalia in children. *South Afr Med J* 57:47-50, 1980.

CHAPTER **15**

Unexpected Ovarian Tumor Discovered at Vaginal Hysterectomy

JOHN J. MIKUTA, M.D.

CASE ABSTRACT

Because of pelvic pressure, a feeling of falling out, backache relieved by lying down, and a progressive genital prolapse, a vaginal hysterectomy and repair was recommended to a 54-year-old, markedly obese female (270 lb., 5 feet 2 inches) who was 2 years beyond her last menstrual period.

Immediately following vaginal removal of the uterus it was evident that there was a 7-cm thick-walled ovarian cyst present that had not been diagnosed preoperatively. The tumor was unilateral and free of any visible or obvious adhesions to surrounding organs.

DISCUSSION

This patient represents the typical kind of situation frequently faced by gynecologists when the examination of the pelvis cannot be done with sufficient accuracy to identify all problems that may be present. Such difficulty may be created by obvious situations, as in this patient, where excessive weight accompanied by short stature would create a significant problem in determining what was present in the pelvis. An additional factor may be the presence of significant amounts of fecal matter in the rectum or sigmoid which may make identification of the pelvic organs very difficult. This particular situation can be obviated by cleansing enemas or laxatives prior to the office pelvic examination.

In a situation where it is impossible to identify what is going on in the pelvis, it is advisable to carry out ultrasonography in an effort to localize the possibility of any uterine or adnexal enlargements, and it is quite possible that in a patient such as described here a cystic lesion of the size identified at the time of operation would have been quite readily found.

A second aspect is the performance of an examination under anesthesia just prior to the carrying out of either a vaginal operation, be it a simple dilatation and curettage or a vaginal hysterectomy, or a vaginal repair. The same thing would apply to examination immediately prior to the performance of an exploratory laparotomy, in order to determine if something may be present which was not identified at the time of the preoperative office examination.

In the situation presented here, the tumor which was discovered did not provide any stigmata suggestive of malignancy, such as external papillary projections or any significant adhesions, and apparently was cystic rather than solid. However, the presence of any ovarian enlargement in a postmenopausal woman must be looked upon as a possible neoplasm until proven otherwise. This has been emphasized by Barber and Graber as the postmenopausal palpable ovary syndrome (PMPO). In the presence of easy mobility of the ovary and possibly the tube as well, a salpingo-oophorectomy via the vaginal approach could readily be done in order to determine the nature of the tumor. Care must be taken to avoid rupture of the cyst. There are times when it is difficult to perform a salpingo-oophorectomy through the vagina even when the ovary is of normal size. However, clamping across the mesovarium and using one hemostat as a handle will allow the surgeon to remove the ovary and then decide whether removal of the tube is an absolute necessity.

While the surgeon in this instance is waiting for the pathologist to provide a report on the removed ovary, it would be advisable to remove the opposite ovary. Since any ovarian enlargement in one ovary in the postmenopausal woman should be construed as evidence of possible neoplasia, the potential for this in the opposite ovary would be greater when such activity is found on the other side.

In general, at the time of vaginal hysterectomy in a woman of menopausal or postmenopausal age, because of the high mortality associated with ovarian carcinoma, it is advisable that gynecologists make an effort to remove the ovaries at the same time. Because the tube is so rarely involved with malignancy, it is not really necessary to remove the tube at the same time.

We have proceeded thus far on the assumption that the cyst that was removed was benign. However, in the event that there was some question as to whether the cyst contained some malignant areas, the surgeon would be faced with different choices. First, I think it should be noted that if there is any question about the accuracy of the histologic frozen section diagnosis then it may not be necessary to proceed directly to making a decision about additional treatment at this time. On the other hand, if there is no question that a carcinoma is present, the gynecologist may then proceed in one of two ways.

The first of these would be to complete the vaginal procedure as planned; then, if the patient's condition was satisfactory and if appropriate discussion had occurred prior to the operation that allowed for a deviation from the initially planned procedure, the gynecologist should enter the abdomen through an appropriate incision which would allow complete exploration of the remainder of the pelvis, the upper abdomen, and the subdiaphragmatic areas. On entering the abdomen, washings should be obtained from the pelvis, the lateral gutters, and subdiaphragmatic areas using heparinized saline solution. This would provide additional information as to the possible extent of any malignant cells and is necessary for proper staging. Completion of any pelvic operations as indicated could then be done, such as removal of the opposite adnexa, removal of the tube or tubes, etc. In addition, two more portions of the operation should be carried out—namely, omentectomy and exploration and biopsy of retroperitoneal nodes, particularly on the side of the tumor and also in the area of primary spread of the ovarian malignancy, mainly to the common iliac and para-aortic nodes.

If the patient's condition does not permit or if there is a question about the appropriate informed consent regarding further surgery, it may be necessary to complete the vaginal portion of the operation, allow the patient to recover from the anesthetic, and then recommend to her the additional surgery that may be necessary.

Selected Readings

Aure JC, Hoeg K, Kolstad P: Clinical and histologic studies of ovarian carcinoma, a long term follow-up of 990 cases. *Obstet Gynecol* 37:1, 1971.

Bagley CM Jr, Young RC, Schein PS, et al: Ovarian carcinoma metastatic to the diaphragm, frequently undiagnosed at laparotomy. *Am J Obstet Gynecol* 38:921, 1971.

Barber HRK, Graber EA: The PMPO syndrome (postmenopausal palpable ovary syndrome). *Obstet Gynecol* 38:921, 1971.

Creasman WT, Rutledge FN: The prognostic value of peritoneal cytology in gynecologic malignant disease. *Am J Obstet Gynecol* 10:773, 1971.

Knapp RC, Friedman EA: Aortic lymph node metastases in early ovarian cancer. *Am J Obstet Gynecol* 119:1013, 1974.

Munnell EW: The changing prognosis and treatment in cancer of the ovary: A report of 235 patients with primary ovarian carcinoma. 1952-1961. *Am J Obstet Gynecol* 100:790, 1968.

Piver MS, Shashikant L, Barlow JJ: Preoperative and intraoperative evaluation in ovarian malignancy. *Obstet Gynecol* 48:312, 1976.

Smith JP, Delgado G, Rutledge FN: Second-look operation in ovarian carcinoma postchemotherapy. *Cancer* 38:649, 1975.

CHAPTER **16**

The Postmenopausal Palpable Ovary Syndrome

HUGH R. K. BARBER, M.D.

CASE ABSTRACT

A 58-year-old patient, 4 years after the menopause and not taking estrogens, has recently noted some bloody vaginal discharge. Because of some painful cervical stenosis a "comfortable" endometrial biopsy could not be done, and the patient was admitted for fractional diagnostic curettage. The curettings were minimal in quantity and not grossly suspicious. The uterus was not enlarged, but the right ovary was found to be clearly palpable, although the left was not.

DISCUSSION

The menopause is peculiar to the human race, and with it comes the cessation of cyclical hormone activity within the ovary. Nevertheless, sometime after the uterine responses cease, primordial follicles can still be found in the cortex and ovulation may continue for a short time. In the normal course of events, the postmenopausal ovary shrinks and becomes densely fibrous, the external convolutions increase, and its appearance can be likened to that of a very small walnut.

Anatomy

The ovaries are dull white, almond-shaped structures located in the uterine adnexa. Ovarian size varies with age. During the reproductive period, the ovaries are approximately 3.5 cm in length, 2 cm in breadth, and 1.5 cm in thickness (6). Postmenopausally, the ovaries decrease in size by approximately 0.5 cm in each dimension (3).

Ultrastructure

The menopausal ovary tends to atrophy and shrink when the Graafian follicles and ova disappear. The tunica albuginea becomes very dense and causes the surface of the ovary to become scarred and shrunken. The cortex is marked with increased thinning as well as numerous corpora fibrosa and corpora albuginea with areas of dense fibrosis and hyalinization. The ovary shows varying degrees of avascularity. The ultrastructure indicates a great increase in fibroblasts and connective tissue throughout, especially in the cortex where germinal structures are largely absent (4). The advanced follicles, identified in postmenopausal ovaries, are usually undergoing atretic changes. Although there is a great increase of atretic follicles in postmenopausal ovaries, normal-appearing follicles are occasionally found; granulosa cells, however, are smaller. Any observed corpus luteum is usually undergoing atresia. The luteal cells appear vacuolated with an increase in the dense bodies and lipofuscin droplets. An infiltration of connective tissue can be observed in the atrophying corpus luteum. At the same time that the ovarian cortex is becoming very atrophic, the medullary region with stromal or interstitial cells is more abundant and usually active. Groups of functional stromal cells may be found throughout the postmenopausal ovary, especially around the hilar region. On occasion, single cells or smaller clusters of very active cells are apparently near the atretic follicle or corpus luteum. The stromal cells show similarities with Leydig's cells of the testes. Guraya (5) reports that stromal cells are usually controlled by pituitary gonadotropes. When stromal cells atrophy, they revert back to fibroblasts. It appears that there is an abundance of active stromal cells in the postmenopausal ovary and that these cells may be producing androgens.

In early 1971, one of the postmenopausal patients whom I had been following for some time came in for a routine pelvic examination. I palpated what appeared to be a normal-sized premenopausal ovary and was struck by the fact that it had not been present on her previous examination. In this age group, it was obvious that nothing should be stimulating the ovary to produce any functional changes, and any enlargement had to be due to a new growth. I advised the patient to take cathartics for a couple of days, followed by an enema, and return in 1 week for another pelvic examination. The same findings were present at the repeat examination. I elected to have the patient admitted to the hospital, examined under anesthesia, and the plan was to explore her to see if the ovary appeared to be the size of a premenopausal ovary. On exploration, I found a normal premenopausal-sized ovary that had been completely replaced by ovarian cancer. The ovary measured approximately 3 to 3.5 × 2 × 1.5 cm. Within the next several months, I had the opportunity to operate on three other women with similar pelvic findings, and each had an early cancer of the ovary (1).

The literature suggests that a pelvic examination should be done every 6 months. This routine should help to detect early changes in the ovary. Despite the protocol for regular examinations, the chance of detecting an ovarian neoplasm during routine pelvic examination in an asymptomatic woman is only 1 in 10,000 examinations. It is obvious that the detection rate is very low. In most instances, doctors judge any ovarian cyst under 5 cm as of little significance. This concept must be challenged, especially in the postmenopausal woman.

Although we may accept the axiom that the ovary may be too old to function but never too old to form a tumor, we are lulled into a sense of false security if the mass has not reached the size of 5 cm. Until recently, it was felt that the common epithelial ovarian cancer practically never occurred before age 40 years and it peaked by age 60 years. However, recent figures show that at age 25 years there is an annual rate of 3 per 100,000 females; at age 60 years, 40 per 100,000 women; and the rate continues to climb (9). If we accept the premise that a cancer starts as a derangement within the cell and progresses from atypia to dysplasia on to in situ

and then to invasive cancer, there is a greater possibility of making an early diagnosis when any change is detected in the ovary in the postmenopausal patient. Early cancer is not a tumor in the sense that a mass is not necessarily present. A volume of tumor must be present before a mass can be detected. As a matter of fact, the earliest that a tumor can be detected by any means is when it reaches a cubic centimeter; by that time, the cancer contains 10^9 or a billion cells with the potential to metastasize and to kill. Therefore, even though it is small in size, it is not truly an early cancer. However, by better education of the public and profession, earlier diagnoses are being made, and hopefully in the future an early diagnosis will be achieved through a serologic assay.

Diagnostic Sign. One diagnostic sign of early cancer in the ovary of a postmenopausal patient has proved both valuable and consistent (7). Stated simply, it means that the palpation of that which is interpreted *as a normal-sized ovary in the premenopausal woman represents an ovarian tumor in the postmenopausal woman* (1). This suggestion may appear to be insignificant in terms of the total problem, but it has been my experience that all such palpable findings have proved to be a new growth; they were not necessarily malignant, but none were functional or dysfunctional. It is my opinion that the postmenopausal palpable ovary is a most significant finding, and hopefully this observation will alert the gynecologist and the primary care physician to its importance. It is unfortunate that we do not have a registry to collate the material. This has been taken under consideration, but because of the proliferation of registries, it was decided not to pursue it at this time.

The postmenopausal palpable ovary (PMPO) syndrome (2) is a misnomer, and it is unfortunate that a more descriptive term had not been chosen when this observation was published. It is to be emphasized that it does not mean that anything that is palpated in the adnexa is abnormal in the postmenopausal patient. Every gynecologist has been able to palpate an ovary that measures 2 cm in a very thin, relaxed patient with poor abdominal musculature and who has an elastic and distensible vagina. It must be re-emphasized that the PMPO is simply the palpation of that which in the premenopausal woman is interpreted as a normal-sized ovary, represents an ovarian tumor in the postmenopausal woman. Expediency in carrying out the exploration is the choice of management when the PMPO is diagnosed.

Several points can be enumerated to support this thesis. There is no such thing as physiologic enlargement of the postmenopausal ovary. A physiologic cyst can arise only from the nonrupture of a Graafian follicle (follicle cyst) or from cystic degeneration of a corpus luteum (lutein cyst). There are no follicles or lutein cysts in the postmenopausal ovary, simply because there are no follicles or corpora lutea. The only thing that will cause the postmenopausal ovary to enlarge is to have excessive stimulation from something such as Pergonal or clomiphene during the time that follicles are still present and I find it difficult to imagine any physician prescribing these drugs in the postmenopausal patient.

The other cause for growth must be a neoplasm, which is not necessarily malignant. It just means that it is not functional or dysfunctional.

By strict definition, menopause means the cessation of menses. It has a definite end-point unlike the climacteric, which includes physiologic, psychologic, and anatomic changes and has no sharp end point. Traditionally, a woman who is amenorrheic is considered menopausal. However, chemically and anatomically, these changes occur over a period of time. Although they are considered to be quite rapid, it takes approximately 3 to 5 years for the terminal picture to be achieved. The conclusion must then be drawn that if an ovary is palpated 3 to 5 years after the clinical menopause, it is a pathologic ovary until proved otherwise, regardless of its size.

Incidence.   Cancer of the ovary is the most frustrating problem that the gynecologist faces. It is on the increase and has a very high death rate. It is badly neglected by both patient and physician. Ovarian cancer is now the leading cause of death from gynecologic cancer in the United States. The figure that is impressive is that ovarian cancer makes up only 24% of all gynecologic cancers but accounts for 47% of all gynecologic cancer deaths. Of newborn girls, 1.4% or 1 in 70 will develop ovarian cancer during their lifetime (8). The tragic feature of ovarian cancer is that 70% to 80% have advanced to stages 3 and 4 by the time it is diagnosed. Therefore, the treatment of ovarian cancer is usually directed to the far advanced

patient or to the terminal care of the patient with advanced or recurrent cancer of the ovary. The challenge presented by ovarian cancer is that more than 11,000 patients will die from ovarian cancer each year in the United States and that the results in 1980 are no better than they were in the previous three decades. By our aggressive approach to diagnosis and therapy, these patients are living longer and hopefully more comfortably, but there has been no improvement in the overall 5-year survival at this point.

It is important to look at the ovarian cancer incidence rates and distribution of cases by age. The incidence of ovarian cancer starts to rise at age 40 years with an annual rate of 10 per 100,000 women, and rises to a peak at about age 77 years when the rate is about 52 per 100,000 women, and then drops at age 80 years to a rate of about 45 per 100,000 (8). It plateaus at this point and remains steady for the remainder of life. It is essential that these figures and the distribution of this curve be kept in mind at the time of making the decision of whether to retain ovaries at the time of hysterectomy in women over age 40 years. Since the incidence of ovarian cancer is on the increase in the highly industrialized nations, an effort must be made to achieve earlier diagnosis than in the past or to practice prophylaxis by removing ovaries at the time of the surgery in women over age 40 years. Currently in the United States there are more than 650,000 hysterectomies being performed annually, and most of these are in women over age 40 years. It is obvious that some cancers of the ovary could be prevented among these women if oophorectomy were done at the time of hysterectomy.

It is recommended that the patient described in the case presentation should have the benefit of an expedited examination under anesthesia and, if the previous impression of a normal-sized, premenopausal ovary is identified, should be explored. When the abdomen is opened, aspirations from the pelvis should be taken for cytology and a careful abdominal exploration followed by inspection and palpation of the abdomen. Total hysterectomy, bilateral salpingo-oophorectomy, appendectomy, and, if the pathology report indicates invasion, an omentectomy should be carried out. Although splitting and obtaining a biopsy specimen of the ovary may be justified in detecting early cancer in the premenopausal patient, the ovaries should be removed without biopsy in the postmenopausal patient.

If more women are to be saved and we are to diminish the mortality from ovarian cancer, we must become more liberal in our indications for operation. It is suggested that the palpation of what appears to be a normal-sized ovary for a patient 3 to 5 years after menopause is indicative of an ovarian tumor and should be investigated immediately. These cases should not be followed and re-evaluated but rather subjected to proof as to the presence or absence of an ovarian tumor. To wait until one feels a solid tumor mass of up to 5 cm and expect a cure is an exercise in fancy and futility.

It is difficult to make a decision on management of a patient who is in the menopause and has fibroids. All too often, an ovarian neoplasm is followed under the false impression that it is a fibroid. Ovarian tumors can enlarge, grow against the uterus, and both the uterus and ovary can rise from the pelvis as a midline mass. Therefore, if the ovaries cannot be palpated as separate entities from the fibroids, it is in the patient's best interest to examine her under anesthesia. The decision as to whether to explore the patient must be made on the findings at that time.

References

1. Barber HRK, Graber EA: The PMPO syndrome (postmenopausal palpable ovary syndrome). *Obstet Gynecol* 38:921, 1971.
2. Barber HRK: The postmenopausal palpable ovary syndrome. *Compr Ther* 5:58, 1979.
3. Busse W (ed): *Changing Concepts: Age through the Ages. Therapy and Therapeutics of Aging.* New York, Medcom Press, 1973.
4. Costoff A: An ultrastructural study of ovarian changes in the menopause. In Greenblatt RB, Mahesh VB, McDonough PG (eds): *The Menopause Syndrome.* New York, Medcom Press, 1974.
5. Guraya SS: Interstitial gland tissue of mammalian ovary. *Acta Endocrinol* 72 (Suppl 171):72, 1973.
6. Kistner RW: *Gynecology, Principles and Practice,* ed. 2. Chicago, Year Book, 1971.
7. Rutledge F, Boronow RC, Wharton JT: *Gynecologic Oncology.* New York, John Wiley & Sons, 1976.
8. Silverberg E: *Gynecologic Cancer: Statistical and Epidemiological Information.* Professional Education Publication. New York, American Cancer Society, 1980.
9. U.S. Department of Health, Education, and Welfare: *End Results in Cancer.* Public Health Service, National Institutes of Health, Report No. 5, Bethesda, MD, 1976, p. 177.

CHAPTER 17

Pregnancy with Bleeding Corpus Luteum

RAY V. HANING, JR., M.D.

CASE ABSTRACT

Possible ectopic pregnancy was considered in a 20-year-old primigravida with progressively disabling right lower quadrant discomfort of 2 days' duration. The patient's last menstrual period had occurred 7 weeks previously, and a pregnancy test was positive. There was considerable fullness in the left adnexa and the cul-de-sac. A positive culdocentesis was obtained which brought forth some 20 cc of unclotted blood. Prompt laparotomy was performed and approximately 1000 cc of blood was discovered in the pelvis. The uterus was softened and enlarged, the fallopian tubes were within normal limits, and there was a 2.5-cm actively bleeding corpus luteum on the left ovary. A few interrupted stitches were placed through the corpus luteum, but the bleeding was not controlled. The corpus luteum was excised from the ovary, and a few mattress sutures of 3-0 chromic catgut placed in the ovarian cortex promptly controlled the bleeding. The incised margin of the ovary was closed with some interrupted 3-0 chromic sutures.

DISCUSSION

Background

Progesterone in pregnancy is secreted by both the corpus luteum and the syncytotrophoblast cells of the placenta. In the early stages of pregnancy, removal of the corpus luteum results in loss of the pregnancy unless an exogenous source of progesterone is supplied. Later in pregnancy, a sufficient proportion of total secreted progesterone arises in the placenta to allow the pregnancy to continue even after removal of the corpus luteum of pregnancy. Relaxin is another corpus luteum product which appears to be important in cervical ripening and which may have other yet unknown beneficial effect. Relaxin cannot currently be replaced if luteectomy occurs, making it important to preserve the corpus luteum if possible at all stages of pregnancy. Once luteectomy has occurred, the following critical questions arise: (a) At what stage does the pregnancy become independent of corpus luteum progesterone? and (b) what type and dose of progestational agent should be administered if the pregnancy is still dependent on corpus luteum progesterone?

Removal of the corpus luteum and any accessory corpora lutea (accessory corpora lutea are present in approximately 20% of pregnancies) prior to the seventh menstrual gestational week (fifth week after conception) results in spontaneous abortion. In the seventh week, some pregnancies are maintained and some are lost. After the seventh week, most pregnancies are independent of the corpus luteum (1, 2). Substitution therapy with 200 mg per day of progesterone in oil prevented pregnancy loss after luteectomy but resulted in a serum progesterone concentration of 80 ng/ml, a value approximately four times that observed in control patients without luteectomy (2, 3). No details were provided in that study on the long-term result in the progesterone-treated pregnancies since termination of pregnancy was performed 7 days after luteectomy when initial maintenance of pregnancy had been demonstrated. To allow for errors in dating of the pregnancy, progesterone replacement therapy should be considered in all patients luteectomized prior to the beginning of the ninth gestational week. This guideline provides approximately 1 week of treatment beyond the time when all pregnancies were maintained without progesterone replacement (in the small number of luteectomy cases evaluated) to prevent loss of some viable pregnancies which have not yet become independent of the corpus luteum for one reason or another (i.e., a late ovulation in the pregnancy cycle). Not all progestational agents are safe for use in pregnancy. Ethisterone and danazol are known to produce masculinization of the external genitalia of the female when administered in the first trimester of pregnancy. All progestational agents are now required to bear a warning against possible teratogenic effects if used in pregnancy. Even progesterone injection, USP, is required to be dispensed with patient labeling warning against possible teratogenic effects. However, a study of congenital malformations among offspring exposed in utero to progestins showed no evidence for a teratogenic effect of either progesterone or 17 alpha-hydroxyprogesterone caproate in the doses used (4). Because only progesterone itself can be considered chemically identical with the progesterone secreted by the corpus luteum, the author recommends the use of intramuscular progesterone in oil as the progestational agent of choice for treating luteectomized patients.

Progesterone Treatment in Luteectomized Pregnant Women

Replacement progesterone should be considered for women luteectomized prior to the eighth gestational week. Replacement in those luteectomized in the eighth week may be desirable to prevent loss of some pregnancies not yet independent of the corpus luteum. The replacement dose is 50 to 200 mg of progesterone in oil per day. Progesterone in oil is irritating to the injection site, and no more than 100 mg should be administered intramuscularly in a single injection. Thus, when doses over 100 mg/day are given, the dose must be divided so that no more than 100 mg is given in a single site. The use of progesterone itself has the advantage that progesterone blood levels can be monitored by radioimmunoassay and the dose adjusted to provide physiological concentrations of progesterone in the venous blood (20 mg/ml or greater). Its disadvantage is the need for daily injections to achieve and maintain physiologically signigicant progesterone levels. Another advantage of progesterone is that since it is the same molecule secreted by the placental cells, it is less likely to affect fetal development than a chemically foreign molecule. After the ninth week, the progesterone injections can be discontinued. Demonstration of fetal cardiac activity after the eighth week of pregnancy is the most reliable means of demonstrating the continued viability of the pregnancy.

Surgical Approaches Designed to Avoid Luteectomy. Laparoscopy and laparotomy in such cases can be utilized to visualize the bleeding site and to rule out a ruptured ectopic pregnancy. Large quantities of blood (including some large clots) can be evacuated at laparoscopy by use of accessory puncture cannulas without valves and a 60 cc catheter tip syringe pressed firmly against the rubber gasket of the accessory puncture cannula. Using a blunt grasping forceps, large clots can be cut to a small enough size to fit through these 5 mm diameter cannulas under suction applied by the syringe. If the bleeding has stopped spontaneously or if the bleeding can be stopped using either monopolar or bipolar coagulation, laparotomy is unnecessary as long as the peritoneal blood and blood clots can be evacuated. Gavage of the bleeding site and the pelvis with warmed isotonic saline can help to confirm cessation of bleeding and also to rinse the last of the blood into the cul-de-sac where it can be removed by suction.

If for one reason or another laparotomy becomes necessary, the blood and blood clot should be removed. If the corpus luteum bleeding has stopped spontaneously or if it can be stopped surgically, luteectomy is unnecessary. Due to the friability and vascularity of the corpus luteum, the use of irrigation to visualize the bleeding site along with good light and surgical loupes to achieve magnification often allows identification of the bleeders accurately enough to permit direct coagulation. Indirect coagulation should be tried if the use of a hemostat is necessary. If multiple small sites of bleeding resist coagulation, brief packing with a warm isotonic saline moistened pack for up to 10 minutes may provide control. The use of sutures and hemostats should be avoided, where possible, since they cut through friable tissue and provoke bleeding from the laceration and/or the needle puncture sites. If sutures must be used, try 6-0 absorbable suture on an atraumatic needle and gentle technique.

Preventing Corpus Luteum Hemorrhage. Aspirin and other drugs which can reduce platelet activity or produce anticoagulation should be avoided in periovulatory and post-ovulatory women if possible. This includes such simple measures as substitution of acetaminophen for aspirin in treating headache.

References

1. Csapo AI, Pulkkinen MO, Ruttner B, et al: The significance of the human corpus luteum in pregnancy maintenance. I. Preliminary studies. *Am J Obstet Gynecol* 112:1061-1067, 1972.
2. Csapo AI, Pulkkinen MO, Wiest WG: Effects of luteectomy and progesterone replacement therapy in early pregnant patients. *Am J Obstet Gynecol* 115:759-765, 1973.
3. Haning RV Jr, Choi L, Curet LB, et al: Interrelationships among human chorionic gonadotropin (hCG) 17-estradiol, progesterone, and estriol in maternal serum: Evidence for an inhibitory effect of the fetal adrenal on secretion of hCG. *J Clin Endocrinol Metabol* 56:1188-1194,1983.
4. Resseguie LJ, Hick JF, Bruen JA, et al: Congenital malformations among offspring exposed in utero to progestins, Olmsted County, Minnesota, 1936-1974. *Fertil Steril* 43:514-519,1985.

CHAPTER **18**

Bilateral Ovarian Mature Teratomas in a Young Woman

JAMES L. BREEN, M.D., F.A.C.O.G., F.A.C.S.
JULIAN E. DeLIA, M.D., F.A.C.O.G.

CASE ABSTRACT

A 7-cm cyst of the left ovary was found in a 22-year-old, para 1 woman. It was persistent and tender and at surgery was identified as a mature teratoma which replaced much of the ovary. A similar smaller cyst was found in the opposite ovary.

DISCUSSION

Bilateral mature teratomas were found in a young woman of low parity. Due to the low incidence of ovarian cancer found in this age group, a low transverse incision was performed. Management consisted of bilateral oophorocystectomies with preservation of ovarian tissue. Particular attention was directed at utilizing surgical techniques which would ensure minimal interference with tubo-ovarian function and future fertility.

Introduction

The patient presented in this case represents a fairly common clinical situation as seen in patients with mature teratomas. Preoperative evaluation and surgical management will vary according to the patient's age, physical findings, and reproductive desires. Three specific surgical decisions had to be addressed in this patient: (a) type of abdominal incision, (b) intraoperative management, and (c) procedures to prevent future infertility.

Choice of Incision

A significant percentage of pelvic surgeons adhere to the principle that low vertical incisions must be utilized in evaluating all adnexal masses. This type of incision allows for easier exploration of the upper abdomen and will permit cephalad extension, should it be necessary. On the other hand, most patients prefer the cosmetic advantages of a low transverse incision (Pfannenstiel). Surgical advantages of this incision include a lower infection and dehiscence rate and less postoperative discomfort. Ultimately, the incision selected must be adapted to the operative procedure envisioned, considering the various diagnostic possibilities, most notably, ovarian malignancy.

The lowest incidence for malignant ovarian neoplasms occurs during the second to fourth decades of life. In childhood, one-third of ovarian neoplasms are malignant. After age 40 years, there is an increasing incidence of ovarian cancer, with 70% of ovarian malignancies occurring after 50 years of age.

Of all ovarian tumors, the mature teratoma is most amenable to a preoperative diagnosis. Approximately 50% of these neoplasms will have radiographic evidence of their nature on a simple scout film of the abdomen. In addition, although immature elements or other germ cell tumors can coexist with mature elements in these tumors, these malignant varieties most commonly occur under the age of 18 years, with less than 5% occurring in patients over 18 years (1, 3, 4).

Judgment is required on the part of the surgeon to determine the need for additional studies or examinations, prior to laparotomy, to aid in determining the nature of the adnexal disease. In general, studies that are helpful in the differential diagnosis of a pelvic mass include a complete blood count, urinalysis, liver function tests, sedimentation rate, serum chorionic gonadotropin and alpha-fetoprotein (tumor markers) roentgenography of the chest and abdomen, intravenous pyelography, barium enema, upper gastrointestinal series, liver scan, pelvic ultrasonography, and proctosigmoidoscopy. Elaborate preoperative studies will not be necessary in most instances of unilateral or bilateral masses occurring in reproductive-aged patients, similar to the one presented. Ultimate test selection, however, will be modified by the patient's age, history, and physical examination (7).

Mature teratomas have physical findings that are characteristic of both benign and malignant ovarian tumors. Their mobility, smoothness, cystic nature, and unilaterality suggests benignity. The large percentage (25%) that present acutely with torsion also suggests a mobile benign tumor. At times, however, their solid character, bilaterality, and large diameter are suggestive of malignancy.

The final decision as to which incision to use can be made following a careful pelvic examination in the operative room, while the patient is under general anesthesia. Indeed, it should be a routine practice to re-evaluate or confirm previous pelvic findings prior to making an incision for the treatment of pelvic masses. One may find that the situation is different from that noted previously. We feel, given a patient with the findings outlined in this case presentation, that a low transverse incision would be acceptable. Always remember that a transverse incision can be made much larger by converting it to a Cherney incision.

Intraoperative Management

Immediately upon entering the abdomen an evaluation is made to see if ascitic fluid is present and what is the status of the abdominopelvic cavity serosal surfaces. Until the exact nature of the tumor is known, ascitic fluid or peritoneal washings should be collected, as these will be important in the proper clinical staging if the ovarian tumors are malignant. Once the exact nature of the tumor is determined, the above may not be necessary.

The exploration of the upper abdomen should precede the pelvic exploration. Particular attention is paid to the diaphragmatic surfaces, liver, gallbladder, kidneys, bowel surfaces, and periaortic nodes.

With this completed, the bowel can now be gently packed away from the pelvis and the pelvic organs examined visually and manually

to determine the nature of the tumor. The gross characteristics of most ovarian tumors should be familiar to the surgeon (2).

Mature teratomas are frequently found anterior to the uterus—a condition that may be due to the low specific gravity of the sebaceous material within the cyst or to the fact that its germ cell origin makes it, from an embryologic standpoint, a midline tumor. They are usually globular or ovoid with a great range in size but average 6 to 10 cm. The dense capsular wall is smooth, yellowish-white, and has fine vascular markings.

The key to the diagnosis of type and the determination of the benign or malignant nature of the tumor often will depend on the appearance of its contents after it is opened in the operating room. It is a good principle not to rupture or open any tumor prior to its removal, to prevent intra-abdominal spill.

The treatment of choice for mature teratomas is an oophorocystectomy with the preservation of as much ovarian tissue as possible. The capsular ovarian fragment, even if small, will contain germ cells. Its importance for future reproduction has been repeatedly documented. There are three exceptions to ovarian conservation, i.e., torsion with loss of viability, rupture, or malignancy. In later years, in a patient with her fertility completed, a total abdominal hysterectomy and salpingo-oophorectomy is acceptable therapy.

The patient presented was desirous of future fertility and had bilateral disease. Every attempt should be made, in such a patient, to excise benign solid tumors and cysts carefully, provided the remaining portion of the ovary can be preserved with an adequate blood supply.

The ovary should be well isolated from surrounding structures and packed, to prevent possible spill of the tumor's contents into the abdominal cavity. Spontaneous rupture of the teratoma or its rupture during removal will allow the sebaceous material and other contents to enter the peritoneal cavity. This material is irritating to the peritoneum and is capable of producing a chronic granulomatous response. If this occurs, lavage the peritoneal cavity with water or saline.

A shallow linear incision of the ovarian capsule is made far from the mesovarium and is of sufficient length to allow for removal of the tumor. The tumor is then carefully shelled out from the remaining ovary. Bleeding, which is most prominent in the hilar region, may be controlled either by fine suturing of individual vessels, delicate electrocautery, or by running a horizontal mattress suture close to the hilum. Two rather broad flaps of ovarian tissue will remain. Care should now be taken to reapproximate these flaps to achieve a repair free from abraded or raw edges.

The excised cyst should now be opened to verify its nature before addressing the opposite ovary. The contents of a mature teratoma are usually liquid, but on cooling the sebaceous material tends to solidify. The majority are unilocular and contain a mural projection or dermoid process (Rokitansky's protuberance) within which the majority of primary tissue elements are found. Identification of hair, teeth, and other elements is common. Occasionally, the exact nature may have to await a frozen section or permanent histologic evaluation. These tumors are known to occur in a mixed form with immature elements or other germ cell tumors present which bear poor prognoses. In situations where some confusion exists, it is best to continue along the conservative route and not extirpate the reproductive organs in a young woman. One must maintain the willingness to reoperate, pending adequate histologic evaluation of the tumor on permanent sections.

In this patient the management of the opposite ovary was dictated by finding a cyst present on close inspection. This cyst should have been managed as outlined above.

Not as clear is the management of the opposite ovary when it appears normal in the presence of a contralateral mature teratoma. Bilaterality of this tumor ranges from 10% to 20%. The finding of small foci of a mature teratoma on bivalving normal ovaries prompted the recommendation that routine wedge resections or bivalving should be performed to exclude occult bilaterality, whether the ovary appeared abnormal or not. The harmful effects, however, of ovarian wedge biopsy have been noted in several studies of patients who had the procedure for polycystic ovarian disease (9). The high incidence of peritubal and periovarian adhesions noted has virtually rendered this aproach obsolete in polycystic ovarian disease except in the rare case refractory to medical management.

Doss et al. (5), in a study of 213 cases of mature teratoma, have provided data to support a conservative approach to the contralateral ovary. In this series no occult tumors were found when the opposite ovary appeared grossly normal. Ovarian investigation by surgical means was no more sensitive than the surgeon's eyes and hands. Although it cannot be denied that the inspection and palpation may occasionally miss a small occult tumor, necessitating reoperation, we feel the risk of reoperation to restore fertility is greater in patients treated with wedge of a normal ovary.

Prophylaxis of Adhesions

A significant number of women presenting with infertility will give a history of prior pelvic surgery. Pelvic adhesions and anatomic distortion are undesirable sequelae of gynecologic surgery regardless of the indication for the initial surgery. These are particularly disconcerting when the patient is desirous of retaining her reproductive capacity. Since adhesion formation seems to be the result of trauma, major emphasis should be placed on the use of techniques which minimize adhesion formation.

The advent of gynecologic microsurgery has considerably improved the outcome of adnexal surgery. Although no comparative studies exist to date that demonstrate the advantage of microsurgical techniques versus macrosurgical techniques for various benign ovarian diseases in the human, animal studies have shown a 5-fold increase in adhesion formation when traditional macrosurgical techniques are utilized (6). When one is confronted by a patient with the physical findings and reproductive desires similar to our case, it is imperative to avoid tubal distortation and postoperative adhesions. These sequelae will be minimized by using microsurgical principles utilized in infertility surgery.

The etiology, prevention, and experimental and clinical experience regarding postoperative adhesions were recently reviewed by Levinson and Swolin (8). Although it is unreasonable to suggest the use of magnification in ovarian tumor surgery, other principles can be adopted with potentially rewarding results. These include:

1. Careful washing of surgical gloves to remove talc and the use of lint-free swabs and packs.

2. Elimination of sponging by use of irrigation and suction instead.

3. Gentle handling of tissue by avoiding the use of instruments that traumatize tissue.

4. Use of pinpoint electrocautery, bipolar tips, or very fine suture ligatures for hemostasis.

5. Elimination of raw surfaces by careful reapproximation of cut surfaces.

6. Use of fine nonreactive sutures with atraumatic needles for the ovarian repair (6-0 Dexon or Vicryl can be used without magnification).

7. Avoidance of prolonged drying of tissue.

8. Reduction of tissue inflammation with intraperitoneal and systemic medications (antibiotics and anti-inflammatory agents).

Currently, insufficient data exist to support broad-scale usage of the above techniques in ovarian tumor surgery. In theory, however, the time spent will be rewarded by a lowered incidence of iatrogenic infertility in the patient with benign disease.

References

1. Breen JL, Bonamo JF, Maxson WS: Genital tract tumor in children. *Pediatr Clin North Am* 28:355, 1981.
2. Breen JL, Jaffers WJ: *Atlas of Gynecologic Pathology*. Philadelphia, F. A. Davis, 1968.
3. Breen JL, Maxson WS: Ovarian tumors in children and adolescents. *Clin Obstet Gynecol* 20:607, 1977.
4. Breen JL, Neubecker RD: Malignant teratoma of the ovary. *Obstet Gynecol* 21:669, 1963.
5. Doss N, Forney JP, Vellios F, et al: Covert bilaterality of mature ovarian teratomas. *Obstet Gynecol* 50:651, 1977.
6. Eddy CA, Asch RH, Balaceda JP: Pelvic adhesions following microsurgical and macrosurgical wedge resection of the ovaries. *Fertil Steril* 33:557, 1980.
7. Johnson GH: Pelvic mass and the diagnosis of carcinoma of the ovary. *Clin Obstet Gynecol* 22:903, 1979.
8. Levinson CH, Swolin K: Postoperative adhesions: Etiology, prevention and therapy. *Clin Obstet Gynecol* 23:1213, 1980.
9. Toaf R, Toaf ME, Peyser MR: Infertility following wedge resection of the ovaries. *Am J Obstet Gynecol* 124:92, 1976.

CHAPTER 19

Ovarian Tumor Too Large to Be Delivered Through a Small Pfannenstiel Incision

ABE MICKAL, M.D., F.A.C.O.G., F.A.C.S.

CASE ABSTRACT

A persistent large ovarian tumor was found in a 27-year-old patient, and removal was recommended. Laparotomy began through a small Pfannenstiel incision, but once the abdomen was opened, it was evident that the incision was too small to permit intact delivery of the tumor.

DISCUSSION

"Pray before surgery but remember God will not alter a faulty incision."

Arthur H. Keeney

Abdominal Incisions

Moynihan (2) in 1914 stated:

"Too great care cannot therefore be exercised in the proper choice of incision and of the means of its securest closure. If a difficult manipulation is performed through an opening which cramps the surgeon's hand the wound edges will be bruised, perhaps soiled with escaping fluids, indeed, so great damage may be done that proper healing of the wound is impossible."

It is axiomatic in surgery that the best operation for any patient is one that best meets the needs of the clinical problem and at the same time minimizes the operative risk. This begins and ends with the proper incision which will allow adequate exposure for the exercising of the appropriate surgical technique and skills in the management of the problem at hand. Unfortunately, at times the desire of the patient for cosmetic effect buffered by the surgical confidence of the surgeon results in an improper incisional approach being occasionally made.

The two basic styled incisions for abdominal surgery are the vertical (longitudinal) and the transverse. A brief review (1, 4) of these incisions follows:

1. Vertical: (a) Midline—all components of the abdominal wall are incised vertically including the linea alba. (b) Paramedian (right or left)—this is similar to the midline in that the components of the abdominal wall are incised vertically, but the rectus sheath is entered and the muscle is displaced laterally.

2. Transverse: (a) Pfannenstiel (bikini cut)—a small semilunar incision following the transverse fold demarcating the mons pubis and the inferior portion of abdominal wall. The anterior sheath of the rectus is incised transversely with separation of the rectus to allow a transverse incision of the peritoneum. (b) Cherney—the skin incision at the level of the anterior superior spines. The external oblique muscles are bluntly but carefully separated. Then the pyramidalis muscles are separated from the rectus and pushed inferiorly. The tendinous insertion of the rectus is severed from its attachment to the symphysis. Transversalis fascia and peritoneum are then incised transversally. (c) Maylard—the same technique as for the Cherney with the exception that the rectus muscle bundle is incised transversally. Three tendinous inscriptions divide the rectus into four muscle bundles; the lower is the longest and the site for the incision of the region of the semicircular line of Douglas.

The use of the Pfannenstiel incision has become popular in gynecologic surgery because of its acceptance by the patient as well as its cosmetic effect and good healing qualities. I prefer this incision whenever possible. Its most likely contraindication is the limitation of exposure. This does not pose a serious problem when dealing with benign disease. However, when one encounters a larger than expected ovarian tumor or a pelvic malignancy, then the limitation imposed by the Pfannenstiel incision assumes more serious proportions.

The basic considerations for abdominal incisions (3) in gynecologic surgery are:

1. Flexibility of the incision
2. The operative needs of the patient
3. The elective or emergency nature of the problem
4. The condition of the patient
5. The size of the patient and thickness of the abdominal wall
6. Cosmetic effect

Ovarian Tumors in a 27-Year-Old Patient

In addition to considering the management of a large tumor through a Pfannenstiel incision, we should also consider the most common ovarian tumors found in this age group.

Woodruff (5) states that 85% of all true ovarian neoplasms arise from the stromoepithelial tumors, primary epithelial. The scope of this presentation does not warrant a thorough review of the entire classification of ovarian tumors, so only those tumors that reach large proportions and are prevalent in this age group will be summarized briefly as follows:

1. Serous cystadenomas and cystadenocarcinomas; (a) Fifty percent occur in women under the age of 40 years. (b) About 30% of serous tumors are malignant.

2. Mucinous cystadenomas and cystadenocarcinomas: (a) Malignant potential of these tumors is less than that of the serous. (b) They are bilateral in 8% to 10% of cases. (c) These are generally the largest ovarian neoplasms, and the larger the tumor the more likely it is of the mucinous type.

3. Benign cystic teratoma (dermoid): (a) These comprise 12% to 15% of all ovarian neoplasms. (b) It is uncommon for malignant degeneration to occur in a primarily benign cystic tumor.

4. Other ovarian masses that may reach large

proportions in the third decade of life: (a) Inflammatory (tubo-ovarian abscess), (b) malignant teratoma, (c) sarcomas (stromal or teratoid), (d) dysgerminoma.

How to Avoid an Improper Incision

Some of the aspects of this problem have been alluded to. If the following procedures had been carried out and evaluated, then the appropriate incision would most probably have been made and the dilemma encountered could have been avoided:

1. Careful history, especially as related to age, parity, menstrual, and present complaints.

2. Careful physical examination, including breast, abdomen, vaginal, and rectovaginal repeated as needed for confident identification of the problem and approaches for its solution.

3. The following diagnostic aids should be employed as needed to achieve the best possible understanding of the clinical picture. Basic tests should include (a) complete blood count and sedimentation rate if indicated, and (b) urinalysis. Additional helpful and confirmatory tests are (a) ultrasound of pelvic organs, (b) x-ray of chest and abdomen, (c) barium enema and a proctoscopic examination if warranted, (d) intravenous pyelogram, and (e) electrocardiogram.

The diagnostic aids that are available today should be of great help in preoperative evaluation as related to abdominal and pelvic masses. These aids are only supportive of and not a substitute for a good history and physical examination. Ultrasonography can give relatively accurate dimensions and configuration of masses in a large majority of cases.

Outline of Possible Solutions

The problem posed is that of a Pfannenstiel incision for an ovarian mass that is presumably too large to be removed through the original incision. It is presumed that all aspects of the surgical procedure have been fully discussed with the patient and an understanding was reached regarding the minimum or maximum extent of surgery. When one encounters such a problem, there are certain steps that should be employed routinely:

1. Full inspection of entire pelvis, especially the opposite adnexa.

2. Careful gross inspection and evaluation of the tumor as to its pathologic and malignant

potential as well as any adhesions to adjacent viscera, etc.

3. Cytology of cul-de-sac fluid.

4. Consultation with pathologist if needed.

5. If the mass is considered benign, then: (a) extend the incision laterally to its fullest extent to enable total delivery of the mass if possible. (b) If the above does not suffice, then transect the tendinous insertion of the rectus abdominus muscle (Cherney). This will greatly enhance the opening and permit greater exposure. I have on occasion used a Maylard incision as well with good results. (c) If one is dealing with a large cystic benign mass, then prior to resorting to ''a'' and ''b'', I have done the following on several occasions:

(1) Inspect the pelvis and the mass to ensure freedom from adhesions.

(2) Gently place a medium or large-sized Deaver retractor blade underneath the mass for stability.

(3) Apply gentle traction with the Deaver retractor to assist in delivery of the mass. This works better than the hand and occupies much less space. The Deaver acts in this way much like an obstetric forceps.

(4) If all the above fail, then carefully pack the entire incision with lap squares to totally seal off the peritoneal cavity, to prevent spillage of the contents of the mass into the abdominal cavity.

(5) Carefully place a purse-string suture using small atraumatic needle (Dexon 3-5, or intestinal 3-0 chromic). Apply no pressure with the Deaver during this procedure.

(6) Puncture anterior surface of cyst within purse-string, after the opposite ends of the purse-string suture are lifted to elevate the cyst wall and prevent spilling, as illustrated in Figure 19.1.

(7) The suction tip is inserted into the puncture site, and the cyst is decompressed to a size that allows easy delivery through the incision. The Deaver can be helpful there if needed.

(8) To prevent spillage, the purse-string suture is tied fast as suction is removed.

(9) The remaining surgical procedure is carried out as indicated, and copious irrigation of the abdominal cavity is recommended. I have carried out this procedure prior to enlarging markedly the Pfannenstiel incision when I was confident of the benign nature of the cyst.

6. If the problem encountered does not fall within the scope of the management procedures previously discussed and the ovarian mass is solid or semisolid and not amenable to drainage, then an inverted T is made. The longitudinal part is not done until the full potential of the transverse incision has been reached. Admittedly, this is not the preferred route, but the well-being of the patient must be the primary concern. Patients are concerned about the appearance of their incisions, but they usually are receptive and understanding if adequate dialogue is achieved. They are apt to be very tolerant when they know that decisions were made in their overall best interest and with good clinical judgment, thoughtful deliberation, and consultation.

My Approach in This Case

I hope that I have adequately evaluated the patient and her problem, using ultrasound and repeated evaluations to reach a sound clinical decision with regard to the probable nature of the mass and the best incisional approach to its management.

As previously stated, I am very fond of the Pfannenstiel incision and would use this approach unless contraindicated by size or potential malignancy of the tumor. A brief outline of my abdominal incisional approaches to ovarian tumors is:

1. In benign cystic disease: Pfannenstiel incision—if this proved to be too small it would be enlarged or the purse-string aspiration technique used for decompression.

2. Solid large tumors—benign or of questionable malignancy: Cherney or vertical, depending on the clinical evaluation as to the most appropriate approach to this patient's problem.

3. Obvious ovarian malignancy: vertical incision.

It has been stated that the mark of a good surgeon is his closure of the incision. Unfortunately, many times this important aspect of the surgical procedure is relegated to the least experienced member of the surgical team. Greater emphasis should be placed on the following surgical principles, including the closure: (a) gentle handling, (b) secure good hemostasis, (c) maintain good blood supply, (d) debridement of all dead tissue, (e) avoid large pedicles with necrotic tissue, (f) obliterate dead space, (g) avoid hematomas, (h) choose suture materials to meet the needs of the tissue in-

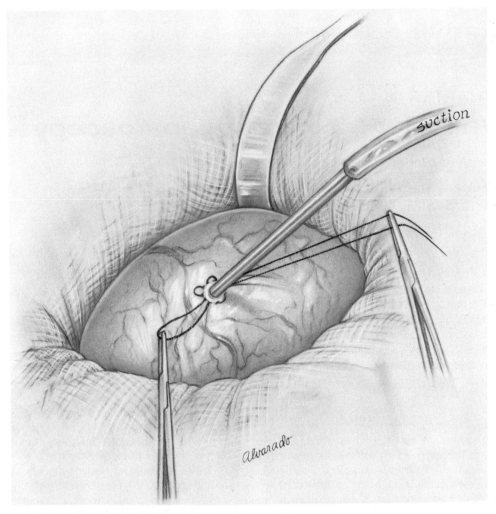

Figure 19.1. A purse-string suture has been placed, and after the opposite ends of the purse-string have been elevated to prevent spilling, the cyst is punctured by a trochar to which suction is attached.

volved, (i) drain through separate stab wounds, and (j) close wound securely but without tension.

The true diagnosis of ovarian neoplasm usually cannot be ascertained without adequate histopathologic studies. Cancers of the ovary are extremely difficult to diagnose early and treat effectively. In 1977 the fifth leading cause of cancer deaths in females between the ages of 35 and 74 years of age was cancer of the ovary. This is a reminder that all ovarian neoplasms must be treated respectfully and the best way to accomplish this is with an incision that gives complete exposure so that the necessary sur-

gical procedure can be accomplished adequately.

References

1. Kermit E: In Benson RC (ed): *Current Obstetrics and Gynecologic Diagnosis and Treatment*, ed. 3. Los Altos, CA, Lange, 1980.
2. Moynihan BGA: *Abdominal Operation*. Vol. I. Philadelphia, WB Saunders, 1914.
3. Nora PF: *Operative Surgery: Principles and Technique*, ed. 2. Philadelphia, Lea & Febiger, 1980.
4. Sabotta J, McMurrich JP: *Atlas of Human Anatomy*. Vol I. New York, GE Hechert, 1936.
5. Woodruff JD: Diseases of the ovaries. In Benson RC (ed): *Current Obstetrics and Gynecologic Diagnosis and Treatment*, ed. 3. Los Altos, CA, Lange, 1980.

CHAPTER **20**

Vascular Injuries at Laparoscopy

L. RUSSELL MALINAK, M.D.
JAMES M. WHEELER, M.D.
GREG SIMOLKE, B.S.

CASE ABSTRACT

A 28-year-old infertility patient complaining of secondary dysmenorrhea was scheduled for diagnostic closed laparoscopy. The insufflation needle was inserted without incident. When the trocar was introduced, however, the patient coughed. Upon removal of the trocar from the sleeve, a spurt of bright red blood was briefly evident through the sleeve. The anesthetist reported a rapid rise in pulse rate, and a precipitous decline in blood pressure. The gynecologist's working diagnosis was that of injury to a major blood vessel at time of insertion of the laparoscopic trocar.

DISCUSSION

Laparoscopy has been increasingly utilized as a diagnostic and therapeutic method in gynecology. Although generally considered a minor operation, laparoscopy is associated with morbidity and mortality. The most dramatic and serious complications of laparoscopy occur in the rare event of vascular injury. Although the prevalence of vascular injuries is unknow, the incidence has been evaluated in several studies. The injuries have been categorized into minor and major vessel trauma. Loffer and Pent (8) reported the incidence of all vascular injuries as 6.4 per 1000 laparoscopies. The Royal College of Obstetricians and Gynecologists reported that great vessel injuries occurred in 9 per 10,000 laparoscopies (2). In a French survey of 100,000 laparoscopies, 31 major vessel injuries were reported, for an incidence of 3 per 10,000 (10). Penfield (11) reported that great vessel injuries are equally common in the aorta and the common iliac vessels and that vascular injuries were as likely due to insertion of the Verres insufflation needle as the sharp trocar. Additional clinical information regarding great vessel injury during laparoscopy has been pub-lished in individual case reports (1, 5, 7, 9, 12, 16). In our experience of 1000 laparoscopies in the evaluation of infertility, there have been no injuries to the great vessels.

The lesser vessels most commonly injured during laparoscopy are the inferior epigastric artery and vein in the anterior abdominal wall, and the vessels located within the mesosalpinx (most commonly injured during tubal sterilization procedures). In our series, the middle sacral vessels have been injured in two patients, for an incidence of 2 per 1000.

Prior to discussion of prevention of vascular injuries during laparoscopy, a review of the pertinent vascular anatomy of the female pelvis is warranted. The umbilicus serves as the reference point for insertion of the laparoscope in clinical practice. Its position in relationship to the great vessels, however, is highly variable; thus, the umbilicus is a potentially dangerous landmark. Also, bony landmarks have been utilized to determine the location of the aortic bifurcation; the bifurcation normally overlies the fourth lumbar vertebra, which topographically corresponds to a line drawn between the summits of the iliac crests. As with the umbilicus, however, the variability in the relationship of the bony landmarks to the bifurcation make them unsatisfactory routine landmarks for laparoscopy. Indeed, the bifurcation is at L-4 in 75% of cases, and is within 1.25 cm above or below the iliac crests in 80% of women. In 9% of patients, the aortic bifurcation lies above L-4 (3), thus providing a further degree of safety from laparoscopic vascular injuries. An extra degree of hazard, however, is present in the 11% of patients whose bifurcation lies below the L-4/L-5 disc space (3). With this degree of variability in anatomic landmarks, the most reliable way to determine the location of the aortic bifurcation is to palpate it, which is possible in all but the most obese of patients. Besides injury to the aorta, other great vessels may be injured; these include the inferior vena cava, the iliac arteries and veins, and the femoral vessels. Due to its posterolateral relationship to the aorta, the inferior vena cava is less likely to be injured during laparoscopic procedures. The internal iliac artery bifurcates into an anterior branch that courses medially, and thus could be injured during midline insertion of instruments. This vessel lies rather deep in the pelvic basin, however, and the laparoscope would have to be thrust more than 6 cm in order to reach it. Similarly, the femoral vessels are rarely injured due to their lateral course and depth in the pelvis.

The most common minor vessels injured are the middle sacral and epigastric vessels. The middle sacral vessels are injured when the angle of insertion of laparoscopic instruments is overly acute; they are the only fixed midline vessels below the aortic bifurcation that are vulnerable to injury. The epigastric vessels, lying lateral to the borders of the rectus muscles, are usually not injured when instruments are inserted into the midline. These vessels and their branches are most commonly injured when second and third punctures are used to introduce additional instruments into the pelvis.

Prevention of vascular injuries at laparoscopy requires thorough knowledge of pelvic anatomy as described above. Of equal importance is the use of proper surgical technique. The surgeon should first recognize patients who are at greater than usual risk for laparoscopic complications: (a) those who are obese or very thin, (b) those who have an android pelvis or an especially pronounced sacral promontory, and (c) those who have had multiple lower abdominal operations. In thin patients, the aorta may lie within an inch of the anterior abdominal skin (4); the distance from the abdominal skin to the aorta is one half of that from the skin of the back to the aorta (15).

To minimize vascular injury, it is important for the surgeon to utilize certain principles in surgical technique. General endotracheal anesthesia is preferred for routine diagnostic laparoscopy. Short-acting, depolarization muscle relaxants allow adequate pneumoperitoneum. Proper positioning of the patient is essential. The patient's longitudinal axis should be placed parallel to the length of the operating table and the pelvis should be placed flat against the table surface in order to avoid medial displacement of the lateral pelvic vessels. A modified dorsal lithotomy position, avoiding over abduction of the hips, will produce less tension on the vessels below the bifurcation, allowing them to follow the curve of the sacrum. Following proper positioning of the patient, the stomach and bladder must be emptied. The uterus, with the aid of an intrauterine cannula, is deflected downward into the depths of the pelvis. The anterior abdominal wall is gently elevated during insertion of the Verres insufflation needle. The use of towel clips or strong "squeezing" to lift the anterior abdominal wall is unnecessary and may produce abdominal wall hematomas. If there is concern that viscera are adherent to the abdominal wall, pneumoperitoneum can be obtained by inserting the Verres needle at the left subcostal margin in the midclavicular line (14). Pneumoperitoneum increases the distance between the anterior abdominal wall and the great vessels. Laparoscopic instruments are inserted at a 45 degree angle to the abdominal wall, aiming at the center of the true pelvis. Direction of insertion must not stray from the midline, lest the more lateral iliac and femoral vessels be threatened. In response to the first American report of a major vessel injury during laparoscopy, Hulka (4) suggested that an assistant stand at the head or foot of the table to assure the surgeon of a midline insertion plane.

In avoiding surgical complications there is no substitute for experience. Physicians who have performed fewer than 100 laparoscopic procedures have almost four times the complication rate (14.7 per 1000) as those with greater experience (3.8 per 1000) (13).

Vascular injuries during laparoscopy will occasionally occur even though the surgeon takes all possible precautions. The most important step following injury is early diagnosis. If a vessel is perforated with the Verres needle, there will often be a prompt return of blood. If bleeding occurs directly into the peritoneual space, vital signs will change abruptly, and abdominal distention may be noted as the hemoperitoneum progressively enlarges. If bleeding dissects through the retroperitoneal space, the findings are more variable, as the hemorrhage may transiently tamponade. In the event of direct injection of insufflation gas into a vessel, air embolism, with resultant cardiac arrest, may develop. If vascular injury is suspected, insufflation must be halted immediately, and the Verres needle left in place to help localize the vessel entered.

Laparotomy must not be delayed when major vessel injury is diagnosed or strongly suspected. As the vertical lower abdominal incision is being made, an indwelling bladder catheter should be placed. The surgeon must communicate his concerns immediately to the anesthesiologist, suggesting Trendelenburg position and left lateral tilt in order to maintain cerebral blood flow and float any gas emboli away from the conducting system of the heart. A central venous line should be expeditiously placed via the internal jugular or subclavian route; aspiration of this line will remove any air within the right atrium. Blood is drawn for baseline chemistries, clotting studies, and type and crossmatch. O-blood should be requested *statim*. While awaiting any blood, volume expansion should be initiated with lactated Ringer's solution, albumin, or Hespan. A vascular surgeon should be paged immediately, and a major vascular instrument tray should be requested.

A prompt vertical midline incision is made to expedite entry into the peritoneal cavity and to allow access to the aorta and vena cava, should compression of these vessels be required. The surgeon can expect a sudden rush of blood and loss of vital signs when the anterior parietal peritoneum is opened, as any effect of tamponade is withdrawn. In the presence of massive hemorrhage, the first priority upon entering the peritoneal cavity is compression of the aorta. Aortic occlusion is accomplished by manual compression or cross-clamping with a vascular clamp. The inferior vena cava is never crossed-clamped, as it will tear, and greatly complicate the situation. Then,

using a hand-over-hand technique of clearing the collected blood with laparotomy sponges, the area of bleeding is identified and compression applied manually. If blood is not present in the peritoneal cavity, retroperitoneal hemorrhage is likely. In this situation, the posterior peritoneum may be distended and colored blue to purple due to retroperitoneal hematoma, obscuring the site of injury. Blood is evacuated to allow discovery of the damaged vessel. Once the injury is identified, compression is applied while the patient is stabilized.

When fluid resuscitation has produced stable vital signs, repair of the injury may proceed. It is critical to know the duration of tissue hypoperfusion--especially distal to the vascular injury. Thus, if more than 10 minutes are required to establish stable vital signs, vessel compression should be intermittently relaxed to allow distal perfusion.

Arterial injuries are more common than venous injuries during laparoscopy. Injuries to small arteries, such as the middle sacral or inferior epigastrics, may be treated by simple ligation of the vessels and are unlikely to cause severe hemorrhage. Management by laparoscopic cautery may be adequate.

Among the various possible injuries to the larger pelvic arteries and abdominal aorta, three are of principal concern to the laparoscopist. The first, a small perforation with the Verres needle may stop bleeding due to spasm of smooth muscle in the arterial wall. Nevertheless, the perforation should be reinforced with 4-0 nylon or Prolene over a Dacron bolster. The posterior wall of all injured arteries should be dissected free and inspected in order to rule out a backwall injury. The second, a laceration secondary to lateral movement of an instrument that has perforated a vessel, is more serious. Lacerations are usually reparable by a running full thickness suture of 4-0 nylon or Prolene. The worst arterial injury is transection. The artery proximal and distal to the injury is clamped and the damaged segment excised. A Dacron graft is used to replace the damaged segment. Each end is sewn with a double-armed 3-0 nylon. Small branches are ligated, whereas significant arteries may be sewn into the graft. The graft is first flushed with backflow by releasing the distal clamp; a 25 gauge needle is inserted into the graft to release any trapped air. The proximal clamp is then released, returning blood flow distally. The graft and distal vessel are injected with a heparinized solution to minimize clot formation distally. If the limb remains cold, intra-arterial injection of a fibrinolysin such as urokinase should be performed. Bleeding will occur at the anastomotic sites for a few minutes. If prolonged, this bleeding can be controlled by topical thrombin. During all vascular procedures, the time of vessel occlusion should be carefully noted.

Venous injuries are less amenable to suture repair due to their relatively thin vessel wall. Furthermore, due to the risk of lacerating tributaries, the great veins cannot be mobilized and inspected posteriorly to rule out a backwall injury. Vessels proximal and distal to the injury should be compressed so that the anterior wall can be opened to inspect the posterior wall for injury. Primary closure with 4-0 monofilament permanent suture may be attempted. If bleeding persists, however, ligation of the inferior vena cava (below the renal veins) or other great veins is indicated.

Following vascular repair, the remainder of the abdomen and pelvis must be thoroughly inspected to rule out concomitant injury. Particular attention should be paid to the mesentary of the bowel, the bowel itself, and the pelvic ureters, which can also be injured by laparoscopic procedures. Elective procedures such as appendectomy should be avoided; however, there exists room for the surgeon to exercise clinical judgment based on the patient's previous and immediate condition.

In the recovery room, careful attention is given to the neurovascular condition of the distal extremities. The need for prophylactic versus complete anticoagulation is individualized. If the injured vessel was completely occluded for more than 10 minutes, it is advisable to induce complete anticoagulation with intravenous infusion of heparin. If partial occlusion during vessel repair allowed intermittent flow to the extremities, thrombosis is less likely and prophylactic subcutaneous heparin can be used.

After 4 to 6 weeks, Doppler-directed flow studies are indicated in patients who required a significant vascular repair or have a discernable difference in their distal pulse pressures.

Arteriography is indicated only if stricture, leakage, or pseudoaneurysm formation at a repair site is suspected.

Vascular injuries are among the most dangerous complications the gynecologic surgeon can encounter. With prompt diagnosis, expedient laparotomy, control of bleeding, and fluid resuscitation prior to definitive vascular repair, morbidity and mortality from these rare complications can be minimized.

References

1. Bartsich EG, Dillon TF: Injury of superior mesenteric vein: laparoscopic procedure with unusual complication. *NY St J Med* 81:933, 1981.
2. Chamberlain G, Brown JC (eds): Gynaecological laparoscopy: The report of the confidential inquiry into gynaecological laparoscopy. London, The Royal College of Obstetricians and Gynaecologists, 1978, p. 114.
3. Goss CM (ed): *Gray's Anatomy*, 27th edition. Philadelphia, Lea & Febiger, 1959, p. 684.
4. Hulka JF: Major vessel injuring during laparoscopy (letter). *Am J Obstet Gynecol* 138:590, 1980.
5. Karam K, Hajj S: Mesenteric hematoma Meckel's diverticulum: a rare laparoscopic complication. *Fertil Steril* 28:1003-1005, 1977.
6. Katz M, Beck P, Tancer ML: Major vessel injury during laparoscopy: Anatomy of two cases. *Am J Obstet Gynecol* 135:544, 1979.
7. Kurzel RB, Edinger DD Jr: Injury to the great vessels: A hazard of transabdominal endoscopy. *South Med J* 76:656-7, 1983.
8. Loffer F, Pent D: Indications, contraindications, and complications of laparoscopy. *Obstet Gynecol Surg* 30:407-427, 1975.
9. McDonald PT, Rich NM, Collins GJ Jr, et al: Vascular trauma secondary to diagnostic and therapeutic procedures: Laparoscopy. *Am J Surg* 135:651-5, 1978.
10. Mintz M: Risks and prophylaxis in laparoscopy: A survey of 100,000 cases. *J Reproduc Med* 18:269, 1977.
11. Penfield A: Trocar and needle injuries. In Philipps J (ed): *Laparoscopy*. Baltimore, Williams & Wilkins, 1977.
12. Peterson HB, Greenspan JR, Ory HW: Death following puncture of the aorta during laparoscopic sterilization. *Obstet Gynecol* 59:133-3, 1982.
13. Phillips J, Keith D, Hupka J, et al: Gynecologic laparoscopy in 1975. *J Reproduc Med* 16:105, 1976.
14. Phillips J (ed): *Laparoscopy*, Baltimore, Williams & Wilkins, 1977, pp. 91-92.
15. Semm K: Risks and dangers in laparoscopy. In *Atlas of Gynecologic Laparoscopy and Hysteroscopy*. Philadelphia, WB Saunders Co, 1977.
16. Shin CS: Vascular injury secondary to laparoscopy. *NY St J Med* 82:935-6, 1982.

CHAPTER 21

Laparoscopy with Unexpected Viscus Penetration

ALAN H. DeCHERNEY, M.D.

CASE ABSTRACT

Diagnostic closed laparoscopy was planned for a 26-year-old infertility patient. Insufflation of gas through the Verres needle was apparently uneventful, but after the operator had introduced the laparoscope into the abdomen, she found she was viewing a mucous membrane of a large cavity strongly resembling the interior of the stomach. The anesthetist reported that gas was now coming from the patient's mouth, even though the trachea had been intubated.

DISCUSSION

Perforation of an intra-abdominal viscus by the Verres needle in preparation for laparoscopy is a common occurrence of little serious consequence. The diagnosis is made either by eructation or flatus occurring during the procedure. This is dependent as to what part of the gastrointestinal tract is perforated, with the stomach yielding eructation and the colon leading to flatus production. If the diagnosis of the perforation of the viscus is made when only the Verres needle has penetrated the organ, one should remove the Verres needle and proceed with the laparoscopy after reinsufflation through another site. The surgeon must keep in mind, though, that this perforation might be the result of adhesions of the viscus to the anterior abdominal wall, and not just the result of a random puncture. Proceeding with open laparoscopy might be a wise choice at this juncture. Another alternative would be using the "needlescope" so as to advance the needle to insufflate and inspect at the same time.

Once the laparoscope is in place, the site of puncture by the Verres needle should be inspected, but usually this does not require any further surgical intervention. Its frequency cannot be identified. Puncture of the bladder by the Verres needle also requires the same conservative approach as would apply to any other viscera.

The approach for a needle perforation is not the case when the trocar penetrates an intra-abdominal viscus. Unfortunately, this is a more commonly diagnosed entity, since it is often difficult to tell if only the Verres needle has penetrated a viscus, but it is easy to tell that the trocar has penetrated a viscus. When the laparoscope itself is introduced one views a mucousal surface. Once this occurs and has been identified, the gynecologist should *leave the laparoscope in place*, do a laparotomy, identify the defect, and close that defect in an appropriate manner after the laparoscope has been removed. The laparoscope was left in place to seal the puncture, and also to allow identification of the site of trauma.

Bowel should be repaired by a purse-string or double-layered suture closing if the laceration is less than one-half the diameter of the lumen of the bowel. If the laceration exceeds one-half the diameter of the lumen (as it might since these lacerations sometimes are oblique) then a segmental resection and anastomosis should be performed. Also of tantamount importance is the maintenance of the blood supply to the traumatized area; if the mesenteric blood supply is interrupted by the puncture, then a resection must be done no matter what the size or the length of the laceration. It is appropriate to have a general surgeon as a consultant in this type of surgery.

The trocar or Verres needle may go through

the bladder. Routinely, the intraumbilical puncture site is too high for this to occur. In this happenstance the second puncture may go into the bladder, the operative field being obscured by massive pelvic adhesions. Occasionally this must be confirmed by cystoscopic examination, but in any event, if the defect leaks urine into the peritoneal cavity, the bladder should be repaired in a purse-string or two-layered suture fashion. It is appropriate to have urologic consultation if this occurs.

There are ways by which these complications can be prevented, and certainly most important is patient selection. Patients who have had previous bowel surgery should have an open laparoscopy rather than a closed laparoscopy. On the other hand, it is difficult to tell which patients who have had previous pelvic surgery should have an open laparoscopy. An alternative to the routine procedure is to use a small gauge laparoscpope such as the needlescope, with a 2 to 3 mm diameter endoscope in order to identify intra-peritoneal structures before the incision is made, and actually advance the needle and insufflate under direct visualization.

Any patient that has had a bowel or stomach perforation by the trocar should be treated in the same manner as anyone who has had bowel surgery, including nasogastric tube, prophylactic antibiotic coverage and a prolonged period of putting the intestine to rest. The same goes for laceration of the bladder—the Foley catheter should be left in for the full 7 days, and the patient should be placed on prophylactic antibiotics.

Verres needle perforations require no special postoperative orders other than observation for the development of either chemical or bacterial peritonitis, of which the patient must be advised. It requires no increase in usual hospital stay.

CHAPTER 22

Bowel Burn with Laparoscopy

RICHARD M. LACKRITZ, M.D.

CASE ABSTRACT

During the performance of a laparoscopic tubal resection and coagulation, as the first side was being completed using a standard three burn technique, the anesthetized patient gave a little cough, and the small bowel brushed the electrode as the tubal coagulation was being accomplished. Although at the moment the operator thought he saw a small white patch on the serosal surface of the small intestine, he was unable to visualize it when he had completed the tubal resection and thermocoagulation of the other side.

DISCUSSION

The incidence of gastrointestinal complications of laparoscopy is usually reported as between 0.1% and 0.3% (1, 4). As the rate is quite low, most surgeons fortunately will not have to deal with this dangerous situation. The growing popularity of tubal clips and rings should decrease the chances of a bowel burn. But since even mesosalpingeal bleeding is often controlled by coagulation, intestinal thermal injuries will undoubtably continue to occur.

Intestinal burns may or may not be recognized at laparoscopy. In the largest series reported, eight of 10 women injured suffered thermal bowel burns of the terminal ileum (3). The remaining two patients had rectosigmoid damage. Five of the 10 injuries were unrecognized at laparoscopy and subsequently required resection of a portion of ileum. Of the five recognized cases, one woman was immediately explored and the serosa of the damaged ileum was oversewn. The other four patients were followed without surgery, and all did well.

The etiology of thermal injuries is unknown but probably occurs by one of two mechanisms: Either a spark jumps from the grasping forceps during the coagulation, or the heated tubal tissue or laparoscopic forceps brushes directly against the bowel, causing a burn.

Most patients with recognized thermal injuries will have less than 1 cm. of damage and can be followed expectantly (3). Larger lesions probably mandate exploration once the diagnosis is made. In a retrospective study by Thompson and Wheeless (2), five patients with unrecognized thermal injuries to the intestine presented in similar ways. Signs and symptoms of bowel injury appeared between 3 and 7 days postoperatively. All did well for the first 2 days after surgery. Subsequently, the patients appeared to suffer from acute pelvic inflammatory disease. They developed nausea, anorexia, low-grade fever (99 to 101 degrees F), and colicky lower abdominal pain. Antibiotics did not improve their symptoms, and all soon developed ileus and obvious peritonitis. Leukocytosis was common, and ileus was noted on flat plates of the abdomen. When these patients were explored, the extent of the primary injury was found to be between 5 mm and 4 cm in diameter. Fortunately, all did well after resection of the damaged area of bowel.

When exploration is necessary, the bowel should be resected at about 5 cm to each side of the lesion, as intestinal damage may be more extensive than confined solely to the site of the burn. The surgeon should avoid suturing or oversewing of potentially necrotic intestinal tissue (3).

Nearly all patients with *small* recognized intestinal burns can be managed expectantly. If they develop symptoms similar to salpingitis and do not respond to antibiotics, exploration is mandatory; if treated by timely bowel resection and anastomosis, the prognosis should be good.

Therefore, in the patient described or any patient in whom a thermal gastrointestinal injury is suspected, hospital admission should be ordered. As others suggest (3, 4), we recommend intravenous feeding for 3 to 4 days, antibiotic bowel prep, as well as systemic antibiotics. If no symptoms occur by then, the patient can probably go home. Those who will need surgery will have begun to develop symptoms not unlike early appendicitis with peritoneal signs. Within a day or two they will develop more severe symptoms similar to patients with a ruptured appendix, and the need for exploration becomes obvious. At surgery, multiple cultures, appropriate antibiotic coverage, and bowel resection should usually result in a satisfactory outcome. Adequate drainage is mandatory, especially in those patients who have a pelvic abscess. Signs and symptoms of pelvic thrombophlebitis may occur as with any pelvic abscess, and appropriate anticoagulation should be started in those cases.

References

1. Cunanan RG, Courey NG, Lippes J: Complications of laparoscopic tubal sterilization. *Obstet Gynecol* 55:501, 1980.
2. Thompson BH, Wheeless CR: Gastrointestinal complications of laparoscopic sterilization. *Obstet Gynecol* 41:669, 1973.
3. Wheeless CR: Thermal gastrointestinal injuries. In Phillips JM, et al (eds): *Laparoscopy*. Baltimore, Williams & Wilkins, 1977.
4. Wheeless CR, Thompson BH: Laparoscopic sterilization: Review of 3600 cases. *Obstet Gynecol* 42:751, 1973.

CHAPTER 23

Unilateral Pelvic Abscess Following Removal of Intrauterine Device

ABE MICKAL, M.D., F.A.C.O.G., F.A.C.S.

CASE ABSTRACT

A 34-year-old divorced para 2 had been wearing an intrauterine device (IUD) for 2 years but was annoyed by persistent uterine tenderness and menorrhagia, although there was no history of fever. She requested permanent sterilization. At surgery, her physician removed the intrauterine device, performed a dilatation and curettage (D & C), and through the laparoscope performed a bilateral tubal coagulation. Five days later the patient was seen in the emergency room with considerable pelvic discomfort, chills and fever (103 degrees F), and tachycardia (pulse 110). The uterus was quite tender, and it was evident that an adnexal fullness was present on the right side. The patient was given a prescription for ampicillin, 500 mg four times daily, and sent home.

One week later, her symptoms were unimproved, although her temperature rarely exceeded 101 degrees F, and there was a distinct adnexal mass on the right side. The ampicillin was continued; when seen again 2 weeks later, the right adnexal mass was estimated at 6 cm in diameter and was exquisitely tender, but there was no fullness or bulging of the cul-de-sac. There was chronic low-grade body temperature which reached its highest point at 8 p.m. (101 degrees F). The patient requested that she be seen by a consultant. A consultation was arranged. The consultant confirmed the above findings, discontinued the ampicillin and placed the patient on chloromycetin, 250 mg four times a day. Her fever disappeared within 2 days and a leukocytosis and elevated sedimentation rate gradually subsided. The mass persisted, and 1 month later the patient was taken to surgery for laparotomy.

DISCUSSION

Was Pelvic Inflammatory Disease Present at the Time of Initial Surgery?

There are numerous reports in the literature regarding the effect of an IUD on intrauterine and tubal infections. Taylor et al. (12) reported unilateral tubo-ovarian abscess in IUD wearers. The reason for the unilaterality of this is due to imbedding of the IUD on the uterine wall producing an infection at this site. This infection spread to the corresponding tube and ovary by direct extension or by lymphatic spread. Since this report there have been similar reports regarding unilateral tubo-ovarian abscesses in IUD wearers (8, 10). The final answer to the exact impact of the IUD on tubo-ovarian disease is not as yet in. Edelman and Berger (3), in November of 1980, reported that their study did not support the concept that wearers of the IUD were more likely to have unilateral tubo-ovarian abscesses. They also concluded that further studies would be required to define more completely the relationship between IUD use and pelvic inflammatory disease.

Burkman (1) reported the results of case control studies in 16 hospitals in nine cities in the United States regarding the association of IUDs and pelvic inflammatory disease. There were 1447 patients in the pelvic infections group and 3453 patients in the control group. Some of the conclusions reached in this study were:

1. There was an increased association for women aged 25 years or less and for non-black women.
2. Recent insertion or reinsertion of an IUD was associated with an increased risk for pelvic infection, but duration of use was not.
3. The pelvic infection persisted several months after removal of the IUD.
4. The type of IUD does not markedly influence the risk.
5. The risk is greater when the IUD is compared to other forms of contraception or no contraception.
6. First episode hospitalization for pelvic infection is twice the baseline figure of IUD users. This is of great economic as well as health significance.

The association of an increased pelvic inflammatory disease rate with or without abscess formation has been fairly well substantiated. The original article in by Taylor et al. in 1975 (12) implicated all types of IUDs in the development of pelvic infections or tubo-ovarian abscesses. The discontinuance of the IUDs with multifilament tails was of some value in reducing the risk of ascending infection, but a major problem still persists. Smith and Soderstrom (11) examined removed sections of fallopian tubes during sterilization and found a nonbacterial salpingitis rate of 47% in IUD users compared to less than 1% in nonusers. Eschenbach et al (4) reported in 1977 that, of 500,000 cases of pelvic infections, 110,000 occurred in women with an IUD in place.

All of the previously mentioned information illustrates the fact that the IUD is a potential focus of infection. There should be a good doctor-patient dialogue and understanding of the IUD and its related problems and benefits. Many other factors may also predispose an individual to the development of pelvic infections. These factors include the sexual activity of the individual, multiplicity of sex partners, personal life style and environment, history of previous pelvic problems, status of pelvic organs at time of IUD insertion (cervicitis, etc.), age and parity, and insertion problems (perforations, complete, or incomplete).

The Centers for Disease Control in Atlanta held a symposium on pelvic inflammatory disease in June, 1980. A brief summary of this meeting by Golden (6) was reported as follows:

1. In women who develop salpingitis, 20% become infertile.
2. Those who can conceive have a 6- to 10-fold increased risk of ectopic pregnancy.
3. In 1976, 35% of women in this country who used no contraception were involuntarily sterile, indicating the magnitude of the infertility problem.
4. One-half of the deaths from ectopic pregnancies can be attributed to the ectopic gestation resulting from scarring from bouts of salpingitis. (Deaths from ectopic gestations account for 11% of the maternal deaths in the United States.)
5. Direct and indirect costs of pelvic inflammatory disease amount to about $2 billion per year.

Powers (7) reported 204 ectopic pregnancies between 1974 and 1978. Twenty-one women (10.3%) had an IUD in place at time of diagnosis, and 18 (8.8%) had used IUDs in the past. It was interesting to note that only 27 (13.2%) patients had a record or history of salpingitis. Seventy-seven (37.7%) were nulliparous, and 66 of the 127 parous patients had only one delivery. The largest age group was between 25 and 29.

In summarizing the question relating to infection with the IUD, one must conclude:

1. Since most IUD wearers are young and of low parity, the long-term impact of the IUD on the future reproductive capacity has not been fully assessed or reported.
2. There is an increased risk of pelvic infection. It may be subclinical and well within the tolerance of the individual to deal with it provided there is no superimposed infection or trauma.
3. There is a definite increased risk of ectopic pregnancies.
4. In young women, nulliparous or of low parity, the IUD may not be the contraceptive of choice. I do not recommend the IUD for young, single, or nulliparous patients except in unusual circumstances.

Surgical Procedures Done on This Patient

After removal of an IUD, D & C, and laparoscopic tubal sterilization, this patient developed complications—namely, a tubo-ovarian abscess. Therefore, one questions the advisability of doing all these procedures at the same time and in the order in which they were done.

My feeling is that the time to remove the IUD was when the patient was seen in the office and all aspects of the problem were discussed. This was not an emergency admission, and the patient would have been a better candidate for a diagnostic D & C for menorrhagia. Many IUDs are removed in the office without problems. The menorrhagia could have been a result of the IUD, and the removal may have been of some aid in determining this effect. A D & C would have been indicated for a final diagnosis on this patient's bleeding problems at the time of her hospitalization for the tubal sterilization 1 or 2 weeks later.

The need for antibiotics should also be determined at the time of the office visit and IUD removal. If on examination, the patient had signs and symptoms of pelvic infection (leukocytosis, cervical-uterine pain, adnexal tenderness, etc.) then a 5- to 6-day course of oral antibiotics may be indicated. (I use either doxycline hyclate (Doxycycline), 100 mg bid, or erythromycin stearate (Erythromycin), 500 mg tid.

This patient with persistent uterine tenderness was taken to surgery for the removal of the IUD, D & C, and laparoscopic tubal sterilization. No mention was made of short-term prophylactic antibiotics, and in my opinion they should have been used. All antimicrobial agents that have been used prophylactically have shown fairly good results. On the Louisiana State University Ob-Gyn Service at Charity Hospital we have more experience with cephoxitin sodium (Cefoxitin) and ticarcillin sodium (Ticarcillin), principally because we have had investigational studies related to these drugs. Metronidazole (Flagyl), doxycycline hyclate, and the second and third generation cephalosporins have been reported as being equally effective.

Laparoscopic Tubal Sterilization: First and Last. Another area of consideration in this patient is the chronologic order of procedures performed. There is no question that a subclinical salpingitis exists in most IUD wearers. However, the vast majority of IUD patients undergo laparoscopic tubal sterilization without major complications. This indicates that cauterization of the fallopian tubes seldom causes a pre-existing salpingitis to flare up, or if it does, the body's host defense mechanisms can usually cope with it. When a laparoscopic tubal cauterization is done, the avenue for direct spread of an intrauterine infection to the ovaries is usually sealed off. If one contemplates doing a removal of an IUD and D & C and tubal sterilization, then doing the laparoscopic procedure first may reduce the chances for tubo-ovarian infection.

If I were to choose the order in which these procedures would be done then I would do the following: (a) office removal of IUD and short term oral prophylactic antibiotics, 3 to 4 days; (b) tubal sterilization, and D & C when admitted to hospital in 2 weeks.

Postoperative Follow-up. The patient was seen with the following presenting symptoms in the emergency room on the fifth postoperative day with considerable pelvic discomfort, chills and fever (103 degrees F), tachycardia (110), tender uterus, and adnexal fullness on the right side.

All of the above findings warrant immediate admission and evaluation of the patient for a possible tubo-ovarian abscess, with appendicitis to be ruled out. One of the major problems in treating moderate to severe pelvic infection with or without abscess formation is inadequate treatment. The fault lies equally with the patient and the physician. The patient delays in seeking help and the doctor, unfortunately, is disenchanted with the so-called "PID" (pelvic inflammatory disease) patient. This implied diagnosis does much to detract the physician from actively and aggressively evaluating and treating the patient. We are seeing less of this neglect now as compared to 10 to 20 years ago, because sections of infectious diseases are being established in obstetrics and gynecology departments with marked emphasis on improved care and management of patients with pelvic infections. Postgraduate courses in pelvic infections and antibiotic therapy have also contributed to this improvement.

The best time to cure or alter the destructive course of inflammatory disease is at the time of original attack. Hospital cost is admittedly high, but inadequately treated infections are far more expensive and devastating to the individual's reproductive system.

One other possible consideration in the etiology of the patients' postoperative morbidity is bowel injury at the time of laparoscopic tubal cauterization. The fact that the patient's clinical course did not progressively worsen would indicate that bowel injury did not likely occur, but it must be part of the differential diagnosis.

Choice of Antibiotics. Ampicillin trihydrate is a good oral antibiotic, but it alone is not adequate treatment for a patient presenting as this patient did in the emergency room. One week later, the patient was still febrile (101 degrees F) with a distinct adnexal mass. Admission to the hospital was again justified but not done. Ampicillin trihydrate was continued, and the patient was not seen for 2 weeks. In neither instance was the best interest of the patient served. A delay of seeing such a sick patient for 2 weeks is also not appropriate management.

It must again be restated that in gynecologic and obstetric infection we are dealing with polymicrobial organism (aerobes, anaerobes, and *Chlamydia trachomatis*), especially the *Bacteroides* species. Treatment should always be directed at all groups of organisms with special emphasis on the anaerobes. Their eradication early in the treatment phase is directly proportional to the speed of recovery and response of the patient. Specific coverage for *Chlamydia trachomatis must* be part of the treatment of pelvic inflammatory disease.

My Plan of Management

1. Admit to hospital when first seen in the emergency room on the fifth postoperative day.
2. Complete evaluation: interval history, physical examination including bimanual, rectovaginal, complete blood count, urinalysis, x-ray of chest and flat plate of the abdomen, culdocentesis with culture.
3. Parenteral intravenous fluids supplementing oral fluids.
4. Antibiotics directed at polymicrobial nature of the disease. Coverage must be adequate for aerobes, anaerobes, and chlamydial infection. The majority of pelvic infections are polymicrobial and must be treated accordingly: Cefoxitin sodium (Mefoxin) 2 gm by intravenous piggyback every 6 hours with doxycycline hyclate 100 mg intravenously every 12 hours. Metronidazole (Flagyl) 500 mg every 6 hours can be added as the third drug of choice if needed.
5. Ultrasound of pelvic area: This is of diagnostic help in 70% to 75% of cases and offers good follow-up on progression or regression of the disease signs.
6. Daily monitoring of vital signs.
7. If response is noted with antibiotic regimen, then continue therapy as long as progress is noted.
8. Laparoscopy would be reserved as an added diagnostic aid when and if needed. The clinical response of the patient would be a determining factor. Cultures from the fallopian tubes and cul-de-sac should always be taken at time of laparoscopy.
9. If the patient's response is poor or condition deteriorates, then physical re-evaluation is done involving chest, kidneys, abdomen, pelvis, and extremities.
   (a) Add antibiotics for more intensive anaerobic coverage-clindamycin phosphate (Cleocin phosphate) 600 mg every 6 hours intravenously, or chloramphenicol sodium succinate (Chloromycetin) 2 gm stat, then 1 mg, then 1 gm every 6 hours intravenously, or metronidazole (Flagyl) 500 gm every 6 hours intravenously. Any of the above can be combined with cefoxitin. Tobramycin sulphate or amikacin sulphate (Amikin) may also be added if indicated. Double or triple agent antibiotic therapy is often needed in severe infection.
   (b) Supportive conservative treatment is continued as long as the patient is responding and progress is being made.
10. If after 8 to 10 days of therapy the patient is improved but an adnexal mass 8 to 10 cm persists and is identifiable by careful rectovaginal examination and ultrasound, then exploratory laparotomy is resorted to.

Surgery is indicated in patients who are not responding to aggressive medical management as indicated by the vital signs, abdominal pain and distention, and/or a progressively enlarging adnexal mass. It is better to explore the abdomen and remove an early unruptured tuboovarian abscess and preserve the remaining organs than await rupture and do a more extensive surgical procedure.

Surgical Procedure Done on Patient. A right tubo-ovarian, unruptured abscess was removed. Culture of the abscess was positive for enterococcus and *Bacteroides fragilis*.

The culture reaffirms the problem of anaerobic organisms in pelvic infections and the need for antimicrobials to cover the aerobic and especially anaerobic organisms. If this patient had been admitted on the fifth postoperative day when her symtoms warranted admission, it is presumed that proper antibiotic therapy may have at that time prevented the ultimate development of a frank tubo-ovarian abscess.

All patients with an initial diagnosis of tubo-ovarian abscess do not necessarily have a discrete abscess. This is a working and presumptive diagnosis and can only be proven by laparoscopy or laparotomy, especially early in the disease process when rupture or leaking of the abscess has not occurred. The clinical impression of an adnexal mass (abscess) may be only an acute salpingo-oophoritis with adhesions to omentum or bowel giving rise to an ill-defined mass, often referred to as a tubo-ovarian complex. Many tubo-ovarian abscesses begin in this manner, with the ovary becoming later invaded by bacteria at an ovulatory site or by lymphatic or hematogenous spread. Early and aggressive conservative management with broad-spectrum antibiotics may be effective in treating the original infection before a true abscess develops. When dealing with pelvic infections with a questionable mass, it is best to consider the most potentially dangerous aspect of the problem and work in that direction rather than to minimize the situation. Too often the disease process develops faster than anticipated and we then must "catch up" and try to stem the tide.

On the Louisiana State University Ob-Gyn Service (5) we have clinically diagnosed 247 tubo-ovarian abscesses between the years 1970 and 1979. Aggressive conservative management was instituted while at the same time preparations were made for surgery if it became indicated. We operated on 57% of these patients, and the other 43% were discharged as relatively cured after medical management. Unfortunately, we do not have adequate follow-up data on the fate of patients who were admitted with a clinical diagnosis of tubo-ovarian abscess and responded to aggressive medi-

cal management. In spite of this inadequate follow-up, I still believe that this is the proper approach to patients presenting with this problem. The sooner the patient is admitted and treated the less the incidence of surgery, whereas the reverse of this is also true. The longer the duration before treatment, the higher the incidence of surgery. Those medically treated are made aware of their conditions and counseled regarding the future of the reproductive organs as well as being hopefully educated toward improved personal care and concern.

There is a changing philosophy toward surgery for tubo-ovarian abscesses. We, along with many others (2, 9) have changed from an outright surgical approach after adequate medical management to a more aggressive medical management with surgery being reserved only for those patients who do not respond or in whom the disease process is not controlled. It has been our policy to remove only the infected organs, but it is difficult to adhere to this policy when surgery is done for ruptured abscesses with free pus in the pelvis or abdomen. There should be no hesitancy on the part of the gynecologist in removing unilateral tubo-ovarian abscess or severely diseased adnexa. This is an excellent time for full pelvic inspection and bacteriologic studies of the diseased organs, as well as cultures from the cul-de-sac and the ostia of the opposite fallopian tube. This is especially advocated in young patients, those of low parity, and patients who desire future pregnancies. The advances being made in antibiotic therapy, especially with regards to anaerobes, provide moral and therapeutic support in our managemnt of patients with unilateral or bilateral tubo-ovarian disease problems. We need no longer feel that we may as well remove everything while we are there to prevent recurrence. The better understanding that now exists regarding organisms and their behavior as well as our improved bacteriologic techniques aided by adequate aggressive medical management warrants our conservative surgical approach, especially in those young patinets desirous of future pregnancies. The success of in vitro fertilizations demands that we counsel our patients about its potential and the possibility of preserving the uterus and an ovary if clinical conditions warrants. In such cases, the removal of diseased and distorted fallopian tubes and the preservation of the uterus and ovary is justifiable. This is also a good opportunity for cultures of the pelvic structures and institution of appropriate therapy. In some cases, aspiration of ovarian abscess and preservation of ovary is indicated. The risk is well worth taking by the conscientious physician who has developed a good rapport and dialogue with his patients.

References

1. Burkman RT: Association between intrauterine device and pelvic inflammatory disease. *Obstet Gynecol* 57:269, 1981.
2. Cunningham FG, Mickal A: Pelvic infection. In Benson RC (ed): *Current Obstetric and Gynecologic Diagnosis and Treatment*. Los Altos, CA, Lange, 1980.
3. Edelman DA, Berger GA: Contraceptive practice and tubo-ovarian abscess. *Am J Obstet Gynecol* 138:541, 1980.
4. Eschenbach DA, Harvisch JP, Holmes KD: Role of contraception and other risk factors. *Am J Obstet Gynecol* 128:838, 1977.
5. Ginsberg DS, Stern JL, Hamod KA, et al: Tubo-ovarian abscess: A retrospective review. *Am J Obstet Gynecol* 138:1055, 1980.
6. Golden: International Symposium of Pelvic Inflammatory Disease, I and II. *Am J Obstet Gynecol* 138:845, 1980.
7. Powers DN: Ectopic pregnancy: A five year experience. *South Med J* 73:1012, 1980.
8. Richart RM: Ovarian abscesses in IUD wearer: Problem-patient conference. *Contemp Ob-Gyn* 17:141, 1981.
9. Rivilin ME, Hunt JA: Ruptured tubo-ovarian abscesses—is hysterectomy necessary? *Obstet Gyencol* 50:518, 1977.
10. Scott WC: Pelvic abscess in association with intrauterine contraceptive device. *Trans Pacific Coast Obstet Gynecol Soc* 45:43, 1978.
11. Smith MR, Soderstrom R: Salpingitis: A frequent response to intrauterine conception. *J Reproduc Med* 16:159, 1976.
12. Taylor ES, McMillan BE, Greer BE, et al: The intrauterine device and tubo-ovarian abscess. *Am J Obstet Gynecol* 123:338, 1975.

CHAPTER **24**

Bilateral Chronic and Symptomatic Salpingitis: Should Hysterectomy be Performed?

HOWARD W. JONES, JR., M.D., D.Sc. (Honoris Causis)

CASE ABSTRACT

Bilateral, symptomatic, and recurrent pelvic inflammatory disease had been identified in a 26-year-old unmarried nulligravid patient who was contemplating marriage and wondering about her future fertility. The patient was disabled by chronic pelvic pain and tenderness, worse around the time of her menstrual period, and there had been frequent febrile flare-ups during the preceding year. Bilateral persistent, tender adnexal masses were identified, somewhat fixed in position and measuring 5 to 7 cm in diameter. Laparotomy, with probable salpingectomy and possible hysterectomy, was recommended. Preoperatively, the patient expressed her plan to marry someday and was visibly upset about her potential loss of fertility. She inquired whether it was necessary that her uterus be removed and whether or not she might be a future candidate for in vitro fertilization.

DISCUSSION

If it is necessary because of disease to remove the fallopian tubes, conventional wisdom has held that a total hysterectomy should also be done. This "incidental" hysterectomy is based on the simple concepts that with no tubes reproduction is impossible; that the uterus can therefore serve no reproductive purpose; that in later years it can only be the source of difficulty, such as from functional bleeding, cancer of the uterus, cancer of the corpus, cancer of the cervix, etc.

All of this has now changed. Reproduction is possible without fallopian tubes and, with the use of donor eggs, reproduction is also possible without ovaries. For patients without tubes the possibility of pregnancy by in vitro fertilization approaches, but, at present, does not equal the expectancy of pregnancy occurring during any one menstrual cycle. The natural inefficiency of reproduction per cycle is overcome in normal reproduction because with normal tubes the opportunity to become pregnant repeats itself thirteen times each year. For

the best possibility for pregnancy from in vitro fertilization, the ovaries need to be available either for laparoscopic harvest or for ultrasound guided harvest and seem to produce eggs better if not involved in the consequences of extensive surface peritoneal inflammatory reaction.

At the time of surgery, when in vitro fertilization is contemplated for sometime in the future, there are special considerations. The ovaries, of course, should be preserved if possible. Salpingectomy should be carried out by removal of the tube in the standard method, but the traditional method of using a deep cornual wedge, with the removal of the interstitial portion of the tube, should no longer be employed. There have been reports of ruptures of the uterus during pregnancy at the site of cornual excision (3). This risk seems to increase when the procedure is carried out bilaterally. Therefore, in removing the tube from the uterus, either no wedge or a very superficial wedge should be used, enabling the approximation of the serosal surfaces in a delicate surgical fashion.

After removal of the tubes attention should be given to removing, insofar as possible, any periovarian adhesions so that the surface of the ovary is as normal as possible. In addition, if the ovary tends to be low in the cul-de-sac, the subsequent harvest of eggs by laparoscopy can be made much easier by ovarian suspension: by shortening the utero-ovarian ligament and, if necessary, severing it and reinserting it at the site of the excised tube, or even higher into the insertion of the round ligament (1) (Fig. 24.1). If future transvaginal ovum retrieval for in vitro fertilization is planned, the utero-ovarian ligaments should be reattached at a point low on the back of the uterus.

In addition, if the uterus tends to sag, a necessary and important part of the operative procedure should be suspension of the uterus by shortening the round ligaments according to the method of Gilliam (2) or by some modification thereof.

In the event that the ovary is largely destroyed or so intimately involved in the inflammatory process or its residua that it is no longer savable, this does not mean that in vitro fertilization is impossible in this patient, even if both ovaries are so involved. Therefore, hysterectomy may not be indicated, even if both ovaries are removed. If the uterus is normal, reproduction is theorectically and practically possible, provided that the patient is willing to accept a donor egg.

The practical point of the recent considerations is that it is incumbent upon the surgeon to be aware of the newer reproductive technologies and to discuss these possibilities at length with the patient prior to any operation which might involve an ''incidental'' hysterectomy.

As with all infertility surgery, routine antibiotics are indicated and should be used in a prophylactic manner if no organism can be identified, but obviously if pus is encountered at the time of operation, a culture should be taken and the antibiotic therapy modulated depending upon the bacteriological findings.

There are very few circumstances in contemporary surgery where drainage of the abdomen is indicated. Even with a ruptured

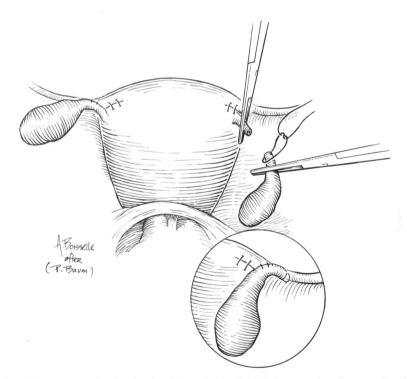

Figure 24.1. Diagram showing bilateral salpingectomy. Right utero-ovarian ligament has been clamped and cut to insert at lower right. Notice how ovary has been suspended by suturing it to the round ligament. If future transvaginal ovum retrieval is planned, the utero-ovarian ligaments should be reattached low on the back of the uterus.

tubo-ovarian abscess with the removal of the adnexa, aspiration and irrigation of the peritoneal cavity drainage is not helpful and, indeed, should be avoided unless there is some urgent indication for it, as, for example, a raw oozing area or an unremovable abscess which was drained. In short, the objective of the surgery should be to leave the pelvis as clean as possible, with the thought that subsequently the ovaries could be approached for the purpose of harvesting mature eggs.

References

1. Garcia JE, Jones HW Jr, Acosta AA, et al: Reconstructive pelvic operations for in vitro fertilization. *Am J Obstet Gynecol* 153:172-178,1985.
2. Gilliam DT: Round-ligament ventrosuspension of the uterus: A new method. *Am J Obstet Gynecol* 41:299, 1900.
3. Mohlen J, Schortle B: Cornual resection as prophylaxis against interstitial pregnancy: Is it necessary or dangerous? A review of the literature. *Eur J Obstet Gynecol Reproduc Biol* 17:155, 1894.

CHAPTER 25

Ruptured Ectopic Pregnancy in an Infertility Patient with Coexistent Chronic Pelvic Inflammatory Disease

CELSO-RAMON GARCIA, M.D., F.A.C.S., F.A.C.O.G.
PHILLIP C. GALLE, M.D.

CASE ABSTRACT

An emergency laparotomy was performed on a 28-year-old, nulligravid, infertility patient because of suspected ruptured ectopic pregnancy. At laparotomy, the diagnosis was confirmed, in addition to the presence of many adhesions from previous pelvic inflammatory disease. The opposite tube was thickened and clubbed, and the fimbriated end was occluded.

DISCUSSION

Ectopic pregnancy continues to challenge the gynecologic surgeon. The patient described presents several interesting concepts in the management of ectopic pregnancies. It also provides an opportunity to review the role of immunization, postoperative human chorionic gonadotropin (hCG) surveillance, hysterectomy, steroids, and adjuvants to prevent adhesion formation, and incidental appendectomy.

Diagnosis

The key to the management of the patient with an ectopic pregnancy lies in early diagnosis. To do this, one must maintain a high index of clinical suspicion to attain an early diagnosis. With more sensitive pregnancy tests, ultrasound, and endoscopy, an early diagnosis is facilitated. Schwartz and DiPietro (12) found that with the use of serum beta subunits of hCG, a negative result ruled out an ectopic pregnancy in 100% of their cases. A problem arises when a patient presents with abdominal pain and a positive hCG assay. One must be cautious in the interpretation of ultrasound. It is difficult at times to distinguish an early intrauterine pregnancy from a pseudogestational sac

(9, 16). For this reason, definitive diagnosis of intrauterine gestation can be established only when fetal movement or fetal heart activity is present. Kadar and Romero (8) have combined both ultrasound and serum hCG in distinguishing intrauterine from ectopic pregnancies. If an intrauterine sac is identified and the serum hCG is above 6500 mIU/ml, they report that this can be taken as positive evidence of an intrauterine pregnancy and there is no need to wait for the appearance of fetal heart activity. Even when the serum hCG was above 6500 mIU/ml, but the gestational sac was not demonstrated, the incidence of an ectopic pregnancy was 94%. Therefore, we recommend that if a gestational sac is not visualized, repeat ultrasound and close follow-up are essential.

Although there are no long-term prospective studies on culdocentesis, we believe that it rarely influences management. Moreover, it could increase the risk of intraperitoneal contamination with vaginal or other flora. A positive culdocentesis would not exclude an etiology of less significant intraperitoneal bleeding which might be managed with laparoscopy, nor does a negative test preclude further diagnostic procedures.

While aggressiveness in intensity and

promptness of the diagnostic review should be emphasized, the least invasive approaches should be selected relative to the patient's condition. Certainly, a laparoscopy should not be performed when a patient is in shock, nor probably in the situation where ultrasound and other findings clearly support the diagnosis of a ruptured tubal pregnancy. However, the enigma remains since, despite accepting the above alert attitudes, one still encounters the clinical situation in which the diagnosis of a ruptured tubal pregnancy is made and not necessarily confirmed at the time of emergency laparotomy. Conversely, a chronic ectopic subsequently may be encountered since its presence was not diagnosed early enough.

Management

Subsequent management may vary depending on the patient's age, her desire for future fertility, and other gynecologic data, such as a history of abnormal cytology, menstrual dysfunction, or pelvic infections—in addition to location and severity of the ectopic and the condition of the patient. When an ectopic pregnancy is suspected, the patient or couple should be informed of the range of treatment modalities which include conservational tubal surgery or extirpative surgery, which might include salpingectomy, salpingo-oophorectomy, salpingectomy with tubal ligation, and even hysterectomy. Through such an informed status, the patient can assume a more active role in her management. She should be cautioned that even with conservational surgery, the risk of another ectopic remains elevated.

In the patient who desires future fertility, only conservational surgery allows the best opportunity to preserve reproductive function. Microsurgical techniques, copious saline heparin irrigation and suction, and meticulous hemostasis using bipolar coagulation are paramount. With a ruptured ectopic, the procedures employed include teasing or extraction of the products of conception, linear salpingostomy, or tubal resection, depending upon the location of the pregnancy. A periosteal elevator is frequently employed to separate the products of conception from the endosalpinx. Steroids, antibiotics, and other adjuvants are beneficial to prevent adhesions. There are a series of unruptured ectopic pregnancies which have been treated through a laparoscopic approach (4, 7). This requires a patient, experienced, and able laparoscopic surgeon with an armamentarium of special instruments and equipment, including equipment for significant suctioning and lavage of large quantities of saline in addition to coagulating and cutting cautery. Moreover, this alternative approach may only delay the need for a laparotomy where the compressing fingers can easily control bleeding and avoid the anxieties of bleeding and the prospect of additional unintended damage to the adnexa.

The unruptured ectopic presents a compromised organ, but the ruptured ectopic offers an even poorer prognosis dependent on the degree of damage related to hemorrhage and disruption of the oviduct. If tubal reconstruction can be accomplished, it is advisable. It should be emphasized that even in the presence of a "normal"-appearing contralateral tube, it is impossible to rule out occult tubal pathology.

In the patient who is hypovolemic and unstable, secondary to blood loss, there is little controversy as to the best management. Here, the main objective involves obtaining prompt hemostasis, fluid and electrolyte replacement, and appropriate blood transfusion. Stabilization of the patient may not be feasible until bleeding is controlled. Prompt intervention is essential to control the bleeding. If the gestation is located in the distal portion of the tube or with a tubal abortion, removal of the pregnancy tissue and securing adequate hemostasis may be all that need be done. When the ruptured segment presents in the midportion with the distal portion of the tube and fimbria intact, the products of conception and damaged portion of the tube may require resection, leaving as much normal tissue as possible if conservation is desired. After a period of convalescence, an elective procedure can be scheduled. Resection and anastomosis have been suggested, but the patient's condition and the anatomic distortion of disruption may not support such opportune reconstruction. Those that are done may not be successful because of the luminal and anatomic discrepancies precluding a meaningful anastomosis.

Special Clinical States

Controversy arises in the patient with an ectopic tubal pregnancy and tubal pathology of the contralateral tube who, at the time of laparotomy, is medically stable. Vehaskari (15) concluded that at the time of surgery, if the contralateral adnexa justifies the diagnosis of sterility, one should preserve the tube containing the ectopic, and restoration of the contralateral tube may be advised. In his series, the percentage of patients who became pregnant was 48%, who had at least one delivery postoperatively was 35%, and who had a recurrence of an ectopic was 8.2% in the group that had normal-appearing adnexa and salpinectomy, compared to respective rates of 49%, 30%, and 16% in the group that had either ipsilateral salpingectomy and restoration of the contralateral tube or a tubal abortion and both tubes spared. There are series in which surgery on the contralateral tube is undertaken at the time of the primary surgery, but these are in unruptured ectopic pregnancies (5, 13).

In order to outline the management of a ruptured ectopic pregnancy and coexistent chronic pelvic inflammatory disease with a hydrosalpinx, we will consider several aspects. Most authors, including ourselves, recommend delaying other infertility surgery (3, 14). Rarely, an exception might be entertained in the patient with *minimal* intraperitoneal bleeding and *minimal* tubal disruption in the isthmic, cornual, or ampullary segment. In such a patient, one might remove the ectopic by techniques which will preserve as much of the tube as feasible, and then repair the tube. It is probably best not to operate on the occluded contralateral tube. If the patient were not to establish a subsequent pregnancy within 6 months to 1 year, an elective laparotomy could be considered without the pressures and untimely factors surrounding unscheduled emergency surgery. Tubal surgery performed as an emergency yields poorer results of varied success. The adnexal structures are often edematous and hyperemic, posing a suboptimal time for reconstruction as well as predisposing to adhesion formation.

In the patient described, if the adnexum was markedly edematous with tubal disruption and sanguineous tissue along with substantial intraperitoneal bleeding, we would resect the damaged portion of tube. At a later date, if still deemed pertinent, both the after-effects of the inopportune ectopic gestation and pre-existing adnexal disease may be corrected. This could involve either an anastomosis or tubal reimplantation together with a cuff ampulloplasty on the contralateral tube.

In the situation where the patient is not interested in future fertility, management would again depend on the hemodynamic status and the extent of coexistent pelvic inflammatory disease. In the patient with mild chronic pelvic inflammatory disease without evidence of an acute process and in whom the contralateral tube is not patent, we would perform a unilateral salpingectomy, although some might elect a hysterectomy. This would be particularly so if there is extensive pelvic inflammatory disease with extensive adhesions and abscess, or if there is an underlying gynecologic condition, such as severe cervical dysplasia or carcinoma-in-situ. Hysterectomy is indicated and may be required to obtain hemostasis, as is the case in a ruptured interstitial pregnancy. Another indication in which a hysterectomy would be undertaken is in the situation where the patient has removal of both tubes or offers two nonfunctioning tubes. Such an eventuality should have been discussed preoperatively. In a series of 654 ectopic pregnancies, Breen (2) reports seven cases of subtotal hysterectomies and seven cases of total hysterectomies in which the indications were an interstitial or cornual pregnancy or predisposing to a ''functionless uterus.'' However, because of the possibilities offered through an invitro fertilization, the concept of a functionless uterus could be challenged.

The question of an incidental appendectomy at the time of surgery for ectopic pregnancy remains controversial. There are some who state that incidental appendectomy can be performed in appropriately selected patients (6). Others conclude that elective appendectomy at the time of salpingectomy for ectopic pregnancy is a desirable procedure (11), while some feel that elective appendectomy is never acceptable except in the rare instance of a simultaneous acute appendicitis (10). We feel that incidental appendectomy is never justified in the patient who is medically unstable. Moreover, in the patient who is interested in conserving fertility, appendectomy is probably not warranted because of the theoretical risk of possible contamination and adhesion formation.

Adjuvant Therapy

Because of previous pelvic inflammatory disease and intraperitoneal bleeding, the patient should receive antibiotics intraoperatively and continued postoperatively. Steroids might also be considered.

Two important aspects should be mentioned when dealing with ectopic pregnancies. Rhoimmunoglobulin should be given to unsensitized Rh-negative patients. The dose recommended is 50 mg prior to 13 weeks' gestation, and 300 mg for gestations of 13 weeks or greater (1). In patients undergoing conservative surgery, follow-up hCG review should be carried out postoperatively to confirm adequate removal of products of conception in the persistently anovulatory patient.

SUMMARY AND CONCLUSION

For a ruptured ectopic pregnancy in an infertility patient with chronic pelvic inflammatory disease and a contralateral hydrosalpinx, the operative procedure would depend upon the location of the pregnancy, the extent of tubal damage, and the hemodynamic status. If there was minimal intraperitoneal bleeding and minimal tubal disruption, gentle extirpation of the products of conception with assurance of hemostasis would be followed by tubal repair as feasible. If the adnexal structures were markedly distorted by edema and extravasations of blood as well as significant intraperitoneal bleeding, we would resect the damaged portion of tube to control bleeding. At a later date, both the effects of the inopportune gestation and preexisting adnexal disease could be approached. With evidence of intraperitoneal bleeding and prior inflammation, antibiotics would be used intraoperatively and continued postoperatively, but steroids and other adjuvants would be avoided.

Hysterectomy with a ruptured ectopic should be undertaken if the pregnancy is interstitial or cornual, if there also is extensive pelvic inflammatory disease, or if there is a coexisting underlying gynecologic condition. An incidental appendectomy is not justified in a patient who is medically unstable or who is interested in conserving fertility.

References

1. American College of Obstetricians and Gynecologists: *Technical Bulletin 61.* March, 1981.
2. Breen JL: A 21 year survey of 6i54 ectopic pregnancies. *Am J Obstet Gynecol* 106:1004, 1970.
3. Bronson RA: Tubal pregnancy and infertility. *Fertil Steril* 28:221, 1977.
4. Bruhat MA, Manhes H, Mage G, et al: Treatment of ectopic pregnancy by means of laparoscopy. *Fertil Steril* 33:411, 1980.
5. Bukosky I, Langer R, Herman A, et al: Conservative surgery for tubal pregnancy. *Obstet Gynecol* 53:709,1979.
6. Cromartie AD Jr, Kovalcik PJ: Incidental appendectomy at the time of surgery for ectopic pregnancy. *Am J Surg* 139:244, 1980.
7. DeCherney AH, Romero R, Naftolin F: Surgical management of unruptured ectopic pregnancy. *Fertil Steril* 35:21, 1981.
8. Kadar N, Romero R: hCG assay and ectopic pregnancy. *Lancet* 1:1205, 1981.
9. Marks WM, Filly RA, Callen PW, et al: The decidual cast of ectopic pregnancy: A confusing ultrasonographic appearance. *Radiology* 133:451, 1979.
10. McElin TW, Iffy L: Ectopic gestation: A consideration of new and controversial issues relating to pathogenesis and management. *Obstet Gynecol Ann* 5:241, 1976.
11. Onuigbo WIB: Elective appendectomy at salpingectomy for ectopic pregnancy: Is it desirable? *Obstet Gynecol* 49:435, 1977.
12. Schwartz RO, DiPietro DL: B-hCG as a diagnostic aid for suspected ectopic pregnancy. *Obstet Gynecol* 56:197, 1980.
13. Skulj V, Pavlic Z, Stoiljkovic C, et al: Conservative operative treatment of tubal pregnancy. *Fertil Steril* 15:634, 1964.
14. Swolin K: A tubal surgeon's recommendation for the surgical treatment of ectopic pregnancy. *J Reproduc Med* 25:38, 1980.
15. Vehaskari A: The operation of choice for ectopic pregnancy with reference to subsequent fertility. *Acta Obstet Gynecol Scand* 39:3, 1960.
16. Weiner CP: The pseudogestational sac in ectopic pregnancy. *Am J Obstet Gynecol* 139:959, 1981.

CHAPTER 26
Metroplasty

HOWARD W. JONES, JR., M.D., D.Sc. (Honoris Causis)

CASE ABSTRACT

A 26-year-old para 0 gravida 4 had lost her previous pregnancies by premature spontaneous labor between the 16th and 21st week of gestation. With the most recent pregnancy, it was believed that the herniation of the bag of waters through a partially dilated and partially effaced cervix preceded the onset of labor. A palpable sagittal ridge
in the uterine fundus was noted at the most recent delivery and exploration of the uterine cavity revealed a telltale septum, suggesting a uterus bicornis unicollis.

DISCUSSION

The diagnosis of pregnancy wastage, specifically repeated miscarriage, due to an anatomic
defect as in this case, is basically by exclusion.
However, one can suspect repeated miscarriage due to an anatomic defect of the uterus
by the history of each of the events. The typical history of repeated miscarriage due to a
double uterus is that of early midtrimester minilabor. The loss begins by crampy abdominal
pain, bleeding occurs only several hours after
this begins, and the patient delivers a well-
formed fetus after about 6 or 8 hours. Characteristically, the first miscarriage is associated
with a labor somewhat longer than subsequent
miscarriages. Pain is a prominent feature, although in the above case it was noted that there
was herniation of the bag of waters through a
partially dilated cervix. However, the history
is not characteristic of losses associated with
an incompetent cervix. These are not accompanied by pain. Furthermore, in the above history, there is no history of trauma to the cervix
by a previous operative procedure to account
for an etiologic factor for her problem.

Although a minilabor at early midtrimester
with the passage of a well-formed fetus is the
rule, there are exceptions. First trimester abor-
tions do sometimes occur and seem to be the
result of a double uterus as evidenced by the
fact that such patients when operated on will
have term deliveries. Some patients have had
a missed abortion.

When confronted with a patient with repeated miscarriage and a double uterus, even
though the history is characteristic, it is necessary to rule out other causes of repeated miscarriage. Only when this has been done should
operative correction of the difficulty be considered.

Part of the investigation should include a
family history, because if there are miscarriages among first or second degree relatives
on either side of the family, the possibility of
some chromosomal problem must be considered. In the event there is a positive family
history, chromosome study of the husband and
wife is very much in order.

In addition, it is necessary to rule out endocrine and metabolic and infectious problems.
Principal among these is a luteal phase defect
which can be conveniently studied by a timed
premenstrual endometrial biopsy. In the event
such a biopsy is out of phase, attention must
be directed to the various underlying difficulties which can be associated with this disorder.
These would include disorders of other endocrine glands and metabolic problems such as
undernutrition or obesity. The role of infection, particularly in a North American population, is controversial at best. Negative cultures
for such things as *Chlamydia, Ureaplasma
urealuticum*, and other organisms which have
been associated with miscarriage would, at least,
rule out infections as possible etiologic agents.

A number of investigators have suggested that
cervical incompetence is a common occurrence

in patients with a double uterus. For this reason, Shirodkar or MacDonald cerclage has been suggested as an important part of the therapy. However, the evidence for cervical incompetence is circumstantial at best in most cases, and it would seem advisable to treat cervical incompetence only when its presence can be documented. It cannot be a very common association, because unification of the double uterus gives excellent results in the majority of cases without any attention to the cervix.

Surgical reconstruction of the uterus has been standard practice for a number of years. Recently, the removal of the septum by operative hysteroscopy has been introduced. This may prove desirable in selected cases. However, at this writing, the number of patients studied and followed have been insufficient and inadequate to evaluate the procedure definitively.

Metroplasty should probably not be done until at least 3 months have elapsed from the last miscarriage in order to have good, firm uterine tissue with which to deal.

Technique of Surgical Correction

The original Strassman procedure is unsuitable for correcting the defect in a septate uterus. Strassman operated only on the bi-cornuate uterus, as he had worked in an era prior to hysterosalpingography, so that his only diagnoses were made on the basis of bimanual examination and exploration of the endometrial cavity by curette. Tompkins and others have recommended a technique beginning by a sagittal midline incision in the uterus. However, the excision of the septum by wedge is an exceedingly satisfactory procedure and can be recommended. The technique follows:

In order to control bleeding, 20 units of Pitressin diluted in 20 ml of saline may be injected into the myometrium prior to making the uterine incision. This will produce blanching and diminish blood loss during the procedure. Sometimes Pitressin may cause circulatory changes so the anesthesiologist must be alerted when this is being used. In this way the possibility of circulatory changes is greatly diminished (Fig. 26.1).

The uterine septum is surgically excised as a wedge. The incisions begin at the fundus of the uterus. Care must be taken in approaching the endometrial cavity so that the cavity is not transsected. As soon as the cavity is opened on each side, a Kelly clamp may be inserted. As

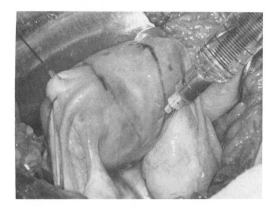

Figure 26.1. Photograph of the exterior of a septate uterus. The wedge to be excised has been outlined with brilliant green. Guy sutures of chromic catgut have been placed on each side at about the insertion of the round ligament. Pitressin is being injected into the myometrium prior to excision of the wedge.

these can be made to touch within the endometrial cavity, incision along the inside of each of the Kelly clamps should assure that the endometrial cavity is not transsected. The original incisions at the top of the fundus are usually within 1 cm (and sometimes even less) of the insertion of the fallopian tubes. However, if the incision is directed toward the apex of the wedge there seems to be little danger of transsecting the tube during its interstitial transit of the myometrium. After the wedge has been removed, major bleeding vessels sometimes can be noted. There seems to be a rather constant vessel near the top of the incision in the region of the tube. This is apparently the main branch of the uterine artery in this area. It is convenient to ligate this with very fine suture material, even though it may not be bleeding due to constriction with the Pitressin. Generally, it is not necessary to ligate other vessels. After the wedge has been removed, the uterus may be closed in three layers with interrupted stiches; 00 chromic catgut on an atraumatic tapered needle is quite convenient. Two sizes of needles are used—a 1/2-inch half-round for the inner and intermediate layers, and a larger needle, 3/4-inch half-round for the outer serosal layers. The inner layer of stitches must include about one-third of the thickness of the myometrium, as the endometrium itself is too delicate to hold a suture and will cut through. The suture is placed through the endometrium/myometrium in such a way that the knot is tied within the endometrial cavity. While the suture is being tied, an assistant presses together the two lateral halves of the uterus with his fingers and with the guy sutures in order to relieve tension on the suture line and reduce the possibility of cutting through. The stitches are placed alternately anteriorly and posteriorly. After the first few stitches are placed and before the first layer is completed, the second layer can be started in order to cut down tension. Indeed, as the operation proceeds, even the third layer can be inserted in the serosa both anteriorly and posteriorly. While for a number of years the 00 chromic catgut stitches have been used in the serosa, more recently finer suture material has been used in order to approximate more precisely the serosal edges of the uterus. Theoretically, this should cut down the opportunity for adhesions to occur to the outside of the uterus, but whether this will make any practical difference in the ultimate end result is problematic. At the conclusion of the procedure, a single incision is visible beginning from the back of the uterus at a position dictated by the depth of the septum and continuing anteriorly to a corresponding position in front. Most often it has not been necessary to detach the peritoneal reflection of the bladder, but in the event there is a particularly deep septum, this may be necessary, and the final incision, therefore, will extend further down on the uterus, both posteriorly and anteriorly. In the event that bladder peritoneum was reflected, this will need to be replaced at this point. At the conclusion, the uterus appears rather normal in its configuration, but the striking feature will be the proximity of the insertions of the fallopian tubes on each side. In placing the final sutures, it is exceedingly important that the interstitial portions of the fallopian tubes not be obstructed by the sutures. The final size of the uterine cavity seems to be unimportant. Many times the reconstructed cavity is quite small compared to a normal uterus. Of more importance seems to be the symmetry. A very small symmetrical cavity seems to function quite normally (Fig. 26.2).

Postoperative films often show small dog ears which are leftover tags from the original bifid condition of the uterus. Such dog ears do not seem to interfere with function. Although the postoperative x-rays after such an operation cannot be considered normal in the sense that they appear like a normal endometrial cavity, they seem to function quite normally.

If Pitressin is used, blood loss from the above procedure is minimal. Diminished bleeding from Pitressin lasts about 20 minutes, and the operation normally can be completed within this period of time.

Healing in the nonpregnant uterus is probably not to be compared with healing after a cesarean section scar because the myometrial healing after a term delivery takes place in a uterus which is undergoing involution. It might be expected that cesarean section scars are less firmly healed than those in the nonpregnant uterus. Nevertheless, most patients who have had surgical reconstruction of a double uterus have been delivered by cesarean section. This can be recommended as a matter of precaution. Such patients have had a long diappointing obstetric experience. They are often in their thirties, and in order to minimize the risk of an obstetric catastrophy, an elective cesarean section prior to the onset of labor seems the most conservative course in order to avoid the possibility of uterine rupture. There seems to have been only one reported example of uterine rupture after metroplasty.

In order to allow the uterine incision the best possible opportunity to heal, a delay in becoming pregnant after surgical reconstruction has generally been advised. The period of delay has been from 6 to 12 months, depending on the age of the patient. However, no difficulties have been encountered, so that this period of delay has been satisfactory. Most patients have waited from 9 to 12 months before becoming pregnant. During this interval, it has been thought inadvisable to recommend oral contraceptives because of the progestational effect on the myometrium and the possibility that healing under this circumstance would be similiar to healing in the postpartum uterus. Therefore, mechanical contraception with diaphragm or condom has been recommended and has proven to be satisfactory as judged by the ultimate end result.

The results of metroplasty in appropriate cases have been very satisfactory. Jones and Rock, in a series of 43 patients, reported 77% of the patients subsequently had a term delivery. Among this series of patients were a total 58 pregnancies, of which 73% went to term. Prior to operation, this same group of patients had had a total of 140 pregnancies with no term

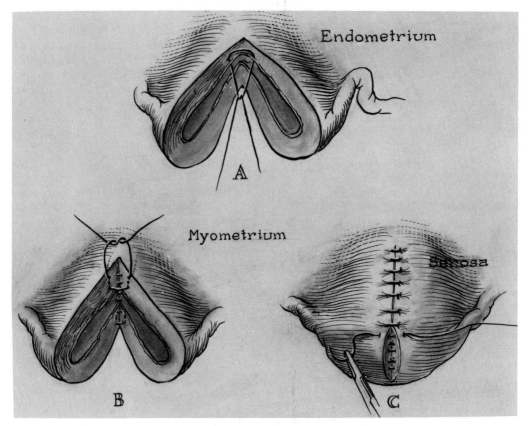

Figure 26.2. Drawings of the placement of sutures following excision of the wedge. *A.* The first layer of internal sutures is placed in such a way that the knot is tied inside of the cavity. Endometrium plus about one-third of the myometrium is picked up in each stitch. *B.* Interrupted stitches, myometrium to myometrium. *C.* Interrupted stitches bringing together the serosal surface and edge of the uterus.

deliveries. Other authors have reported comparable results.

Selected Readings

Jones HW Jr, Rock JA: The clinical management of double uterus. *Fertil Steril* 28:798, 1977.

Ridley JH: *Gynecologic Surgery: Errors, Safeguards, Salvage,* ed. 2. Baltimore, Williams & Wilkins, 1981, p. 252.

Stoot JEGM, Mastboom JA: Restrictions on the indications for metroplasty. *Acta Eur Fertil* 8:79,1977.

Tompkins P: Comments on the bicornuate uterus and twinning. *Surg Clin North Am* 42:1049,1962.

Tulandi T, Arronet GH, McInnes RA: Accurate and bicornuate uterine anomalies and infertility. *Fertil Steril* 34:362,1980.

CHAPTER 27

Endometriosis of the Rectovaginal Septum in an Infertility Patient

JOHN J. MIKUTA, M.D.

CASE ABSTRACT

A 28-year-old patient consulted her gynecologist 3 years after her marriage because of 2 years of involuntary infertility. Her menses were regular and becoming progressively more uncomfortable. The pain would sometimes last longer than the duration of the flow. There was some dyspareunia present, particularly around the time of the menses. There was some nodularity palpable within the cul-de-sac, thought to be in the utero-sacral ligaments. It was recommended that a dilatation and curettage, examination under anesthesia, and laparoscopic examination of the pelvis be performed.

The above procedures were accomplished, and it was evident that, although the tubes were reasonably free, the ovaries were speckled with small implants of endometriosis and the cul-de-sac was virtually obliterated by endometriosis. Rectal vaginal examination suggested extensive involvement of the rectovaginal septum by endometriosis.

DISCUSSION

The objectives of management in this particular patient should be 3-fold:

1. The relief of her symptoms associated with painful menstruation and dyspareunia.

2. The correction of the endometriosis affecting her fertility and menses.

3. The enhancement of fertility by corrective measures.

Generally speaking, the most effective approach in this patient would probably be the surgical correction of the laparoscopic findings. In a patient in whom fertility was not an objective, the use of progestins or danocrine (Danazol) to relieve the symptoms already mentioned would probably be the best initial approach.

Because of the location of the endometriosis and its involvement of the cul-de-sac and extensive involvement of the rectovaginal septum, it is probably advisable that the patient have a bowel preparation prior to the exploratory laparotomy. The use of purgatives and enemas for approximately 72 hours in addition to a clear liquid diet and the use of neomycin

for at least 36 hours prior to surgery would provide an adequate preparation in case of injury or the need to resect a portion of the bowel. If the laparoscopic examination suggested that there was extensive involvement close to the ureters as they come into the pelvis, besides evaluating this with an intravenous pyelogram, placement of ureteral catheters would be helpful in identifying these structures at operation.

The surgical approach should attempt either to remove or destroy the endometriosis which is felt to be symptomatic, and secondly to correct the anatomic changes that appear to be related to the patient's inability to conceive.

The endometriotic implants on the ovary, unless they are of considerable size, would probably be best handled by local fulguration. Lesions greater than 1 cm are probably best resected and the ovary then reconstructed. Other small areas of involvement of the peritoneum that are present can be treated by either excision or fulguration. The peritubal adhesions as well as periovarian adhesions need to be removed so that these structures will be free to have a normal anatomic relation to each other so that the necessary mobility of each structure during the time of ovulation and during the time of fertilization of the ovum would be optimal.

Ideally an effort should be made to remove as much of the disease process as possible from the cul-de-sac and rectovaginal septal area. Again the objectives would be the removal of symptomatic disease as well as the improvement in the mobility of the uterus in relationship to the tubes and ovaries. Surgical excision of the adhesions in the cul-de-sac and in the rectovaginal septum using sharp dissection as needed is the preferred approach. Occasionally an area of bowel wall may have to be resected in order to completely free the rectum from the uterus or the cervix, and the preparation of the bowel makes this a safe procedure. Because of the scarring that is created by the presence of the endometriosis, it may be possible to remove a significant segment of this disease without ever entering the bowel wall itself.

Two other procedures are recommended at the time of endometriosis surgery for infertility. The first of these is a suspension of the uterus, and the second is the performance of presacral neurectomy. The placement of the uterus in an anteflexed and anterior position may prevent the formation of further adhesions in the cul-de-sac and also keep further endome-triosis from forming due to retrograde menstrual flow through the tubes. The presacral neurectomy will be helpful in reducing the amount of dysmenorrhea that may be present, and in the case of recurrence of the endometriosis it will be helpful in preventing the recurrence of pelvic pain and dyspareunia.

In the patient who recovers promptly from surgery of this type and where pregnancy is a desired event, immediate efforts at establishing pregnancy are advisable as compared to suppression of ovarian function. The latter may be carried out in instances where pregnancy is not an urgent issue to allow the tissues more time to heal.

Selected Readings

Andrews WC, Larsen GD: Endometriosis: Treatment with hormonal pseudopregnancy and/or operation. *Am J Obstet Gynecol* 118:643, 1974.

Gray LA: Surgical treatment of endometriosis. *Clin Obstet Gynecol* 3:472, 1960.

Gray LA: The conservative operation for endometriosis: A report of 200 cases. *J Ky Med Assoc* 56:1219, 1958.

Kistner RW: Infertility with endometriosis. *Fertil Steril* 13:237, 1962.

McCoy JB, Bradford WZ: Surgical treatment of endometriosis with conservation of reproductive potential. *Am J Obstet Gynecol* 87:394, 1963.

CHAPTER **28**
Missing Needle

RAY V. HANING, JR., M.D.

CASE ABSTRACT
Following a microsurgical tuboplasty the surgeon had broken scrub, and as the first assistant was preparing to close the peritoneal cavity, the circulating nurse reported the needle count as one missing, a microsurgical needle. A flat plate obtained on the operating room table failed to reveal the needle.

DISCUSSION

Finding the Lost Needle

Standard x-ray techniques are of great assistance in locating or ruling out intra-abdominal location of needles for 6-0 or larger sutures. Microsurgical needles are too small to be visualized by standard x-ray techniques. Even using a Bucky tray and a small field (24 × 30 cm) to cut down on scatter, we were unable to visualize 7-0, 8-0, or 9-0 needles (Ethicon TG140-8, formerly GS9) placed on a patient's abdominal wall at the time of a hysterosalpingogram scout film. We had no trouble visualizing the 6-0, 5-0, or 4-0 needles (Ethicon taper RB-1) or larger needles in the x-ray department (technique: 1.2 mm focal spot, 60 kv, 8 mAs). A portable abdominal flat plate film (35 × 43 cm, focal spot approximately 2 × 2 mm) obtained in the operating room with a grid to cut down on scatter would provide even poorer resolution. This is because an increase in the size of the focal spot increases the size of the penumbra, and as the x-ray field becomes larger, the scatter problem increases, producing still poorer resolution. Although it is possible theoretically to increase the resolution of x-ray techniques by using smaller fields and smaller focal spots, instruments with smaller focal spots are not readily available in the operating room, limiting their utility. The use of multiple small fields presents problems in ensuring that the needle will not be missed between the fields surveyed. Thus, in the operating room, techniques for finding the missing microsurgical needle are realistically limited to visual search of the operative site and the use of strong magnets to locate the needle lost elsewhere. A strong magnet in a sterile drape could theoretically be used to check the superficial areas of the operative field, but, again, such magnets are not readily available in the operating room. Strong magnets are not able to assist in finding a needle which has gained access to the abdominal cavity and which is not superficial in its location. Although the lost needle should be retrieved if possible, the microsurgical needle lost in the operative site is unlikely to be harmful to the patient due to its small size. Thus, the microsurgeon must ultimately make a decision either to stop the search or to continue the search for the missing needle. Such a decision is based on the risk-benefit ratio. If a needle is lost and cannot be found, the patient should be informed of the status of the needle count, the steps that were taken to locate the needle, and the rational for stopping the search at the point where it was stopped.

Prevention of Needle Loss

Since locating the lost microsurgical needle is so difficult, it is useful to discuss techniques for prevention of microsurgical needle loss. There are three possible prospective approaches that can be of use: (1) careful needle handling, (2) careful draping and packing of the microsurgical field to limit access of the dropped needle in the abdominal cavity to only the small microsurgical field itself, and (3) careful measures by the scrub nurse and circulator to make sure that the used needles are stored securely to prevent loss on the instrument table and to make sure that the number of all types of needles used on the case is known so that in the event that the count is 1 missing, it can be immediately determined what size of needle is being sought.

A little recognized problem in dealing with the microsurgical needle is the visual acuity of the scrub nurse. Many people over 40 years of age have begun to lose some ability to accommodate visually. This results in loss of visual acuity for close work, making it difficult for them to see microsurgical needles or suture without corrective lenses such as bifocals. Such individuals should wear appropriate corrective lenses if they are to work with microsurgical sutures.

Needle Handling. The needle should be handled in such a way as to minimize the chance of dropping it or dislodging it from the suture

prematurely. Thus, in addition to receiving it from and passing it back to the scrub nurse always grasped in the jaws of the needle holder or grasped by the suture in a rubber shod clamp, care should be taken not to weaken the fine suture by holding it in metallic clamps or the needle holder. Small rubber shod clamps should be used to hold untied sutures if the needles are still attached, and care should be taken not to place such clamps near the attachment of the suture to the needle as this can promote premature separation of the suture from the needle. Once the needle is back on the instrument table the scrub nurse must take equal care to see that the needle is not lost there since loss on the instrument table will still result in an incorrect needle count at the end of the case. In spite of all these precautions, the occasional loss of a microsurgical needle will continue to occur.

CHAPTER 29

McIndoe Procedure with Rectal Penetration

JOHN D. THOMPSON, M.D.

CASE ABSTRACT

A McIndoe-type construction of a neovagina was being performed on an 18-year-old female with Mayer-Rokitansky-Kuster-Hauser syndrome. The skin grafts from the buttocks had already been taken and sewn to the outside of a rubber covered stent. The surgeon had dissected the tunnel between the urethra and rectum, and was making a special effort to avoid unwanted penetration of the bladder. The dissection had proceeded about one-half the distance from the vulva to the estimated site of the abdominal peritoneum when it was evident that a two-fingerbreadths longitudinal rent had been torn through the anterior wall of the rectum. This was confirmed by a rectal examination.

DISCUSSION

Organs derived from the mullerian ducts in the female include the fallopian tubes, uterus, and most of the vagina. Abnormal mullerian duct embryogenesis with failure of development of the vagina is usually associated with absence of a midline uterus. The uterus is usually represented by rudimentary bulbs on the lateral pelvic sidewalls. Fallopian tubes are attached to these small lateral muscular structures. The ovaries are normal structurally and functionally since their embryologic formation is from the genital ridge. Therefore, such patients are phenotypically female with perfectly normal female secondary sexual characteristics. A normal female body contour with normal breast development occurs at the usual age. The external genitalia are normal female. The karyotype is 46 XX, indicating a normal genetic female.

This condition is known as the Mayer-Rokitansky-Küster-Hauser syndrome. These young girls are usually brought to the physician by their mothers because of amenorrhea. They may

also present themselves later because of difficulty with intercourse. On examination, the vagina is absent except for a small dimple above the hymenal ring which represents that part of the vagina which forms from the urogenital sinus. Other anomalies, especially skeletal and urologic, may be found. Approximately 40% of these patients will be found to have major anomalies of the upper urinary tract, including absent kidney, pelvic kidney, crossed ectopy, and others. An intravenous pyelogram should always be done to assess upper urinary tract structure and function.

The unfortunate embryologic omission of the vagina has stimulated the inventive genius of gynecologic surgeons for almost a century. Although some still advise a nonoperative intermittent pressure technique to create a canal for intercourse, the resulting vagina may be inadequate in depth and caliber. Of all the surgical procedures devised, most gynecologic surgeons now use the Abbe-Wharton-McIndoe operation. The operation consists of three cardinal principles: dissection of an adequate space between the urethra and bladder anteriorly and the rectum posteriorly; insertion of a split-thickness skin graft over a suitable form; and continuous dilatation of the space until the constrictive phase of healing is complete. The first and second principles were advocated by Abbe in 1898. The first and third principles were advocated by Wharton in 1938. All three principles were advocated by McIndoe in 1938.

Dissection of an adequate space is usually not difficult in a patient who has not had previous surgery. However, if scarring from a previous surgical attempt is present, finding a proper plane for dissection may be more difficult. The dissection usually begins with a transverse incision in the vaginal mucosa at the apex of the dimple above the hymenal ring. Using blunt and sharp dissection with scissors, a Kelly clamp and Hegar dilators, one can develop channels on each side of a median raphe (Fig. 29.1). The result is reminiscent of a mullerian duct on each side divided by a midline septum. A finger can be inserted on each side.

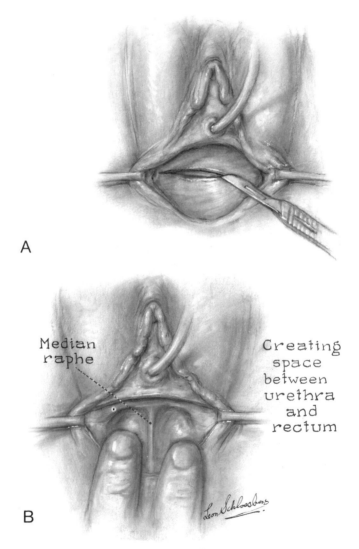

A

B

Median raphe

Creating space between urethra and rectum

Figure 29.1. The McIndoe procedure. *A.* A transverse incision is made in the apex of the vaginal dimple. *B.* A channel can usually be dissected on each side of a median raphe. The median raphe is then divided. Careful dissection will present injury to the bladder and rectum. (Reproduced with permission from Mattingly RF, Thompson JD: *TeLinde's Operative Gynecology*, 6th edition. Philadelphia, JB Lippincott, 1985.)

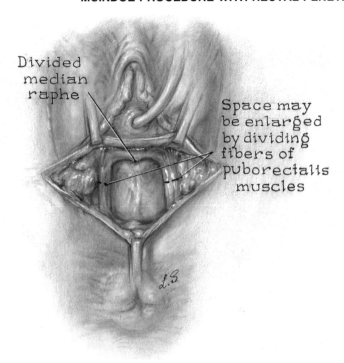

Figure 29.2. A space between the urethra and bladder anteriorly and the rectum posteriorly is dissected until the undersurface of the peritoneum is reached. Incision of the medial margin of the puborectalis muscles will enlarge the vagina laterally. (Reproduced with permission from Mattingly RF, Thompson JD: *TeLinde's Operative Gynecology*, 6th edition. Philadelphia, JB Lippincott, 1985.)

Exerting pressure in a posterior direction will allow the operator to divide the septum between the urethra and bladder anteriorly and the rectum posteriorly without injury to either of these important structures. If the dissection is difficult, a finger may be inserted into the rectum through the anus or an instrument placed through the urethra into the bladder. These simple maneuvers will help the operator determine the proper plane of dissection. The space should be developed superiorly to the peritoneal reflection of the lower cul-de-sac. The transverse diameter of the space can be enlarged by cutting the medial fibers of the puborectalis muscles bilaterally (Fig. 29.2).

For cosmetic reasons, the split-thickness skin graft should be taken from the buttocks. The skin of the buttocks is also thicker. Balsa wood is used for the form since it can be shaped to fit any space size. It should be covered with foam rubber and a rubber sheath before the skin graft is sewed over it. The form should not make undue pressure in any direction, and it should

be larger in the transverse dimension than in the AP dimension.

A penetration into the rectal lumen such as described in this patient is most unfortunate since there is a greater risk of postoperative complications, especially infection. Hopefully, the rectum has been emptied previously with an enema and gross fecal contamination of the operative site will not occur. A broad spectrum antibiotic should be given at once, if not previously administered. The edges of the rectal entry should be carefully delineated and closed with a series of interrupted 000 polyglycolic acid-type (Vicryl or Dexon) sutures. Even though the rectal laceration is longitudinal, it should be closed transversely. The initial mucosal closure should be reinforced by two additional layers of interrupted 000 polyglycolic acid-type (Vicryl or Dexon) sutures, folding the rectal wall transversely over the initial suture line. Dissection should be redirected in the proper plane and the space fully developed. The balsa wood form should be fashioned very

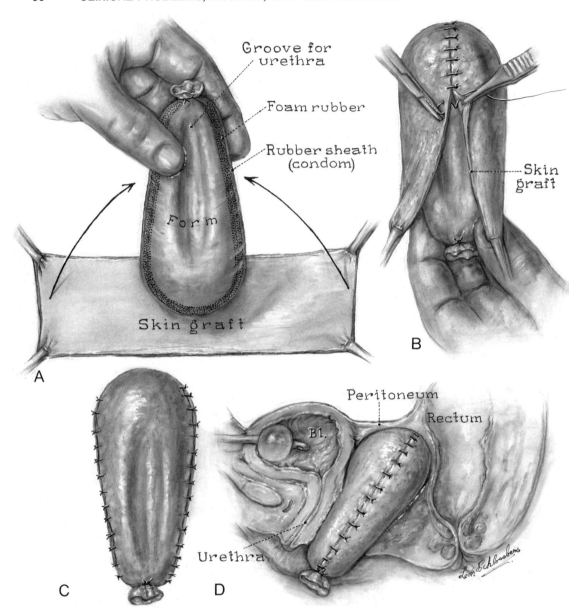

Figure 29.3. *A.* The form may be constructed of a central core of balsa wood covered by foam rubber and an outer rubber sheath (condom). A groove can be made to accommodate the urethra. The outer skin surface should be placed against the form. *(B* and *C)* The edges of the graft are sutured with no. 5-0 polyglycolic acid interrupted sutures. *D.* The form should fit the new vaginal space exactly, without undue pressure at any points. The bladder may be drained suprapubically. (Reproduced with permission from Mattingly RF, Thompson JD: *TeLinde's Operative Gynecology,* 6th edition. Philadelphia, JB Lippincott, 1985.)

carefully to fit in the space without placing pressure on the suture line in the anterior rectal wall. The skin graft should be sutured over the form and the form placed in the vagina (Fig. 29.3) to be left in for at least 1 week before it is removed the first time. The patient is then instructed in the use of the form until the constrictive phase of healing is complete. This usually requires at least 6 months and sometimes longer.

Postoperative care of this patient is similiar to that of any patient following repair of a rectal injury or a rectovaginal fistula. My personal preference is for a liquid diet for several days followed by a low residual diet and stool softeners. The patient may be allowed to eat a regular diet after 3 weeks. Since the rectal injury occurred in healthy tissue, there should be no difficulty with healing and a colostomy should not be necessary. Of course, a colostomy may be required if primary healing does not occur.

If the injury had been sustained in the bladder instead of the rectum, the same general principles would be applicable. The margins of the bladder laceration should be carefully delineated and the bladder mucosa closed securely using interrupted 000 polyglycolic acid-type (Vicryl or Dexon) sutures. The security of the first layer should be tested by instilling 200 cc of a weak methylene blue solution transurethrally into the bladder. Any leakage should be stopped with reinforcing mattress sutures. Two additional layers of interrupted 000 polyglycolic acid-type (Vicryl or Dexon) sutures are used to approximate broad surface to broad surface without tension. Again, the form covered with the split-thickness skin graft should be fashioned carefully to avoid undue pressure on the suture line. In this situation, a transurethral Foley catheter should not be used. In-urethral Foley catheter should not be used. Instead, bladder drainage is provided for at least 2 weeks with a suprapubic catheter. Since the injury occurred in healthy tissue, primary healing should occur.

Selected Readings

Abbe R: New method of creating a vagina in a case of congenital absence. *Med Rec* 54:836, 1898.

Evans TN, Poland ML, Boving RL: Vaginal malformations. *Am J Obstet Gynecol* 54:126, 1981.

Fore SR, Hammond CB, Parker RT, et al: Urologic and genital anomalies in patients with congenital absence of the vagina. *Obstet Gynecol* 46:410, 1975.

Garcia J, Jones Jr HW: The split-thickness graft technique for vaginal agenesis. *Obstet Gynecol* 49:328, 1977.

Griffin JE, Edwards C, Madden JD, et al: Congenital absence of the vagina. *Ann Intern Med* 85:224, 1976.

Ingram JM: The bicycle seat stool in the treatment of vaginal agenesis and stenosis: A preliminary report. *Am J Obstet Gynecol* 140:867, 1981.

Mattingly RF, Thompson JD: *TeLinde's Operative Gynecology,* 6th edition. Philadelphia, JB Lippincott, 1985, Chap 15.

McIndoe AH, Banister JB: An operation for the cure of congenital absence of the vagina. *J Obstet Gynaecol Br Empire* 45:490, 1938.

Rock JA, Reeves LA, Retto H, et al: Success following vaginal creation for mullerian agenesis. *Fertil Steril* 39:809, 1983.

Thompson JD, Wharton LR, TeLinde RW: Congenital absence of the vagina. *Am J Obstet Gynecol* 74:397, 1957.

Wharton LR: A simple method of constructing a vagina. *Ann Surg* 107:842, 1938.

CHAPTER 30
Incarcerated Procidentia

JOSEPH H. PRATT, M.D.

CASE ABSTRACT

A 70-year-old multipara with a long history of genital prolapse had worn an intravaginal Gellhorn pessary for several years. The pessary was spontaneously extruded during an episode of straining at stool about 2 months before the patient was seen. There is now a massive "irreducible" procidentia, associated with some bloody vaginal discharge, the latter apparently arising from some ulcerations upon a very thick and edematous cervix. An attempt at manual replacement of the procidentia was not successful.

DISCUSSION

Gynecologic histories report instances of incarcerated procidentia generally in the older patients. Historically, death was the expected outcome, although some patients did survive when the tissues could be replaced and there were no gangrenous loops of bowel present. Conservative measures included head down positions, cold moist packs, and repeated attempts to squeeze and replace the tissues inside the abdomen. Rarely a ligature was placed about the mass and tightened daily until the distal tissues could be excised. Surprisingly there were occasional survivors.

Total procidentia of the uterus is most generally associated with partial or even complete prolapse of the bladder and is commonly accompanied by either enterocele or rectocele (Fig. 30.1). It is usually found in the older multiparous postmenopausal woman. When such a mass becomes irreducible for days or even months the problem is indeed rare (Fig. 30.2).

Conservative measures include preliminary bed rest, cleansing douches, and intravaginal supports until the edematous tissues subsided, the vaginal ulcerations became less acute, and the procidentia reduced. In any event, vaginal hysterectomy and repair are indicated even if the prolapse cannot be first reduced.

It is the general health of the patient that determines whether one can proceed directly with a definitive operation whose aim is both reduc-tion of the incarcerated tissues and the prevention of its recurrence. Most patients seen with this problem are elderly and many of them are seriously ill with medical problems, physical neglect, and even starvation. These difficulties must be alleviated before subjecting a patient to a major operative procedure. Therefore,

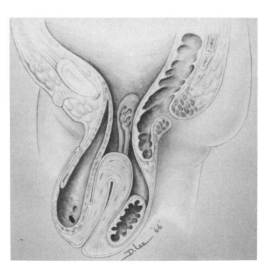

Figure 30.1. When the bladder is completely prolapsed, the urethra points almost vertically upward and the bladder distends *below* the urethra and seldom empties completely. The ureters course up along the bladder and the ureterovesical orifaces can be as they were here some 10 to 15 cm *outside* the introitus. Behind the uterus there may be a very large enterocele and it may contain loops of ileum.

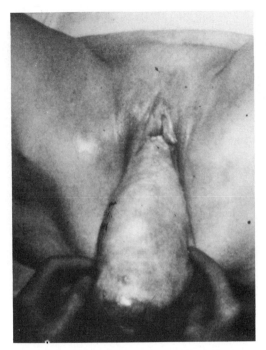

Figure 30.2.   An incarcerated procidentia is shown in a postmenopausal woman.

supportive therapy, attention to the electrolytes, attempts at reduction of the mass by elevation of the legs, cool packs, and pressure would be primary measures.

Malignancy in procidentia is rare in the United States though seen not uncommonly in the Indian population of Central America. The ulcerations of cervix and vaginal mucosa of an incarcerated procidentia are due to wear and tear against the clothing. They are shallow lesions and clean up readily. An endometrial lesion would be incidental to the care of the patient since the mass is to be extirpated in toto anyway.

Since we were not dealing with an emergency situation, a routine preoperative workup including an excretory urogram should be evaluated and the patient then scheduled for a vaginal hysterectomy and repair.

Hydroureter is often present. Identification and protection of the ureters is the most dangerous technical portion of the operation but the ureters are easily identifiable and can be kept away from possible suture damage. We are unable to say whether any hydronephrosis and hydroureters are due primarily to compression and mechanical obstruction of the ureters

against the pubic rami or from angulation around the uterine arteries. In consideration of the increased length of the ureters and their fixation at that length due to the incarcerated procidentia one could postulate that the inability of the ureters to relax and contract is a major factor in the development of hydroureterosis.

Ureteral obstruction to some extent is very common but is relieved by reduction or excision of the mass. A more intriguing problem is the frequent occurence of stones in the prolapsed bladder. The size of these are reported as from pebbles to massive accumulations. Fortunately, they are readily removed by an incision in the base of the bladder which is then closed as the cystocele is repaired.

Technique of a vaginal hysterectomy and repair. Through an anterior elliptical incision whose lowest point was just above the cervix, the bladder is separated from the uterus and the cardinal ligaments. A similar incision on the posterior side of the mass identifies rectum, rectocele, and enterocele and many square inches of superficially ulcerated vaginal epithelium are excised from the enterocele area. Before clamping and dividing the utero-ovarian and cardinal ligaments, both ureters are identified for 6 cm along the bladder base and identified again before anchoring the ligaments to the corners of the vaginal vault. After extirpation of the uterus and edematous tissue of vagina and lateral ligaments, the excess peritoneum of the cul-de-sac enterocele is excised, the peritoneal cavity closed, and the uterosacral, cardinal, and ovarian ligaments then sutured to the vault. A wedge dissected back to rectal fibers and measuring up to 6 cm wide and 6 cm deep of excess vaginal wall is taken from the posterior fornix. The very large cystocele is repaired (replacing the bladder behind the symphysis) and the tissues beneath the bladder were then imbricated in multiple layers, again excising enormous amounts of excess vaginal tissues. (The excess tissue beneath the bladder, after the latter has been freed and replaced behind the symphysis, is utilized as support by imbricating the tissues in multiple layers beneath the bladder. It is assumed that the large bladder will contract to relatively normal capacity once it is in a more normal situation.)

The enormous quantity of vaginal epithelium covering the incarcerated procidentia is reduced by the excision of various wedges or strips. All ulcerated tissues are extirpated, but it is necessary to preserve sufficient vaginal epithelium to construct a vaginal canal. The rectocele is repaired through a midline "V", leaving a vagina estimated at 25% shorter but of a generous 2 fingerbreadth width.

An indwelling catheter may be left in place for up to several outpatient weeks if the patient is unable to void adequately in the postoperative phase.

SUMMARY

The general condition of the patient determines whether an immediate reparative operation can be considered or whether a few days of rest and supportive therapy should precede surgery. However, malignancies are rare and vaginal hysterectomy with repair offers a good prognosis in the patient with an incarcerated procidentia, even if it cannot be reduced preoperatively.

Selected Readings

Chambers CB: Uterine prolapse with incarceration. *Am J Obstet Gynecol* 122:459-462, 1975.

Holden FC: Discussion of Phaneuf's paper, "The place of colpectomy in the treatment of uterine and vaginal prolapse." *Am J Obstet Gynecol* 30:873, 1935.

Pranikoff K, Cockett AT, Walker LA, et al: Procidentia incarcerated by vesical calculi. *J Urol* 127:320-21, 1982.

CHAPTER 31

Evisceration One Year After Vaginal Hysterectomy Without Colporrhaphy

DAVID H. NICHOLS, M.D.

CASE ABSTRACT

While lifting some heavy furniture 1 year after a vaginal hysterectomy (without repair), a 38-year-old obese multipara experienced a sudden "giving way" in the vagina accompanied by sharp pain. Thirty minutes later she noticed some intestine protruding from the vagina and went immediately to the hospital.

The patient, a mild diabetic, had been attempting over the past year to disguise a weight gain by wearing a tight girdle. She regularly has experienced several daily fits of coughing, secondary to a postnasal drip from a chronic sinusitis.

When seen at the hospital, several loops of very dusky bowel were found filling and protruding from the vagina through a 1-inch rent in the vault of a vertically directed vagina. A coincidental full-length rectocele was present.

DISCUSSION

The problem is that of postoperative vaginal evisceration 1 year after a vaginal hysterectomy without repair. That there was a large rectocele and a vertical axis to the vagina at the time of the present admission strongly suggests that these were present but not corrected at the time of the original surgery. In this circumstance, increases in intra-abdominal pressure as might be associated with heavy lifting, coughing, and wearing a tight girdle would be directed to the vaginal vault in an axis parallel to that of the vagina. Were the tissues of the vaginal vault poorly supported, this would over a period of time tend toward eversion of the vaginal vault, or telescoping of the vagina. In the present circumstance, the full strength of these increases in pressure was directed against the site of uterine amputation. The tissue healing and qualities of scar tissue in a diabetic patient are thought to be somewhat less than those of a non-diabetic, and when the patient has a chronic cough, and by habit wears a tight abdominal constricting garment, the increases in intra-abdominal pressure may be more than

the integrity of the vaginal vault can withstand.

The goals of reconstructive surgery are clearly those of relieving symptoms, and restoring anatomy and function to normal. Restoration to normal anatomic relationships had not been accomplished at the time of the original hysterectomy setting the stage for the possibility of increased risk of future symptoms requiring surgical reconstruction. Had the defective vaginal axis and the rectocele been repaired at the time of the original vaginal hysterectomy, a proper upper vaginal axis now directed parallel to the levator plate and at right angles to the direction of intra-abdominal pressure should have been achieved and this surgical catastrophe likely prevented.

Adequate support of the vaginal vault at hysterectomy is clearly an important goal and accomplishment, but when there has been failure to correct a defective vaginal axis, in this case by a full length anterior and posterior colporrhaphy and perineorrhaphy, the patient's pelvis has not been given the assurance of good postoperative equilibrium that it deserves. It is my opinion that the other anatomic abnormalities of her genital relaxation should have been corrected at the time of the original surgical treatment even though they may have been relatively asymptomatic at that time.

Emergency treatment for this patient with vaginal evisceration requires immediate laparotomy with repositioning of the bowel within the abdominal cavity, thorough inspection of the bowel to assure its probable viability, with careful inspection of the base of the mesentery to which the prolapsed bowel had been attached to determine whether a laceration or hematoma was present which might compromise the blood supply of the bowel. This may have occurred secondary to acute traction to the intestine coincident with the evisceration. Lastly, the site of the rent through the vagina must be carefully examined, any necrotic tissue around the vaginal opening excised, the vaginal vault opening effectively closed with long-acting but absorbable suture, and the cul-de-sac of Douglas obliterated. At a future date, the anatomy of the supports of the vagina should be carefully reassessed and any abnormalities corrected by a transvaginal secondary operation, i.e. colporrhaphy and perineorrhaphy when indicated.

In the case described (Fig. 31.1), the patient was taken immediately to surgery where at pelvic laparotomy through a lower midline inci-

sion the bowel was gently drawn back into the abdominal cavity. A dusky segment of ileum measuring 13 inches in length, and located 14 inches proximal to the ileocecal valve, was noted which was without visible peristalsis or palpable pulse along the mesenteric border (Fig. 31.2). The color did not improve after a wait of several minutes. Although there was no rent in the mesentery, the involved section of bowel with its mesentery was excised, and an end-to-end anastamosis of ileum was accomplished using a two layered technique. The edges of the defect in the vaginal vault were trimmed and closed from side to side with interrupted polyglycolic acid sutures. The deep cul-de-sac was obliterated by several purse-string sutures. A suction drain was inserted through a stab wound 3 inches lateral to the abdominal incision. Retention sutures were placed and the abdomen closed in layers. Postoperatively, the course was smooth and unexpectedly benign. There was no temperature elevation, bowel sounds returned promptly, and the patient was discharged in good condition on her sixth postoperative day. Four months later, the patient was readmitted for elective anterior and posterior colporrhaphy and perineorrhaphy, which achieved restoration of a normal vaginal axis, the upper end of which was now horizontally

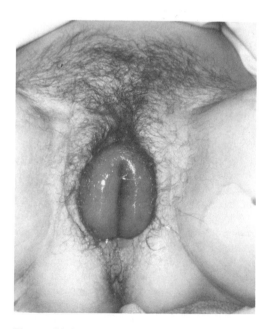

Figure 31.1. Loops of small bowel are shown protruding from the vulva.

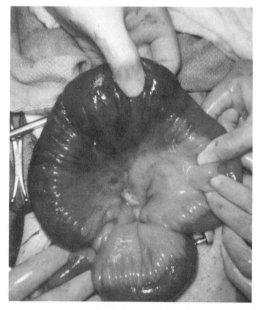

Figure 31.2. The dusky segment of devitalized ileum is shown prior to resection.

inclined and parallel to the levator plate. The patient had stopped smoking with much improvement of her chronic cough, and was no longer wearing a tight girdle, and had begun a voluntary program in weight control with appropriate weight loss. These measures greatly lessen the chance for future recurrence of the evisceration.

CHAPTER 32

Genital Prolapse with Unsuspected Ventral Fixation

JOHN H. ISAACS, M.D.

CASE ABSTRACT

Vaginal hysterectomy with repair is recommended for a 68-year-old multipara with progressive genital prolapse in whom the uterine cervix, bladder, and enterocele protrude well beyond the vulva. The patient thinks she underwent a partial hysterectomy because of abnormal bleeding some 35 years previously, but she does not remember the name of the doctor or the hospital. During transvaginal surgery, when the enterocele sac is opened, it is evident that the uterus extends high within the pelvis. This finding is confirmed when the anterior peritoneal cul-de-sac is opened. It is observed that traction on the cervix produces some dimpling at the lower end of an old midline abdominal scar. What is the next course of action?

DISCUSSION

It is entirely possible that procidentia with unsuspected ventral fixation may defy conscientious efforts to evaluate thoroughly this patient preoperatively. However, certain precautions and considerations may serve to illuminate the situation, and the physician can then be forewarned of potential difficulties.

Mitchell (5) points out that the inexperienced vaginal surgeon should not attempt a vaginal hysterectomy on patients who have a history of previous pelvic surgery or who are suspected of having other pelvic pathology. Although this advice is often given in standard textbooks, this has not been my experience nor the experience of others (3, 4). Nonetheless, if vaginal surgery is to be performed in such cases, careful assessment of the patient's pelvis under general anesthesia prior to surgery is mandatory. Nichols and Randall (6) warn that when uterovaginal prolapse is present, the fundus may occupy a relatively normal position within the pelvis while the cervix becomes elongated and accounts for the prolapse.

Since the patient's previous surgical history is unknown in this case, the physician must depend entirely on the preoperative physical findings and other diagnostic techniques. The initial evaluation requires a thorough pelvic examination, keeping in mind that it is the cervix which often elongates and is the major part of the uterus contributing to the prolapse. Unless the examining physician is aware of this fact, a cursory pelvic examination may give the erroneous impression that the presenting prolapse represents the entire uterus, and the physician may fail to palpate the uterus extending high in the pelvis. Even a large leiomyoma or an adnexal mass well above the elongated cervix may not be detected unless a careful examination is carried out. One technique which may have helped preoperatively in the case presented is to insert a uterine sound into the cervix as shown in Figure 32.1. If the sound can be inserted only a short distance, this substantiates the history of a partial hysterectomy some 35 years previously. Conversely, if the uterus sounds to a depth of 8 to 12 cm, the surgeon is alerted to the possibility that the patient had a previous ventral fixation. If this precaution is taken prior to surgery, the patient can be warned of the problem and of the additional complications that can occur. A pelvic sonogram may also have been helpful in this case. With a full urinary bladder, the sonographic studies would have revealed a mass posterior to the bladder extending to the undersurface of the abdominal

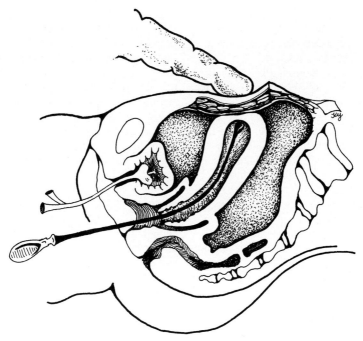

Figure 32.1. A uterine sound is inserted into the uterus. The examiner's hand, placed on the abdomen, could probably palpate the tip of the probe as it is pressed against the uterine fundus.

wall suggesting that the uterus was still present and most likely fixed to the anterior abdominal wall.

Solution to the Problem

In this particular situation, the previous ventral fixation procedure is unsuspected and has to be resolved at the time of surgery. It is helpful if the surgeon knows about the various types of uterine suspension procedures that are and have been commonly performed so that he can be aware of the potential ways that the uterus can be attached to the anterior abdominal wall.

In 1924, Graves (1) described a ventral suspension wherein the fundus of the uterus and the anterior abdominal wall peritoneum were scarified and the fundus was then sutured to the anterior wall peritoneum. This type of ventral suspension was almost completely replaced later in the 1920s by another technique of ventral fixation, in which the round ligaments were used to suspend the uterus. There are a number of these suspension procedures described, including the Gilliam round ligament ventrosuspension of the uterus and the Olshausen suspension.

Basically, these operations pull the round ligaments through the anterior abdominal wall and fix them to the rectus abdominus fascia, as shown in Figure 32.2. Knowledge of these surgical procedures is important for the surgeon since he may then have a better idea of what is holding the uterus to the anterior abdominal wall and how these attachments may be released.

There are several possible solutions to the stated problem, and the technique employed

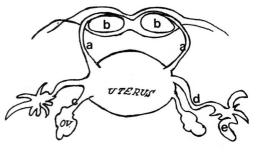

Figure 32.2. The round ligaments (*a*) are brought through the peritoneum and fixed to the fascia of the rectus abdominus muscles (*b*). The ovarian ligaments (*c*) and the fallopian tubes (*d, e,*) are pulled up close to the anterior abdominal wall peritoneum but not attached to it.

depends a great deal on the skill and experience of the surgeon. For the less experienced vaginal surgeon, the wisest choice is to abandon the vaginal approach, open the abdomen, and remove the uterus abdominally; the large enterocele may be partially obliterated via the abdominal route through a series of purse-string sutures closing off the enterocele sac. The cystocele and/or rectocele can be repaired via the vaginal route prior to opening the abdomen.

A second option is to perform a Manchester operation and thereby leave the attached fundus in place. The reader is referred to the excellent description of the Manchester procedure in Wheeless's *Atlas of Pelvic Surgery* (7). If this technique is used, the enterocele sac is resected and the upper edge of the posterior peritoneum is attached to the posterior surface of the uterus after the cervix is amputated. The cystocele is then also repaired. The upper edges of the anterior and posterior vaginal mucosa are then sewn to the raw edge of the fundus where the cervix has been removed. The result is a reconstructed vaginal canal, the prolapsed cervix is excised and the uterine fundus remains in place.

Another possibility, and the one most likely to be undertaken by the more experienced vaginal surgeon, is to continue the vaginal hysterectomy and slowly work up to the round ligaments. A retractor is inserted between the bladder and the anterior surface of the uterus. A second retractor is placed between the rectum and the posterior surface of the uterus. The uterosacral ligaments, cardinal ligaments, and as much of the lower part of the broad ligaments as possible are then progressively clamped, cut, and ligated. If the top of the uterus cannot be reached, one can follow Bonney's advice (2). He suggests that a pair of volsella can be attached to the cervix on each side with one blade of each placed in the cervical canal and the other on the outside of the cervix. Gradually the uterus is then bisected moving superiorly by using a knife or a pair of strong, blunt-pointed scissors. After the uterus is bi-

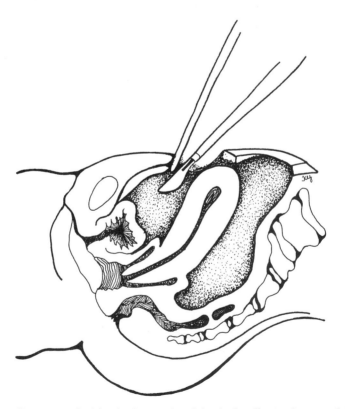

Figure 32.3. A small transverse incision in the anterior abdominal wall over the area of the uterine fixation will expose the round ligaments. The ligaments could then be clamped, cut, and ligated, freeing the uterus from its abdominal attachments.

sected, a third volsellum is applied to one half of the bisected fundus and pulled inferiorly. This will bring the upper part of the broad ligament and the round ligament into view. Clamps can be applied on the one side, and half of the uterus can be cut away.

The other half is treated in a similar fashion. The large enterocele is then excised, the neck of the sac purse-stringed, and the peritoneum closed. Additional sutures into the attenuated endopelvic fascia give support to the vaginal vault. The cystocele is also repaired.

Although the above technique may work quite well in the hands of an experienced vaginal surgeon, it is fraught with danger that includes wounding the bladder, bowel, or ureters or the slipping of a ligature resulting in uncontrollable bleeding. Because of this, my selection, and the one I advise for all but the most experienced vaginal surgeon, is a combined abdominal and vaginal approach. After the anterior and posterior cul-de-sac are opened, the surgeon proceeds superiorly along the uterosacral, cardinal, and broad ligament on each side as high as possible. With such a technique the major blood supply to the uterus is clamped and ligated. When the surgeon progresses superiorly as far as is technically feasible, traction on the cervix can clearly delineate the area on the abdominal wall where the uterus is fixed. The abdomen is then prepped while the patient is still in the lithotomy position, and a small transverse incision is made over the area of fixation. The peritoneum is opened, and the round ligaments are identified close to their fundal attachments. These ligaments are then clamped and ligated, any adhesions can be lysed, and the uterus is then freed from its abdominal attachment as shown in Figure 32.3. The ovarian ligaments and fallopian tubes are identified, clamped, cut, and ligated via this small abdominal incision or they may be clamped and cut via the vaginal route if the uterus descends far enough for the tube and ovarian ligament to be visualized. The uterus is then delivered vaginally. The enterocele is repaired vaginally. The small abdominal incision required to accomplish the above has only minimal effect on the postoperative recovery time, and it reduces the possibility of bowel or bladder damage that may occur if all of the surgery is attempted vaginally.

References

1. Graves WP: *Gynecology,* ed. 3. Philadelphia, WB Saunders, Philadelphia, 1924, p.231.
2. Howkins J, Stallworthy J: *Bonney's Gynaecological Surgery.* Baltimore, Williams & Wilkins, 1974, pp. 242-246.
3. Isaacs JH: Vaginal hysterectomy. In Sciarra J (ed): *Gynecology and Obstetrics.* New York, Harper and Row, 1984, Vol. I:Chap. 19.
4. Käser O, Iklé F, Hirsch HA: *Atlas of Gynecological Surgery,* 2nd ed. New York, Thieme-Stratton, 1985.
5. Mitchell GW Jr: Vaginal hysterectomy; anterior and posterior colporrhaphy; repair of enterocele; and prolapse of vaginal vault. In Ridley JH (ed): *Gynecologic Surgery.* Baltimore, Williams & Wilkins, 1974, p.46.
6. Nichols DH, Randall CL: *Vaginal Surgery,* ed. 2. Baltimore, Williams & Wilkins, 1983.
7. Wheeless CR Jr: *Atlas of Pelvic Surgery,* 2nd ed. Philadelphia, Lea and Febiger, 1987.

CHAPTER 33

Vaginal Hysterectomy with Intrapelvic Adhesions

J. GEORGE MOORE, M.D.

CASE ABSTRACT 1

A 47-year-old multipara, markedly obese, and with mild urinary stress incontinence was troubled by chronic persistent menorrhagia which had been refractory to endocrine treatment and a D & C. There was a history of a Gilliam suspension of the uterus 20 years previously. The uterus, distorted by multiple leiomyomata, was estimated to be 10 to 12 weeks' gestational size and minimally movable. The cervix was in first degree prolapse. Vaginal hysterectomy was initiated. After both anterior and posterior cul-de-sacs had been opened and the cardinal ligament ligated in its entirety on each side, the corpus could not be brought into the wound. Multiple leiomyomata measuring up to 6 cm in diameter were palpable, and it became evident that the uterus was firmly attached by its round ligaments to the anterior abdominal wall. There was some rotational descent of the bladder neck.

DISCUSSION

This is not an uncommon clinical problem in which intraoperative difficulties might be anticipated. Also, postoperative pulmonary problems must be expected in a morbidly obese patient. Therefore, preoperative blood gas studies should be determined and a radial arterial line placed intraoperatively so that pulmonary problems and blood gas determinations can be monitored during and following the surgery.

The degree of prolapse of the cervix is not really indicative of the support of the uterine corpus. Frequently, with relaxation of the lower pelvic supports, the cervix will elongate with the corpus maintaining its well-supported position (3, pp. 74-75). Also, with prior pelvic surgery (especially a uterine suspension) and with extensive postoperative adhesions, the uterine corpus may maintain its intrapelvic position and fixation.

Certainly, with this markedly obese woman, an attempt at vaginal hysterectomy and colporrhaphy was justified. Usually, following ligation and detachment of the cardinal and utero-sacral ligaments together with reduction of uterine size by morcellation, sequential coring out of the myometrium (4, p. 189) or uterine hemisection, the uterus can be brought down into the wound. Once this objective is accomplished the uterine circulation can be secured with progressive bites up the broad ligament on either side and access is thereby gained to the ovarian and/or infundibulopelvic ligaments. Hemisection of the uterus (Fig. 33.1) allows for easier access to the ovarian ligaments and enables safer control in securing the top of the the broad or infundibulopelvic ligaments (Fig. 33.2). This hysterectomy and repair were safely completed by the vaginal route.

A firm attachment of the uterine *fundus* to the abdominal wall (Figs. 33.2 & 33.3) would virtually preclude a safe dissection to release the attachment (3, pp. 74-75) and, consequently, the morcellation procedure would not allow sufficient descent of the uterus and therefore would be of little value. To solve such a patient's clinical problems, i.e., intractable menorrhagia and stress incontinence in the presence of dense fundal adhesions, the hysterectomy should be completed transabdominally

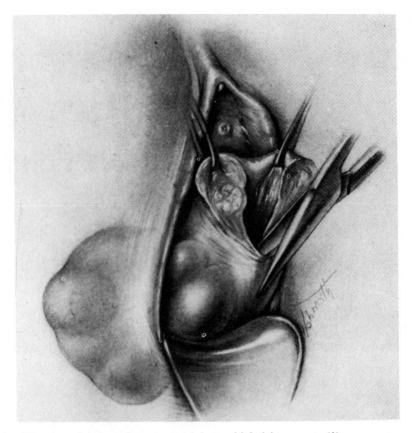

Figure 33.1.   Bisection of prolapsed uterus containing multiple leiomyomata (1).

along with a retropubic urethropexy (MMK or Burch procedure using a nonabsorbable suture such as #00 Prolene) through the space of the Retzius.

With massive obesity, a transverse lower abdominal incision (2) (probably below the abdominal panniculus) should afford sufficient room for the hysterectomy and would also provide optimal access to the space of Retzius. In some instances where the pannicular apron hangs below the symphysis, the lower transverse abdominal incision may even be placed superior to the navel but just above the pubic symphysis. Jackson-Pratt suction drains should be placed laterally on either side in the space of Retzius and in the thick subcutaneous fatty tissue to decrease the chances of a seroma and/or wound disruption.

CASE ABSTRACT 2

Vaginal hysterectomy and repair were contemplated on an obese, 50-year-old multipara with first degree prolapse of a movable and slightly enlarged uterus, a moderate sized-cystocele and rectocele, and chronic menorrhagia. Peritonitis from an appendiceal abscess had been treated surgically by appendectomy and drainage 10 years previously, followed by a prolonged but gradual recovery. There had been no subsequent pregnancy. During surgery, the posterior and anterior cul-de-sacs had been opened, and the uterosacral and cardinal ligaments ligated separately, but when sustained trac-

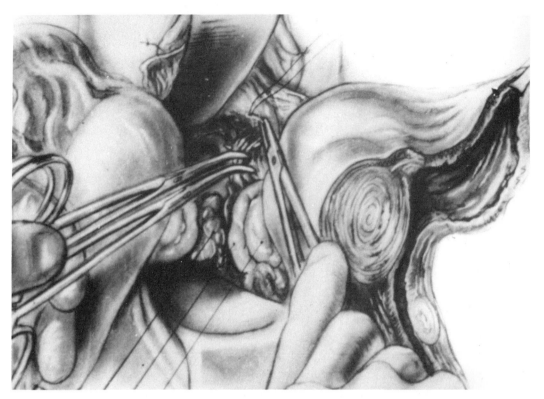

Figure 33.2. Following bisection, the infundibulopelvic ligament of first one side then the other is clamped and ligated (1).

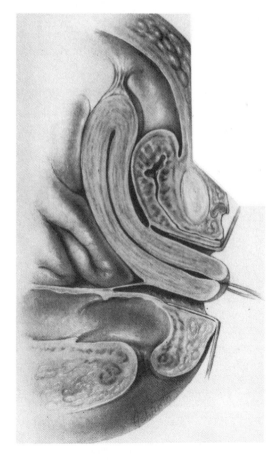

Figure 33.3. Sagittal section of uterus after ventral fixation (1).

tion was applied to the cervix the uterus did not descend as expected. The surface of the uterus was examined digitally, disclosing dense adhesions to it of bowel, and there was a bilateral hydrosalpinx. There appeared to be a 3-cm leiomyoma in the myometrium. Aggressive traction failed to produce further uterine descent.

DISCUSSION

Prior pelvic surgery, history of endometriosis, or a history of pelvic inflammatory disease should always pose the possibility of intra-operative difficulty when a vaginal hysterectomy is contemplated. These features do not unequivocally preclude undertaking a vaginal hysterectomy and, indeed, the vaginal approach would be preferred, just so long as the surgeon is ready and willing to complete the procedure through a transabdominal incision if necessary. The scarring associated with postoperative endometriotic or inflammatory adhesions is associated with pelvic fixation and adherence of the intraperitoneal structures (most commonly bowel) to the uterine corpus, adnexa, and broad ligaments. Under such circumstances, the possibility of injury to the urinary bladder, rectum, and intestine, inability to complete the procedure vaginally and the necessity to complete the procedure transabdominally, should always be explained to the patient when obtaining informed operative consent. As a matter of practice with a planned hysterectomy even when difficulties are not anticipated, these possibilities should always be mentioned to the patient, with documentation in the record.

In this patient, the history of peritonitis fol-

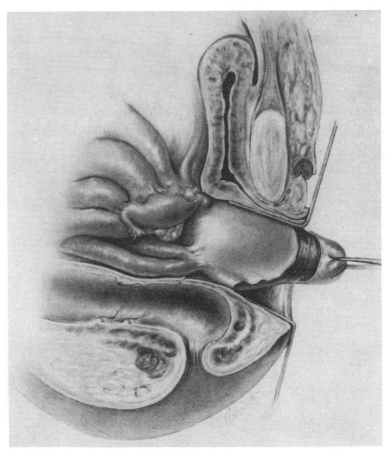

Figure 33.4. Sagittal section during vaginal hysterectomy showing intestinal adhesions to uterine fundus (1).

lowed by an appendiceal abscess and surgical drainage should warn of possible operative difficulties. But other features of the preoperative evaluation might indicate that vaginal surgery could provide the best approach to correcting the clinical problems. With the uterus somewhat prolapsed and only slightly enlarged, a fractional D & C to rule out uterine cancer, and a vaginal hysterectomy to correct the "chronic menorrhagia" is definitely justified. The large cystocele and moderate rectocele are certainly best (and ideally) corrected by an anterior and posterior colporrhaphy. Without extensive pelvic adhesions, fixation, and inflammatory scarring, the procedure has a good chance of proceeding without difficulty. . . . But, alas, it was not meant to be!

Ligation and detachment of the uterosacral and cardinal ligaments and entry into the peritoneal cavity through both the posterior cul-de-sac and the anterior vesico-uterine fold of the peritoneum went smoothly. However, at this point, the uterus did not descend as anticipated, bilateral hydrosalpinx was noted, and dense adhesion of bowel to the surface of the uterus was encountered (Fig. 33.4). The 3-cm myoma is only an incidental finding and would almost certainly not create a problem. Undoubtedly, the chronic inflammatory scarring also led to fixation of the pelvic structures and prevented descent of the corpus, although weakness of the lower uterine supports allowed elongation of the cervix and lower uterine segment (1). At this point, the operator has several decisions to make. First, should an attempt be made to persist in removing the uterus vaginally? If it were a matter of one or two filmy adhesions of bowel to the uterine fundus, they might safely be released. Often with a free space between filmy adhesions, the uterus can be hemisected (after securing the uterine cir-

culation), and the release of adherent bowel can be carried out with better visualization (Fig. 33.1). In this instance, the scars were dense and the bilateral hydrosalpinx would make the management of ovarian ligaments very difficult. The advisability of leaving the chronically inflamed adnexa is also a disturbing question. Hence, the decision is properly made to complete this hysterectomy and bilateral salpingo-oophorectomy through a transabdominal approach.

The second decision relates to the cystocele and rectocele. Can they be corrected through an abdominal approach? No, they are best corrected transvaginally at this time, with an anterior and posterior colporrhaphy. Also, the cardinal ligaments should be anchored to the angle of the vagina on either side, and the detached uterosacral ligaments should be plicated. The vagina should be whipstitched for hemostasis and then the abdominal incision made for a safer approach to the hysterectomy and bilateral salpingo-oophorectomy.

As indicated earlier, contraindications to vaginal hysterectomy noted in the evaluation are only relative. Prior surgery, endometriosis, and pelvic inflammation, pose the possibility of intraoperative difficulty. The experienced vaginal surgeon, however, may be able to complete the surgery vaginally, but he must be prepared to back off and proceed abdominally if safety cannot be assured.

References

1. Benson R: Surgical complications of vaginal hysterectomy. *Surg Gynecol Obstet* 106:527-535, 1958.
2. Maylard EA: Directions of abdominal incisions. *Br J Med* 2:895, 1907.
3. Nichols DH, Randall CL: *Vaginal Surgery*, 2nd ed. Baltimore, Williams & Wilkins, pp. 74-75, p.189.

CHAPTER 34
Dyspareunia Following Acquired Vaginal Atresia

TOMMY N. EVANS, M.D.

CASE ABSTRACT 1

One year following vaginal hysterectomy for uterine prolapse with repair of a cysto-cele and rectocele, an otherwise healthy 48-year-old multipara was unable to have sat-isfactory intercourse because of vaginal atresia. The introitus admitted 3 finger-breadths; the vagina was only 2 inches in depth because of a stricture in the mid and upper vagina that would admit only a fingertip.

CASE ABSTRACT 2

Four years following radiation therapy for a Stage II-B carcinoma of the cervix, a 43-year-old multipara complained of severe dyspareunia. Although there was no evidence of recurrent carcinoma, the vagina was virtually obliterated with a depth of only 3 cm as a result of adherence of the vaginal walls and obliteration of the lumen by rigid cicatrix.

DISCUSSION

Case Abstract 1 describes a far too common complication of vaginoplastic surgery. Acquired vaginal atresia following colporrhaphy is a preventable and serious problem. Generally, meticulous attention to the vaginal dimensions during anterior and posterior colporrhaphy should prevent this complication. Sometimes excessive amounts of vaginal mucosa are excised. It is better to leave a little extra or redundant mucosa than to excise too much, since, afterall, it is not the mucosa that is responsible for restoration of lost pelvic supports.

Endogenous and/or exogenous estrogen may be important in preventing this complication. Postmenopausal women with severe atrophic vaginitis and secondary inflammatory changes are much more likely to develop adhesive vaginitis following vaginal surgery resulting in obliteration of most, if not all, of the vagina. This may be prevented by the preoperative ad-ministration of estrogens for 2 to 3 months followed by postoperative utilization of a Milex or other suitable dilator until healing is complete. Those who have frequent coitus may require the use of a dilator for only a brief period of time or not at all. Particular attention must be devoted to those who are not sexually active during the first few months following surgery, at which time adhesive vaginitis is easily released digitally. This should be repeated monthly until healing is complete. In such situations intravaginal estrogen cream may be a useful supplement to exogenous estrogen.

Case Abstract 2 represents another example of acquired vaginal atresia which is preventable. All patients treated with radiation therapy for carcinoma of the cervix should insert a Milex or similar dilator at least two times weekly for a year or until post-radiation healing is complete. Many of these patients are not sexually active for months after treatment because of decreased libido and for a number of other reasons. Some husbands need to be counseled to

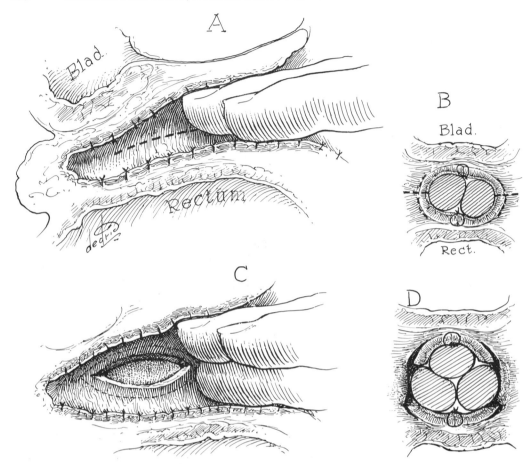

Figure 34.1. Digital examination of the vagina immediately following colporrhaphy discloses an unexpected stenosis in the upper half that will admit but 2 fingerbreadths *(A)*. The sites of the lateral relaxing incisions are indicated by the *dotted lines (B)*. These incisions are made through the lateral wall of the vagina to a depth sufficient to comfortably admit 3 fingerbreadths *(C)*. The vaginal wall is undercut for a centimeter in each direction *(D)*. Any obvious bleeding vessels are clamped and tied, and a firm vaginal packing is inserted. This may be replaced in a day or so by a large vaginal obturator or mold, to keep the cut edges of the relaxing incisions apart until healing and epithelialization are well under way. This is usually by the fifth postoperative day, following which the obturator or dilator may be worn at night for an additional 2 or 3 weeks. Thus, the integrity of the colporrhaphy incisions in the anterior and posterior vaginal walls is not compromised. From Nichols DH, Randall CL: *Vaginal Surgery*, 2nd ed. Baltimore, Williams & Wilkins, 1983, with permission.

eliminate the fear that the cancer is contagious or that intercourse would be painful for the patient. Use of estrogen cream as a lubricant when utilizing the dilator may be helpful.

Management

Management of the acquired vaginal atresia in both of these cases depends upon a number of variables. If the apex of the residual short vagina following surgery is soft and pliable, utilization of progressive dilators comparable to that described by Frank for vaginal agenesis may be adequate. More recently, Ingram has described a technique utilizing progressive dilators and a bicycle seat. When applied to highly motivated patients, these techniques may be useful in both congenital and acquired atresia. However, both the Frank and Ingram methods

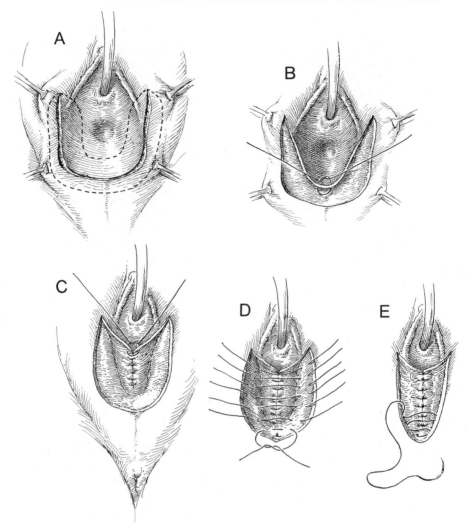

Figure 34.2. Vulvovaginoplasty. The area of softening beneath the urethra identifies the site of the missing vagina. Following through infiltration with 0.5% lidocaine in 1:200,000 epinephrine solution, a U-shaped incision is made and undermined as indicated by the *broken line (A)*. The medial margins of the incision are united by interrupted sutures *(B and C)* and the subcutaneous tissue by a separate layer *(D)*. The lateral incisional margins are approximated separately *(E)*.

require many months of dedicated effort to achieve a satisfactory result.

In other instances of acquired atresia, the use of lateral transverse releasing incisions held open by an obturator or dilator until epithelialized may result in a satisfactory vaginal caliber (Fig. 34.1).

In most instances of acquired vaginal atresia, the best results can be achieved through utilization of the vulvoplasty technique for construction of an artificial vagina described by

Arthur Williams. In Figures 34.2 and 34.3, the progressive steps utilized in performing this operation are illustrated. Following complete healing, the Williams operation should be followed by the use of a large dilator. Supplemental estrogen should be used in the estrogen-deficient patient.

In some patients with extensive cicatrix formation following previous surgery, a vaginectomy with reconstruction of a neovagina with a split-thickness skin graft may be the proce-

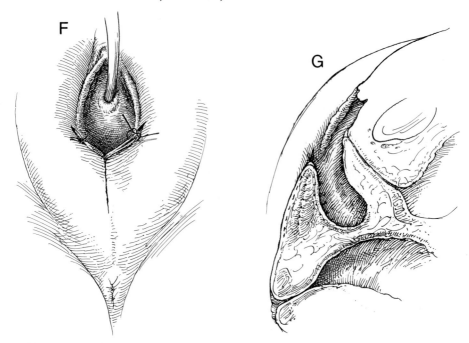

Figure 34.3.   Vulvovaginoplasty at the completion of the operation is shown in frontal view *(F)* and sagittal section *(G)*. From Nichols DH, Randall CL: *Vaginal Surgery,* 2nd ed. Baltimore, Williams & Wilkins, 1983, with permission.

dure of choice. Under these circumstances, as with congenital atresia, incision of the levator musculature bilaterally may reduce the frequency of postoperative vaginal contraction.

Acquired atresia following radiation is best treated by the Williams operation. Vaginal dissections in heavily radiated areas of devascularized tissues may result in a permanent vesicovaginal or rectovaginal fistula.

Selected Readings

Evans TN, Polland ML, Boving RL: Vaginal malformations. *Am J Obstet Gynecol* 141:910, 1981.

Frank RT: The formation of an artificial vagina without operation. *Am J Obstet Gynecol* 35:1053, 1938.

Ingram JM: The bicycle stool in treatment of vaginal agenesis and stenosis: A preliminary report. *Am J Obstet Gynecol* 140:867, 1981.

Williams EA: Congenital absence of the vagina: A simple operation for its relief. *J Obstet Gynaecol Br Commonw* 71:511, 1964.

CHAPTER 35

Vaginal Hysterectomy and Repair with Weak Cardinal-Uterosacral Ligament Complex

DAVID H. NICHOLS, M.D.

CASE ABSTRACT

A vaginal hysterectomy and repair had been performed on a 65-year-old sexually active woman because of progression of a postmenopausal genital prolapse, which recently had become virtual procidentia. The patient was unable to retain a vaginal pessary. After the prolapsed uterus was removed, it was evident that there was practically no cardinal and uterosacral ligament strength which could be used to support the vault of the vagina to restore or maintain vaginal depth postoperatively.

DISCUSSION

When massive eversion of the vagina is the result of a general postmenopausal prolapse, atrophy of most of the endopelvic soft tissue support is often present, and there may be no strong cardinal-uterosacral ligaments to surgically develop for new support of the vault of the vagina. In most instances, the situation can be predicted by the findings at preoperative office evaluation or the examination under anesthesia, when strong uterosacral ligaments are not palpated, and cystocele and rectocele are present and enterocele is frequently absent (Fig. 35.1). This is in sharp contrast to the more common uterovaginal or sliding prolapse, where elongated but strong and hypertrophic uterosacral ligaments can generally be identified along with a significant enterocele. The cervix and vaginal vault in the latter instance slide and descend along the anterior surface of the rectum, producing cystocele but not necessarily rectocele.

Massive posthysterectomy vaginal eversion may follow either abdominal or vaginal hysterectomy, particularly when there has been insufficient attention to the correction of defects in support of the vagina at any of several possible levels. Since a dropped uterus is the result of the genital prolapse, and not the cause,

a simple hysterectomy without effective repair including support of the vaginal vault is likely to be unsuccessful (Fig. 35.2).

There are several factors which may precipitate massive eversion. It may develop from a

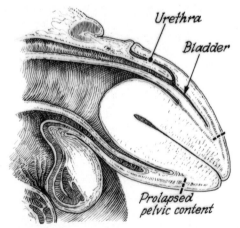

Figure 35.1. Procidentia is present with cystocele, rectocele, and descent of the cul-de-sac. There is displacement of the bladder outside of the pelvis and descent of the vesicourethral junction and proximal urethra and of the anterior rectal wall. The cul-de-sac of Douglas is displaced outside of the pelvis. Reprinted with permission of Northern Chesapeake Publishers, Inc., from Nichols DH: Transvaginal sacrospinous fixation. *Pelvic Surg* 1:10, 1981.

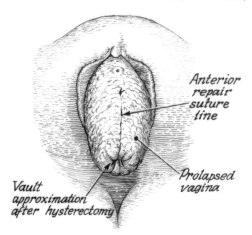

Figure 35.2. A vaginal hysterectomy has been accomplished and the attenuated cardinal and uterosacral ligaments confirmed. Any redundant peritoneum has been resected and the peritoneal cavity closed by high purse-string ligation. A full-length anterior colporrhaphy has been accomplished. Reprinted with permission of Northern Chesapeake Publishers, Inc., from Nichols DH: Transvaginal sacrospinous fixation. *Pelvic Surg* 1:10, 1981.

congenital abnormality in tissue strength, organ position, or innervation. It may also develop in response to sustained increases in intra-abdominal pressure. Obstetric damage to genital supports may be a cause. Although the condition is seen in patients of any age, it is more common among older women and appears to have some association with menopausal atrophy and involutional changes.

In most instances of massive vaginal eversion, however, significant uterosacral ligament strength can be identified preoperatively or intraoperatively. Shortening these hypertrophic ligaments at the time of vaginal hysterectomy is preferred and may be combined with the New Orleans type culdeplasty (3) or one of its modifications (6). This shortening can also be performed following abdominal hysterectomy, although appropriate transvaginal colporrhaphy should follow.

When massive vaginal eversion occurs long after total hysterectomy, cardinal and uterosacral ligaments that had been separated from the uterus but not used in support of the vagina will have usually become atrophic, so that in their weakened and attenuated condition surgical usefulness may be less than effective. This should be evident at surgery, and an alternate

method of support of the vaginal vault elected.

In this era of longer life-span and sustained sexual activity, preservation of coital function is important to the patient, and treatment of massive eversion by surgical procedures that might obliterate the vagina or eliminate its coital function is not desirable. Colpocleisis or colpectomy may give rise to an exceedingly troublesome postoperative urinary stress incontinence (8), and enterocele or pudendal hernia may persist.

The surgical goal should be to re-establish the normal depth and axis of the vagina. The lower vagina curves cranial and posterior, and the upper vagina becomes horizontal and terminates near the hollow of the sacrum.

Various surgical approaches have been employed to treat massive eversion, some transabdominal and some transvaginal. Although ventral fixation or ventral suspension of the uterus or of the everted vagina has been described, it is not without problem. The creation of an abnormal anterior axis to the vagina may limit bladder capacity, producing a troublesome incontinence (1), and expose the unprotected cul-de-sac of Douglas to the full range

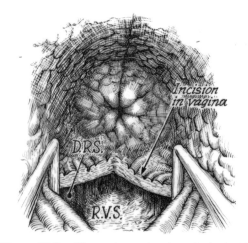

Figure 35.3. The perineum has been incised and an opening made into the rectovaginal space (*RVS*). The full length of the rectovaginal space has been developed to the vault of the vagina by blunt dissection and the full thickness of the posterior vaginal wall incised to a point cranial to the rectocele. The descending rectal septum (*DRS*), which separates the rectovaginal space from the pararectal space, is seen on the patient's right. Reprinted with permission of Northern Chesapeake Publishers, Inc., from Nichols DH: Transvaginal sacrospinous fixation. *Pelvic Surg* 1:10, 1981.

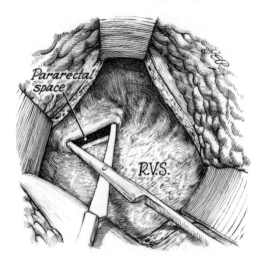

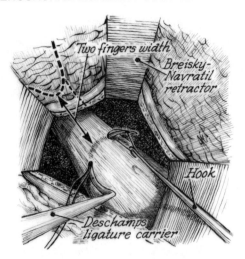

Figure 35.4. The right cardinal ligament and ureter have been displaced anteriorly by a Breisky-Navratil retractor in the twelve o'clock position and the rectum displaced to the patient's left by a retractor in the four o'clock position. An opening is made either bluntly or by using a sharp-pointed hemostat through the descending rectal septum into the right rectal space at the site of the ischial spine. This opening is enlarged by spreading the point of the hemostat or of the Mayo scissors to permit access to the coccygeus muscle which lies in the lateral wall of the pararectal space and contains within it the sacrospinous ligament. *RVS,* rectovaginal space. Reprinted with permission of Northern Chesapeake Publishers, Inc., from Nichols DH: Transvaginal sacrospinous fixation. *Pelvic Surg* 1:10, 1981.

Figure 35.6. The coccygeus muscle and sacrospinous ligament have been penetrated by the blunt end of a long Deschamps ligature carrier at a point one and one-half to two fingerbreadths medial to the ischial spine, safely away from the pudendal nerve and vessels and sciatic nerve. The ligature carrier had been previously threaded with a full uncut length of 52-inch no. 2 polyglycolic acid suture (Dexon). Traction to the hook exteriorizes the suture, and the Deschamps ligature carrier is removed. The end of the suture loop is cut, resulting in two strands of suture material penetrating the ligament. Reprinted with permission of Northern Chesapeake Publishers, Inc., from Nichols DH: Transvaginal sacrospinous fixation. *Pelvic Surg* 1:10, 1981.

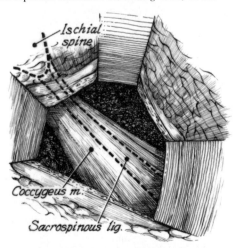

Figure 35.5. The coccygeus muscle containing the sacrospinous ligament (shown by the *dotted lines*) is visible in the depths of the right pararectal space. Reprinted with permission of Northern Chesapeake Publishers, Inc., from Nichols DH: Transvaginal sacrospinous fixation. *Pelvic Surg* 1:10, 1981.

of changes in intra-abdominal pressure with the significant risk of subsequent development of enterocele. Transabdominal attachment of the vault of the vagina to the promontory of the sacrum by fascia or plastic mesh through a retroperitoneal tunnel may effectively support the vault of the vagina, but correction of cystocele and rectocele through the same operative exposure is not possible (7). It is, however, a more physiologic and anatomically correct procedure than ventral suspension.

Transvaginal procedures include fixation of the vagina to shortened strong cardinal-uterosacral ligaments (9), to the fascia of the pelvic diaphragm (2), or to a strong nongynecologic structure such as the sacrospinous ligament (4, 5).

In the case described, appropriate colporrhaphy and transvaginal fixation of the vagina to the sacrospinous ligament is the procedure of choice. The sacrospinous ligament runs from the ischial spine to the sacrum within the sub-

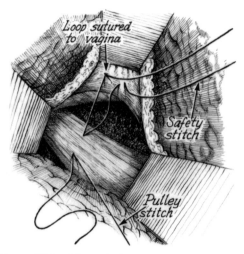

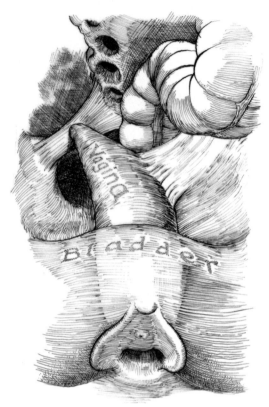

Figure 35.7. The end of one suture is threaded on a free needle, which is sewn through the full thickness of the undersurface of the fibromuscular layer of the vaginal wall, and fixed in position by a single half-hitch. The end of the second piece of suture is stitched to the undersurface of the vagina 1 cm medially. After an appropriate segment of posterior vaginal wall has been excised as part of the posterior colporrhaphy, the margins of the posterior vagina are approximated with a running subcuticular stitch of polyglycolic acid suture until the midportion of the vagina has been reached. The sacrospinous fixation stitches are tied, fixing the vagina to the surface of the coccygeus muscle-sacrospinous ligament, and the posterior colporrhaphy and perineorrhaphy are completed. Reprinted with permission of Northern Chesapeake Publishers, Inc., from Nichols DH: Transvaginal sacrospinous fixation. *Pelvic Surg* 1:10, 1981.

Figure 35.8. A phantom frontal view of the sacrospinous fixation is seen, demonstrating fixation of the vagina to the surface of the right coccygeus muscle and sacrospinous ligament at a point one and one-half to two fingerbreadths medial to the right ischial spine. Reprinted with permission of Northern Chesapeake Publishers, Inc., from Nichols DH: Transvaginal sacrospinous fixation. *Pelvic Surg* 1:10, 1981.

stance of the coccygeus muscle. Its location is readily determined by palpation. Since the surgical anatomy describes the proximity of the pudendal vessels and sciatic nerve beneath the ischial spine, suture penetration of this ligament should occur at a preselected position one and one-half to two fingerbreadths medial to the ischial spine to avoid trauma to the blood vessels and nerves. The ideal instrument for penetration of this ligament is the long-handled, blunt-tipped Deschamps ligature carrier, and the suture of choice is Dexon no. 2. To expose the coccygeus muscle and ligament safely, it is desirable to proceed from an incision in the perineum which opens the rectovaginal space (Fig. 35.3) and is carried through the right rectal pillar into the right pararectal

space (Fig. 35.4), exposing deep within this space the coccygeus muscle containing the sacrospinous ligament (Fig. 35.5). The muscle is grasped by a long Babcock clamp and then penetrated by the blunt tip of a Deschamps ligature carrier threaded with a full uncut length of 54-inch Dexon no. 2, at a point one and one-half to two fingerbreadths medial to the ischial spine, safely away from the pudendal nerve and vessels and the sciatic nerve (Fig. 35.6). The free ends of the suture are fixed to the vault of the vagina (Fig. 35.7) and, when tied, will attach the vaginal vault firmly to this area (Fig. 35.8). The knots should be snug, avoiding any suture bridges. Appropriate colporrhaphy is then completed.

References

1. Hodgkinson CP, Kelly WT: Urinary stress incontinence in the female. III. Round-ligament technic for retropubic suspension of the urethra. *Obstet Gynecol* 10:493, 1957.
2. Inmon WB: Pelvic relaxation and repair including prolapse of vagina following hysterectomy. *South Med J* 56:577, 1963.
3. McCall ML: Posterior culdeplasty: Surgical correction of enterocele during vaginal hysterectomy: A preliminary report. *Obstet Gynecol* 10:595, 1957.
4. Nichols DH: Effects of pelvic relaxation on gynecologic urologic problems. *Clin Obstet Gynecol* 21:759, 1978.
5. Nichols DH: Sacrospinous fixation for massive eversion of the vagina. *Am J Obstet Gynecol* 142:901, 1982.
6. Nichols DH, Randall CL: *Vaginal Surgery*, ed. 2. Baltimore, Williams & Wilkins, 1983.
7. Parsons L, Ulfelder H: *An Atlas of Pelvic Operations*, ed. 2. Philadelphia, WB Saunders, 1968, pp. 280–283.
8. Symmonds RE, Jordan LT: Iatrogenic stress incontinence of urine. *Am J Obstet Gynecol* 81:1231, 1961.
9. Symmonds RE, Williams TJ, Lee RA, et al: Posthysterectomy enterocele and vaginal vault prolapse. *Am J Obstet Gynecol* 140:852, 1981.

CHAPTER **36**

Massive Eversion of a Shortened Vagina

GEORGE W. MORLEY, M.S., M.D.

CASE ABSTRACT

A 45-year-old, sexually active woman has had two previous operations for a troublesome symptomatic prolapse. These include a vaginal hysterectomy with colporrhaphy and repeat colporrhaphy with excision of an enterocele. Three years following the last procedure, and over a period of several months, a recurrent vaginal eversion has developed. The vagina, though totally everted, is but 3 inches in length and cannot be brought to the site of the sacrospinous ligament.

DISCUSSION

This situation poses one of the most difficult problems encountered by those interested in vaginal reconstructive surgery. Fortunately, the "short vagina" syndrome is not a frequent complication of previous hysterectomy—either vaginal or abdominal—or any other previous vaginal surgery; however, when it does occur, it is fraught with a variety of abnormal signs and symptoms and emotional frustrations.

One need not discuss the etiology of this syndrome in any great detail but certainly all who do surgery must be apprised of this possibility in performing gynecologic surgery either transvaginally or transabdominally. This is an "ounce of prevention!"

I have seen a number of these patients who had undergone transabdominal hysterectomy with removal of a portion of the upper vagina for a variety of indications; however, it is much more common in those patients who have previously undergone vaginal surgery. From a therapeutic point of view, there are a variety of ways to approach this complex problem.

A *transabdominal sacropexy* (4) certainly is an appropriate way to manage this problem; however, given a vaginal depth of only 3 inches, something more than just attaching the vaginal apex to the sacrum must be considered. One could open the apex of the vagina after which an extension of the vagina could be fashioned from an absorbable synthetic material utilizing either a polyglycolic acid or a polyglactin 910 mesh. This newly constructed elongated "upper vagina" which can be of varying length is then attached to the presacral ligament as performed during the more conventional transabdominal sacropexy (4). A more permanent foreign body material such as a Mersilene mesh has been used in the past but it has the disadvantage of sometimes becoming infected or occasionally eroding through adjacent tissues or organs. These situations are not only annoying but the foreign body is very difficult to remove or retrieve.

During the postoperative period, the absorbable synthetic material acts as a matrix or scaffolding to which fibroblastic proliferating tissue can attach. This process also stimulates the formation of granulation tissue which carries with it an exuberant blood supply. During the healing period, an appropriately sized obturator is worn in the vagina so as to maintain appropriate depth and caliber. A split-thickness skin graft may or may not be required to cover the granulation bed; migratory epithelialization may occur spontaneously and quite satisfactorily. In either case, the obturator is left in place 24 hours/day for three months except when voiding or evacuating the lower colon or when taking a daily cleansing douche. Ultimately, the obturator can be worn for approximately 8 hours each 24 hour period--either during the day or at night.

A number of gynecologic surgeons have had considerable success with the *sacrospinous or sacrotuberous ligament suspension* (5) for massive eversion of the vagina; however, this simply will not work satisfactorily for this patient since this procedure will not increase the depth of the vagina and the patient will continue to experience dyspareunia. One could instruct the patient on the use of vaginal dilators in an attempt to gain more vaginal depth, then later attach the apex of the vagina to these ligaments. However, this approach is probably of limited value.

A *vulvoplasty* (7) as described by Williams of Great Britain will certainly add depth in this area; however, this will not provide any correction for the basic problem of vaginal eversion. This technique could be used in combination with a sacrospinous ligament suspension possibly using a synthetic nonabsorbable suture and leaving a deliberate suture bridge if the latter were thought possible in this specific case. In performing this type of vulvoplasty, one must have a sufficient amount of vulvar tissue present to fashion what is referred to an a "labioperineal pouch." Finally, the angle of inclination from this procedure is oftentimes more acute than desired. It is recommended that if one chooses to utilize this technique that the author's original description be reviewed prior to performing this unique, creative, and relatively simple operation.

In the appropriately motivated patient, the nonsurgical approach to the treatment of vaginal agenesis as described by Frank (2) certainly might benefit this patient by increasing and improving the vaginal depth and caliber over a period of time. Subsequently, it could be anticipated that a satisfactorily enlarged vagina would be developed, thus making this patient a candidate for a transvaginal sacrospinous ligament suspension as a more permanent correction of this defect. The Frank procedure is certainly simple, safe, cost-effective, and worth a try! Certainly all the hormonally depleted patients should be on estrogen replacement therapy for a protracted period of time. More recently, the Ingram "bicycle seat stool" modification (3) of the Frank procedure has been described and is worthy of review.

In an attempt to exhaust all possibilities, I feel certain that someone might suggest *vaginectomy followed by construction of a neo-vagina*. Personally, from a technical point of view this certainly can be done without any particular difficulty; however, a basic plastic surgical principle must be mentioned which is simply that one should not "throw away" normal viable tissue! It seems to me that this patient's tissue can be used to some advantage and should not be discarded. If, however, one is motivated toward a total replacement of the vagina utilizing the split-thickness skin graft technique then it can be performed without encountering any particular difficulties.

The *myocutaneous flap technique* utilizing the gracilis musculocutaneous tissues (1) is primarily used in reconstructive pelvic surgery following extensive or radical surgical procedures done primarily for gynecologic malignancy. Whereas this approach is another alternative, it appears to be more radical than that usually required to correct this defect surgically. Again, it is another option.

Finally, a combined transabdominal and transvaginal approach to the correction of this abnormality is worthy of mention. Once the vaginal apex has been located through an abdominal entry into the peritoneal cavity, the apex is opened to an ideal caliber. A split-thickness skin graft vaginoplasty of the McIndoe type is then performed. A properly fitting obturator with a split-thickness skin graft attached to the uppermost part of the obturator inserted transvaginally to an approriate depth and then secured externally to the vulvar tissues. The graft itself is provided with an abundant blood supply from the surrounding structures including the surface of the small bowel. This technique has been used quite satisfactorily on pelvic exenteration patients and it provides the patient with very adequate depth. Parenthetically, a modification to the use of the patient's donor site skin has been described by Rothman (6) utilizing peritoneum in place of the skin graft in the construction of a neo-vagina. This certainly has merit but has not been used to date by the author. Fetal amnion has been similarly tried! Either of these approaches would probably require a two-stage procedure but the important required depth would be accomplished by this first step. It is conceivable that no further surgery would be required; however, if necessary, some type of suspension could be used as a second stage procedure.

In summary, one must realize that these problems are not simple ones that can be corrected with any one of the more conventional means. These abnormalities need an individualized approach by someone familiar with these unusual findings so that these unfortunate patients can benefit from his or her previous experience.

References

1. Becker DW, Massey FM, McCraw JB: Musculocutaneous flaps in reconstructive pelvic surgery. *Obstet Gynecol* 54:178, 1979.

2. Frank RT: The formation of an artificial vagina without operation. *Am J Obstet Gynecol* 35:1053, 1938.

3. Ingram JM: The bicycle seat stool in the treatment of vaginal agenesis and stenosis: A preliminary report. *Am J Obstet Gynecol* 140:867, 1981.

4. Mattingly RF, Thompson JD: *TeLinde's Operative Gynecology*, 6th ed. Philadelphia, JB Lippincott, 1985.

5. Nichols DH, Randall CL: *Vaginal Surgery*, 2nd ed. Baltimore, Williams & Wilkins, 1983.

6. Rothman D: The use of peritoneum in the construction of a vagina. *Obstet Gynecol* 40:835, 1972.

7. Williams EA: Congenital absence of the vagina: A simple operation for its relief. *Br J Obstet Gynaecol* 4:511, 1964.

CHAPTER 37

Enterocele, Vaginal Vault Prolapse, and Cystocele Following Vesicourethral Pin-Up Operation

DAVID H. NICHOLS, M.D.

CASE ABSTRACT

A 38-year-old multipara with rotational descent of the bladder neck complained of socially disabling urinary stress incontinence. Pelvic examination disclosed some multiparous relaxation with rotational descent of the bladder neck, some cystocele, an early prolapse of the uterus, and a rectocele. She was treated by the Burch modification of the Marshall-Marchetti-Krantz procedure with complete relief of her troublesome urinary incontinence.

Two years later the patient, although continent, had developed some troublesome pelvic pressure and backache, worse when on her feet. When examined, a vulvovaginal mass was identified as a large cystocele and a second degree prolapse of the uterus with enterocele and rectocele.

DISCUSSION

This patient represents progression of some elements of genital prolapse that were present but untreated at the time of her original surgery. As Burch pointed out (1), there is a 15% incidence of enterocele subsequent to his vesicourethral pin-up operation. A change in the normally horizontal upper vaginal axis to one vertically directed exposes an unprotected culde-sac to the full range of changes in intra-abdominal pressure, favoring the development of enterocele.

For the patient described above, these problems now require a secondary operation, vaginal hysterectomy with colporrhaphy, which might well have been prevented had the culde-sac been specifically obliterated at the time of the original operation. One principle of reconstructive pelvic surgery is that if any part of the symptomatic genital prolapse is to be treated, any coincident parts, though not yet symptomatic, should be treated at the same time (2). Because there is no convincing evidence that coincident "routine" hysterectomy improves the results of the Marshall-Marchetti-Krantz or Burch operation, I would not recommend that coincident "routine" hysterectomy be a part of the original operation unless there was another reason or indication for hysterectomy, i.e., symptomatic leiomyomata or uterine prolapse.

The tendency toward subsequent prolapse is made worse in a patient with coincident chronic respiratory disease such as chronic bronchitis with cough, or who has the habit of regularly straining at stool to achieve an evacuation. Pregnancy itself increases intra-abdominal pressure, and is associated with an increased risk of recurrent stress incontinence when it intervenes following a surgical repair. The first operation to relieve urinary stress incontinence is the one that has the greatest likelihood of success, and the opportunity for surgical relief declines considerably with each subsequent operation. The patient is thus well-advised to postpone surgical repair of the conditions causing urinary stress incontinence until after her childbearing career has been completed.

All of these factors increase intra-abdominal

pressure and favor the development of subsequent symptomatic prolapse.

Since descent of the uterus is the result of a genital prolapse and not the cause, progression of prolapse is frequently seen. Prolapse of the vault of the vagina can occur independently of the presence or absence of the uterus, and not uncommonly may progress to a full vaginal vault eversion.

For the patient described above, if her childbearing career has been completed, the appropriate treatment would be vaginal hysterectomy and colporrhaphy with obliteration of the cul-de-sac (2). Had steps been taken at the time of the original surgery to obliterate cul-de-sac, the rapid progression of subsequent events and thus the need for subsequent surgery might have been prevented.

References

1. Burch JC: Urethrovaginal fixation to Cooper's ligament for correction of stress incontinence, cystocele, and prolapse. *Am J Obstet Gynecol* 81:281, 1961.
2. Nichols DH, Randall CL: *Vaginal Surgery*, 2nd ed. Baltimore, Williams & Wilkins, 1983.

CHAPTER **38**

Vaginal Evisceration Following Pelvic Surgery

CLIFFORD R. WHEELESS, JR., M.D.

CASE ABSTRACT 1

A vaginal hysterectomy without repair had been performed uneventfully upon an obese 35-year-old multiparous woman with second degree prolapse, an asymptomatic cystocele and rectocele, and chronic dysfunctional uterine bleeding. The surgeon described the operation as using the "Heaney technique." The peritoneum had been closed and the vaginal vault left open for drainage, although the cut edge of the vagina had been covered with a circumferential running lock hemostatic stitch. Chromic catgut had been used throughout. Blood loss at surgery was minimal, and no vaginal packing had been used postoperatively.

Although the patient was nauseated postoperatively, she was ambulated the evening of surgery and consumed a regular diet for supper. Nausea and sudden violent vomiting followed. The patient noted a sensation of "something giving way down below" and she returned to bed. When the perineal pad was changed an hour later (10 hours postoperatively), a loop of small intestine was found protruding from the vagina (Fig. 38.1).

CASE ABSTRACT 2

A 20-year-old primigravida, 8 weeks pregnant by dates and examination, was scheduled for therapeutic abortion by suction evacuation of the uterus. The patient was in excellent health and desired an abortion for social reasons. A preoperative hemoglobin was 10.5 gm. Physical findings were unremarkable except for a uterus that was approximately 8 weeks in size. The abortion was performed under general anesthesia. The uterus was sounded to 8.5 cm. The cervical canal was progressively dilated with K-Pratt dilators to the 32 French position. A 10-mm straight suction cannula was introduced without difficulty, although the cervical canal was described as "tight." After the suction was turned on, the operator noted the appearance of blood-tinged amniotic fluid in the plastic curette. The curette was rotated in 180 degree arcs at the same time it was advanced forward and backward within the uterus. Tissue was seen in the curette. The operator advanced the curette out of the cervix and noted significant resistance. His impression was that fetal tissue was preventing the withdrawal of the suction curette. He applied additional traction on the curette and withdrew an obvious segment of small bowel through the cervix into the vagina. The vagina was intact (Fig. 38.2).

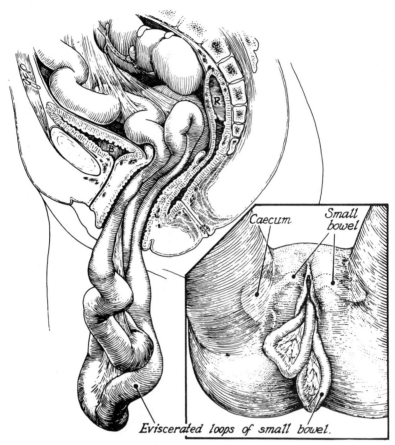

Figure 38.1. Drawing of a sagittal view of the lower abdomen and pelvis plus a perineal view with the patient in the lithotomy position show the vaginal evisceration. The sagittal view in particular emphasizes the point that for complete vaginal evisceration to occur there must be some technique of mobilization of the small bowel mesentery. Otherwise the length of small bowel mesentery is generally insufficient for the evisceration to occur. Reprinted with permission of Northern Chesapeake Publishers, Inc., from Wheeless CR Jr: *Pelvic Surg.*, Vol 2, No. 7, Oct., 1981.

DISCUSSION

Fortunately, vaginal evisceration of the intestine is rare (Fig. 38.1). The literature consists of individual case presentations with an occasional review article; less than 40 cases have been reported (1, 2, 4, 5, 7, 8).

Evisceration usually follows vaginal hysterectomy, usually within the immediate postoperative period. However, there are cases reported years later (2, 4, 5,). It has been reported after abdominal hysterectomy (3, 5) and as a spontaneous sequel to rupture of a large enterocele with and without previous hysterectomy (2).

A contemporary source of vaginal eviscerations has been the suction curettage for termination of pregnancy during which the same intestine is sucked into the eye of a vacuum curette that has perforated the uterine wall and pulled through the perforation in the uterus and out into the vagina (Fig. 38.2 and 38.3).

The etiology of vaginal evisceration, except for that associated with suction termination for that associated with suction termination of pregnancy, is confusing. There has not been one specific pattern of events that can be related in a cause and effect manner.

The anatomy of the small bowel and its mesentery should make vaginal evisceration

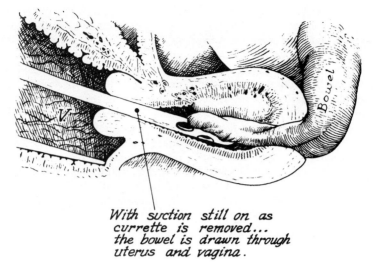

With suction still on as
currette is removed...
the bowel is drawn through
uterus and vagina.

Figure 38.2.   A sagittal drawing showing the suction curette with attached bowel being pulled through the perforated uterus during a termination of pregnancy. The gestational contents have not been removed.

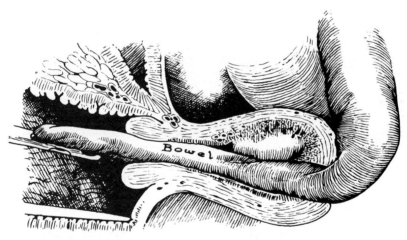

Figure 38.3.   This drawing shows the intestine eviscerated through the cervix out into the vagina. It is at this point that the intestine is most likely to be injured by confusing it with fetal parts.

difficult. Most anatomists describe the mesentery of the small bowel as being from 15 to 20 cm in length (3). Obviously, this distance is insufficient to allow the terminal ileum and/or jejunum to exit the peritoneal cavity through the vaginal cuff or a uterine perforation and eviscerate. There appear to be two possibilities: First, certain individuals could have a mesentery longer than the 15- to 20-cm average. Second, the process involved in evisceration may lengthen the small intestine mesentery by mobilizing it secondary to lacerations in the mesentery at the root of its origin. It is likely that both phenomena occur. Laceration of the small bowel mesentery threatens the continuity of blood supply to the intestine. However, the laceration could occur in such a location as to spare specific vascular arcades within the small bowel mesentery. This may explain why there are successful reports of simply replacing the small bowel into the peritoneal cavity via the vaginal route without performing a laparotomy and the patient recovering without incident. However, a procedure such as replacement of the intestine through the vaginal opening without laparotomy could be a perilous adventure. The overall mortality from vaginal evisceration has been reported at approximately 10% (8). From a review of the literature, it appears that much of this mortality is secondary to peritonitis, possibly related to intestinal necrosis. On the other hand, the morbidity from laparotomy in a modern hospital is minimal. Via laparotomy the intestine can be thoroughly inspected and suspicious areas of compromised intestine resected with primary reanastomosis.

Prevention

Prevention of vaginal evisceration following hysterectomy has several possibilities. Collective series of a significant number of patients for statistically valid results are unavailable. Therefore, the precise etiology of this problem in most cases remains unknown, except for those cases that occurred during termination of pregnancy in which the intestine was pulled through a perforation in the uterine wall. Possibilities for prevention that require discussion should include the following: (a) failure to repair enterocele and cystocele present at the time of hysterectomy (6); (b) the pros and cons of leaving the vaginal vault open at the time of hysterectomy; (c) choice and size of the suture material used in the closure of the vaginal vault and particularly the technique of anastomosis of the stumps of the supporting ligaments of the pelvis to the angles of the vagina.

While vaginal eviscerations have occurred from a variety of clinical and anatomic situations, the majority of eviscerations have occurred in association with poor support of the vaginal cuff, posterior fornix, and cul-de-sac after vaginal hysterectomy (1, 5, 8).

The open vaginal vault is an attractive and tempting possibility for the etiology of vaginal evisceration. However, the open vaginal vault is the technique of many gynecologists, and thousands of hysterectomies have been performed leaving the vaginal vault open without the rare event of postoperative vaginal evisceration. When the vaginal vault is left open, its edge is usually sutured with a running locked catgut suture referred to as ''reefing'' the mar-

gin of the vaginal cuff. At the vaginal angles this ''reefing suture'' usually includes the stumps of the uterosacral and cardinal ligaments and anastomoses them to the angle of the vagina for additional support. In addition, most surgeons (but not all) peritonealize the pelvis by approximating the anterior and posterior peritoneal surfaces. This covers the open vaginal cuff. However, if one returns to the classic anatomic situation where the average length of the mesentery of the small bowel is 15 to 20 cm, evisceration would be virtually impossible unless an additional event occurred to mobilize the intestine for sufficient length to push it through an opening in the vaginal cuff. Therefore, open vaginal cuffs alone are generally insufficient to be the etiology of all vaginal eviscerations. In addition, most vaginal eviscerations reported have occurred after the vaginal cuff has been surgically closed with interrupted catgut sutures.

Choice of suture material may be a factor involved in the occurrence of posterior vaginal evisceration, but, like the open vaginal cuff, an additional factor is usually required to mobilize sufficient intestine to eviscerate out the vagina. If fine absorbable suture material is used (size 3-0 or less), there is the attractive thesis that the anastomosis of the stumps of the cardinal and uterosacral ligaments could break down and set up the anatomic situation for evisceration. In addition, if enough pressure were acutely exerted on the mesentery of the small bowel via a Valsalva maneuver to lacerate the mesentery and thereby mobilize the intestine, evisceration could occur. However, insufficient evidence exists for placing the etiology of vaginal evisceration on choice of suture material. We feel absorbable suture (catgut or synthetic) in sizes of 2-0 to zero represents the ideal suture material for closure of the vagina and reanastomosis of the stumps of the uterosacral and cardinal ligaments to the vaginal cuff. Permanent suture used in this area would not eliminate eviscerations but would add morbidity from suture abscesses.

The method of closure of the vagina could also represent a potential threat for vagina evisceration. All too often the vaginal cuff is closed with figure-of-8 sutures. A figure-of-8 suture, especially if tied tightly, promotes necrosis and healing by second intention. This is not the purpose of the suture in the vaginal cuff. Single sutures tied gently enough to approximate the tissue and provide hemostasis are sufficient. In addition, it is important to plicate the uterosacral ligaments behind the vaginal vault to add additional support and to reduce the tendency toward enterocele formation. We do not feel that the classic McCall's plication of the uterosacral ligaments is necessary in all hysterectomies and, in fact, represents a threat to the ureter if the uterosacral ligaments are plicated for a distance of more than 4 cm. Although the above factors may play a role in this problem, we are impressed that most vaginal eviscerations are associated with significant Valsalva maneuvers, predominantly vomiting, coughing, and lifting heavy objects. Severe vomiting and coughing have been reported in most cases in which evisceration has occurred after hysterectomy. Therefore, prevention must include containing these factors within moderation by eliminating overzealous oral feeding and excessive induction of post-operative coughing. Prevention of evisceration at suction abortion must include the safe utilization of techniques for performing the operation, that is, careful dilation of the cervix and repeated sounding of the uterine cavity.

Early Intervention

The key to the reduction of the severe morbidity and mortality associated with evisceration must be early recognition. Most eviscerations through the vagina are associated with lacerations of the mesentery of the small bowel, and the vascular integrity of the small bowel is at stake (Fig. 38.4, *A* and *C*). In the cases where evisceration is caused by suction abortion, the additional factor of trauma by the suction curette to the surface of the bowel makes early recognition extremely important (Fig. 38.4*B*). Early recognition would allow surgical intervention prior to intestinal necrosis and leakage of intestinal contents into the peritoneal cavity.

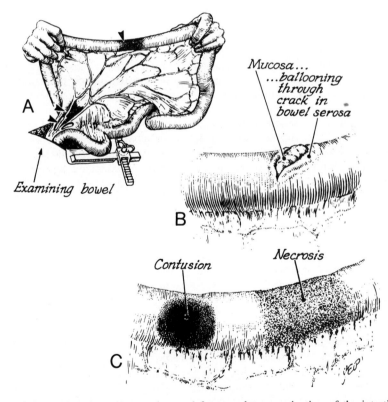

Figure 38.4.   *A.* This drawing demonstrates the need for complete examination of the intestine from the ligament of Treitz to the cecum. Specific areas of laceration within the mesentery should be searched for, and the relationship between the laceration and the vascular integrity of the bowel should be confirmed. *B.* Intestinal enterotomies or tears should be searched for and appropriately repaired. *C.* Areas of contusion and necrosis should be identified.

Appropriate Treatment. Treatment for any evisceration through the vagina should start with pelvic laparotomy. Initial first aid upon discovering the evisceration should be the physiologic protection of the eviscerated loop of intestine by wrapping it in sterile saline-soaked gauze or a sterile towel. The patient should be taken to the operating room immediately where an exploratory laparotomy through a midline incision should be done. A midline incision should be emphasized as we do not feel that the mesentery of the intestine can be inspected adequately through a Pfannenstiel incision. At the time of operation, the intestine should be carefully withdrawn through the defect whether that be the perforated uterus or the vaginal cuff (Fig. 38.5). A complete inspection of the entire intestine and its mesentery from the ligament of Treitz to the cecum is indicated (Fig. 38.4A). The mesentery should be carefully inspected for lacerations and vascular injuries and hemostasis. Suspicious areas of intestine should be resected and reanastomosis performed (Fig. 38.6). If there have been extensive enterotomies in the large intestine with spillage of fecal material into the peritoneal cavity, primary closure should be avoided and the damaged segments of intestine should be exteriorized as the primary procedure. After appropriate healing has occurred, a second procedure 4 to 6 weeks later following a preoperatively prepared intestine can be performed for reconstruction of the bowel and takedown of any exteriorized intestine. We feel there is no role for transvaginal replacement of the intestine into the abdominal cavity without laparotomy because of the possibility of lacerations in the mesentery and undetected injury to the small bowel. This is especially true when evisceration has occurred through the perforated uterus during the performance of a suction abortion. The suction curette could have damaged several pieces of small intestine other than the piece eviscerated through the uterine perforation. When the intestine has been appropriately replaced into the abdominal cavity, inspected carefully, and damaged areas resected, the entire peritoneal cavity should be copiously lavaged with normal saline. A Salem pump nasogastric tube should be inserted into the stomach and left in place until the patient passes flatus or has a bowel movement. The hospitalization of all patients who have sustained enterotomy and probably the entire group of vag-

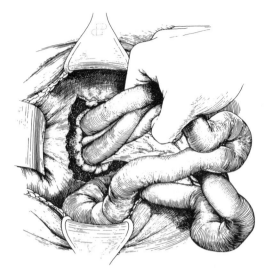

Figure 38.5. Drawing of pelvic laparotomy showing the replacement of the intestine back into the peritoneal cavity through the ruptured vaginal cuff surrounded by the torn peritoneal margins.

inal eviscerations should be covered with broad-spectrum antibiotics. Antimicrobial therapy should be guided by appropriate cultures taken at the time of laparotomy, but therapy should be directed toward the enteric organisms.

In those cases of evisceration associated with termination of pregnancy, it is vital to complete the termination of pregnancy as part of the repair procedure. All too often in the panic of this unexpected and severe complication, attention is directed toward the intestinal problem and away from the potential severe complication of incomplete abortion with retained gestational contents. One solution to this problem is to have a second surgeon immediately perform laparoscopy through the umbilicus and guide the withdrawal of the suction cannula out of the peritoneal cavity and back into the endometrial cavity (Fig. 38.7) where the suction can be resumed and the termination of pregnancy completed (Fig. 38.8). Failure to do this leaves products of gestation within the endometrial cavity and creates potential for all the sequelae of incomplete abortion, i.e., infection, hemorrhage, etc.

Repair of the ruptured vagina or perforated uterus differs. The perforation site in the uterus can be closed with simple through-and-through sutures of absorbable material. However, in the case of the ruptured vagina, careful closure with a well-designed plan of ligament suspension and

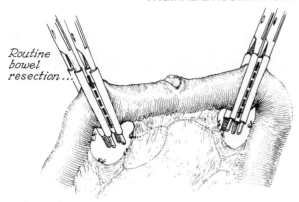

Routine
bowel
resection...

...and
re-anastomosis

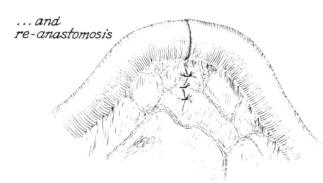

Figure 38.6. Areas of severe intestinal damage and/or vascular necrosis should be surgically resected and a reanastomosis performed.

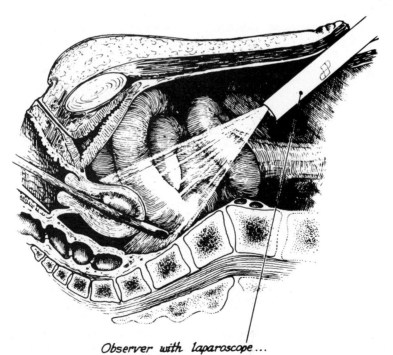

Observer with laparoscope...

Figure 38.7. A sagittal drawing demonstrating the prevention of intestinal evisceration through the uterus and vagina by performing a laparoscopy at the time of perforation of the uterus by the suction curette. The laparoscopist assists the surgeon by guiding the curette out of the peritoneal cavity and back into the endometrial cavity without sucking intestinal contents within the canulla.

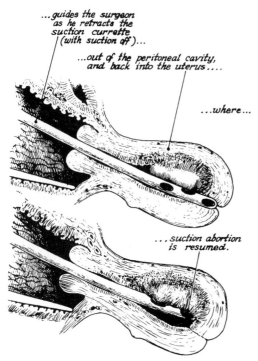

...guides the surgeon as he retracts the suction currette (with suction off)...

...out of the peritoneal cavity, and back into the uterus....

...where...

...suction abortion is resumed.

Figure 38.8. Sagittal drawing showing that once the suction cannula has been withdrawn into the endometrial cavity it is extremely important that the termination of pregnancy be completed. This step must be done even if intestinal contents have been pulled through the uterus and out into the vagina. It can be delayed until the intestine has been appropriately replaced into the peritoneal cavity through the laparotomy incision as shown in Figure 38.2 but must not be forgotten.

obliteration of the cul-de-sac should be made (Fig. 38.9). The suture material should be absorbable, and care should be made to reduce areas of necrosis to a minimum. The opening in the vagina should be excised back to fresh, healthy tissue. The vagina should then be closed with interrupted zero absorbable suture. A separate step to locate and suture the stumps of the uterosacral and cardinal ligaments to the angles of the vagina should be made (Fig. 38.9). In addition, the anterior surface of the rectosigmoid colon should be sutured to the posterior vaginal cuff to eliminate the cul-de-sac (Fig. 38.9). Complete resection should be made of all necrotic tissue along the vaginal cuff and stumps of the supporting ligaments. This is a particularly important step if there has been spillage of fecal material into the peritoneal

cavity. One should not be surprised at the development of a postoperative pelvic abscess if necrotic tissue that has been bathed in the intestinal contents is left within the pelvis postoperatively. Antibiotic therapy will not be sufficient to override this breach in surgical technique. We advocate placing all of these patients on the "mini-dose" heparin schedule of 3000 to 5000 units of heparin subcutaneously twice a day. Those patients who do not have return of intestinal function within 3 to 4 days postoperatively should be given intravenous hyperalimentation. In many of the reported series in the literature, there has been prolonged ileus following vaginal evisceration. If the entire intestine has been completely explored and the surgeon is comfortable as to the vascular integrity of the intestine, prolonged ileus should be treated conservatively with nasogastric drainage and intravenous hyperalimentation. However, if the intestine has been replaced vaginally and there has not been adequate exploration of the intestine, the question of vascular integrity and necrosis of the bowel should be considered. Repeat laparotomy should be considered, and the vascular integrity of the bowel should be ensured.

Although evisceration of the small intestine through the vagina is an extremely serious event, patients have an excellent chance for recovery if intestinal necrosis and peritonitis have not occurred. Moreover, if proper closure of the vaginal vault with elimination of the cul-de-sac and careful approximation of the supporting ligaments to the angles of the vagina is made during the repair process, the likelihood of recurrence is quite small.

The average gynecologist may be in practice for a lifetime and never encounter a case of vaginal evisceration. Because of its rarity, it has been difficult for any one clinic to gain a large volume of experience in treating this phenomenon. Nevertheless, it seems logical to treat vaginal evisceration as one would treat abdominal evisceration following dehiscence of a postoperative abdominal incision. In treating evisceration of the abdominal wall, the surgeon would never consider replacing the intestine through the traumatic abdominal opening or dehiscent wound without a thorough inspection of the peritoneal cavity. This same principle should be observed in vaginal evisceration.

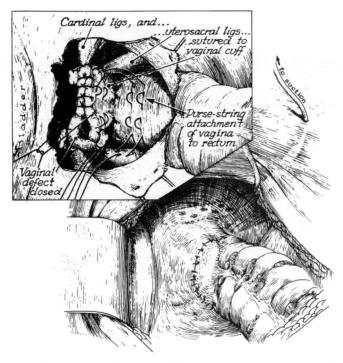

Figure 38.9. The *upper drawing* shows the repair of the ruptured vagina by suturing the vaginal cuff with a single through-and-through layer of size zero absorbable suture. Note that the uterosacral and cardinal ligaments have been identified and are specifically sutured to the angles of the vagina. Three separate rows of zero absorbable suture are placed between the anterior surface of the rectosigmoid colon and the posterior vaginal wall and cuff to eliminate the cul-de-sac. These sutures are placed in a purse-string fashion. The *lower drawing* shows the completed repair with reperitonealization of the pelvis. A suction drain is placed adjacent to the repair.

References

1. Fox WP: Vaginal evisceration. *Obstet Gynecol* 50:233, 1977.
2. Fox PF, Kowalczyk AS: Ruptured enterocele. *Am J Obstet Gynecol* 115:592, 1971.
3. Goss CM: The digestive system. In: Gray H (ed): *Anatomy of the Human Body,* ed. 28. Philadelphia, Lea & Febiger, 1972, chap. 16. p. 1230.
4. Hall BD, Phelan JP, Pruyn SC, et al: Vaginal evisceration during coitus. *Am J Obstet Gynecol* 131:115, 1978.
5. McNellis D, Torkelson L, McElin TW: Late postoperative vaginal vault disruption. *Am J Obstet Gynecol* 111:592, 1971.
6. Nichols DH, Randall CL: Complications of surgery. In: *Vaginal Surgery,* ed. 2. Baltimore, Williams & Wilkins, 1983.
7. Powell JL: Vaginal evisceration following vaginal hysterectomy. *Am J Obstet Gynecol* 115:276, 1973.
8. Rolf BB: Vaginal evisceration. *Am J Obstet Gynecol* 107:369, 1970.

CHAPTER 39

Transvaginal Oophorectomy and Salpingo-Oophorectomy

DAVID H. NICHOLS, M.D.

CASE ABSTRACT

Chronic, socially disabling, menopausal menorrhagia had persisted in a 50-year-old parous patient with no evidence of genital prolapse. The uterus was but slightly enlarged, suggesting the possibility of mild adenomyosis, but the cul-de-sac was free and the uterus was movable. A vaginal hysterectomy was performed and the adnexa inspected. Both tubes were normal, but the ovaries, though movable and free in the pelvis, were found rather high, and some superficial puckered areas of endometriosis were evident. Traction with a sponge forceps to each ovary brought it to the vault of the vagina.

DISCUSSION

Possible oophorectomy coincident with hysterectomy should be given the same consideration whether the uterus has been just removed transabdominally or by the vaginal route (1, 3–5). A decision concerning oophorectomy should be strongly influenced by the estimated risk-benefit ratio. Benefits favoring oophorectomy include potential for neoplastic ovarian disease, endometriosis, and the presumable lack of function in the postmenopausal ovary, whose very retention might increase the likelihood of subsequent ovarian cancer. Risks include the trauma of additional surgery embracing technical difficulties, intraoperative and postoperative hemorrhage, and also loss of ovarian function secondary to castration. Coincident oophorectomy through either the transvaginal or transabdominal preliminary exposure should be considered whenever the anticipated benefits outweigh the risks. An exception should be made in the case of suspected ovarian cancer, where oophorectomy should be performed only through the transabdominal exposure.

Salpingo-oophorectomy should be considered when the infundibulopelvic ligament is long. This is often the case when the uterus prior to hysterectomy has been prolapsed or retroverted. Salpingo-oophorectomy does, however, leave a raw intraperitoneal surface after ligation with the small risk of subsequent bowel adhesion to the raw area. This might precipitate a future volvulus or intestinal obstruction. Oophorectomy alone may be considered when the infundibulopelvic ligament is short, as transvaginal exposure of such an infundibulopelvic ligament may be difficult (6).

The ovary may be grasped with a sponge forceps and brought into the operative field, where the mesovarium can be clamped only under direct vision. Oophorectomy alone permits the tube and its mesosalpinx to fall over the raw area of the ligated mesosalpinx, lessening the chance of subsequent bowel adhesion in this area. When a benign neoplastic ovarian cyst is encountered, freely movable and without adhesions, the ovary should be removed intact, providing that the tumor is of such a size that it can pass unruptured through the vagina. When space is cramped, the mesovarium may be clamped between two forceps and cut and the forceps attached to the ovary used as a gentle handle to deliver the most narrow diameter of the ovary into the vagina. A larger neoplasm requires pelvic laparotomy. Trocar aspiration through the cyst wall to reduce the size should be used but rarely and only when the cyst is unilocular, the wall nonpapillary, and the content serous-like. Spilling of cyst

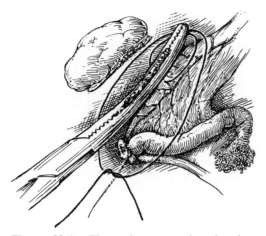

Figure 39.1. The entire mesovarium has been clamped by a Heaney type forceps and the ovary cut free. The mesovarium is penetrated once through its midportion. Each end of the suture is passed around the tip of the forceps as shown and tied at the heel of the forceps, while the latter is being unlocked and slowly removed.

contents may soil the peritoneal cavity, risking possible implantation of even benign tumor cells, especially those of the mucinous cystadenoma. The infundibulopelvic ligament or mesovarium should be securely ligated and under direct vision. Proximity of the ureter should be noted when transfixation ligatures are applied to the infundibulopelvic ligament (2). Ideally, the ligament or mesovarium should be penetrated only once to minimize the risk of slippage or hematoma (3). A useful stitch is shown in Figure 39.1. Polyglycolic acid type suture, 0 or 00, is ideal (Dexon or Vicryl). When salpingo-oophorectomy is being contemplated, primary fixation of the stitch in the infundibulopelvic ligament by penetration with the Deschamps ligature carrier with ligation immediately prior to salpingo-oophorectomy provides penetration of the infundibulopelvic ligament by a blunt needle, lessening the chance of laceration of the ovarian artery. By the elimination of the clamp or forceps, the suture is placed farther away from the nearby ureter, lessening chances of ligating or compromising its integrity. The suture may be tied in the same fash-

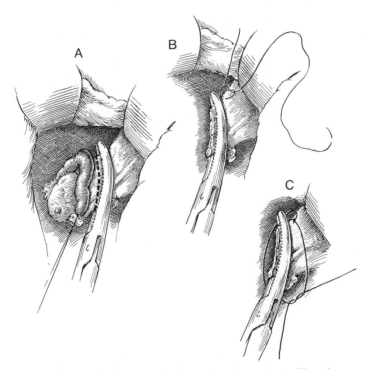

Figure 39.2. The infundibulopelvic ligament is clamped as shown in *A*. The adnexa are removed and a transfixion stitch anchored as in *B* and tied as shown in *C*. Reprinted with permission from Nichols DH, Randall CL: *Vaginal Surgery*, ed. 2. Baltimore, Williams & Wilkins, 1983.

ion illustrated in Figure 39.1, which minimizes slippage. The ovary and tube may then be cut free and removed from the operative field and a separate free tie applied to the infundibulopelvic ligament distal to the fixation stitch. Alternately, the infundibulopelvic ligament may be clamped as shown in Figure 39.2, the adnexa removed, and a fixation stitch placed as shown, which may be followed by a free tie to the ligament stump. Postoperative care should include careful watch for unexpected and concealed intraperitoneal bleeding, which if significant, should make itself known by unexplained tachycardia or postoperative fall in hemoglobin/hematocrit. Severe, steady suprapubic lumbar pain or a palpable intra-abdominal mass are strongly suggestive of retroperitoneal hematoma, and prompt exploratory laparotomy should be anticipated. Estrogen supplementation may be considered, especially if the patient is sexually active and the hormone not medically contraindicated.

If one is preoperatively contemplating oophorectomy, it is well to obtain the patient's permission for this ahead of time; always disclose to the patient postoperatively what was done during surgery.

When considering coincidental elective oophorectomy, one should ask oneself whether it appears that the patient will likely benefit from this procedure or whether circumstances exist under which the need and desirability of subsequent oophorectomy are likely. If the decision has been made to consider oophorectomy or salpingo-oophorectomy, one should assess the technical aspect of the particular problem and determine its feasibility and safety.

If it appears that transvaginal oophorectomy or salpingo-oopherectomy can be performed safely and under direct vision, it should be done. Should surgical exposure present a serious problem, there is no place for risky surgical acrobatics.

References

1. Funt MI, Benigno BB, Thompson JD: The residual adnexa: Asset or liability? *Am J Obstet Gynecol* 129:251, 1977.
2. Hofmeister FJ, Wolfgram RC: Methods of demonstrating measurement relationships between vaginal hysterectomy ligatures and the ureters. *Am J Obstet Gynecol* 83:938, 1962.
3. Nichols DH: A technique for vaginal oophorectomy. *Surg Gynecol Obstet* 147:765, 1978.
4. Nichols DH, Randall CL: *Vaginal Surgery*, ed. 2. Baltimore, Williams & Wilkins, 1983.
5. Ranney B, Abu-Ghazaleh S: The future function and fortune of ovarian tissue which is retained in vivo during hysterectomy. *Am J Obstet Gynecol* 128:626, 1977.
6. Wright RC: Vaginal oophorectomy. *Am J Obstet Gynecol* 120:759, 1974.

CHAPTER 40

Anterior Vaginal Wall Prolapse After Cystectomy

WILLIAM J. HOSKINS, M.D. Capt., MC, USN

CASE ABSTRACT

A female infant born with exstrophy of the bladder underwent bilateral ureterosigmoid-ostomy for urinary diversion at age 1 year. This was later followed by transvaginal cystourethrectomy. At age 22 years, the patient delivered a normal infant vaginally after an uncomplicated antepartum course. One month postpartum there was a marked prolapse of the anterior vaginal wall. This progressed, and at examination 1 month later, a mass including the uterus protruded beyond the vulva and was a source of discomfort to the patient.

DISCUSSION

When the cloaca fails to close anteriorly in the developing embryo the resulting defect is called exstrophy of the bladder (from Greek, meaning "to turn out"). The occurrence of bladder exstrophy is reported to be one in 30,000 to 40,000 live births and is five times more common in males than females (3, 7). The anterior wall of the bladder, the urinary sphincter, urethra, pubic arch, and lower abdominal wall are absent to varying degrees. In the female, there is often abnormally wide separation of the labia and a cleft clitoris. The separation of the pubic bones often leads to a waddling gait when the child begins to walk. This instability of gait rarely persists into adult life. With early involvement of expert urologic, orthopaedic, and plastic surgical treatment, approximately one-third of these patients may have surgical closure of the defect and retain urinary continence. Closure is usually effected in stages including osteotomy to provide firm pubic apposition, bladder closure, reconstruction of the external genitalia and bladder neck reconstruction.

When closure is not possible, urinary diversion and excision of the bladder and urethra is carried out. Although abdominal closure can usually be accomplished without osteotomy, this procedure will usually result in a better ana-tomic result. Genital reconstruction is performed as a later procedure. Historically, direct ureterocolonic anastomosis was the method of choice in urinary diversion for bladder exstrophy; but ascending infections, colonic stenosis, and acidosis are frequent complications. Ideal conduit diversion in the young child is also associated with many long-term complications. One good alternative appears to be formation of a nonrefluxing sigmoid conduit with external drainage for 4 to 5 years followed by colosigmoid anastomosis of the conduit to the rectosigmoid.

Modern surgical techniques in the management of bladder exstrophy have resulted in females reaching adulthood with intact reproductive organs. Gynecologic problems which such patients are prone to develop are (a) uterine descensus with procidentia and (b) anterior vaginal wall defects. Although reports are rare, Damm (1) reported a case of uterine prolapse following a vaginal cesarean section in a patient with a dead fetus and 50 hours of obstructed labor. This patient had undergone excision of the bladder exstrophy at age 2 years. Decarle, in a discussion of a case presentation by Overstreet and Hinman (5) presented two additional cases of uterine prolapse following vaginal delivery in patients who had undergone excision of bladder exstrophy and recommended that these patients be delivered by classical cesarean section to prevent postpartum genital prolapse.

When considering how to effect surgical repair of a patient as described in the abstract, three factors must be considered: (a) Does the patient desire to retain childbearing capacity? (b) Should the repair be accomplished via an abdominal or a vaginal approach? (c) Should one suspend the genitalia anteriorly or posteriorly? Factors a and b are closely related because the applicability of a vaginal approach would be dependent on the patient not wanting to preserve childbearing. If such was the case, vaginal hysterectomy with sacrospinous suspension of the vaginal vault according to the method of Randall and Nichols (6) would be the procedure of choice. The anterior vaginal defect could then be excised and closed. If the perineal body (as is often the case in these patients) was particularly broad, a relaxing perineoplasty might be helpful. This method of repair has the distinct advantage of avoiding an abdominal operation in a patient who probably has extensive scarring and where extensive pelvic disection might disrupt function of the ureterosigmoid anastomosis.

If the patient desires to retain childbearing function, it is unlikely that repair can be effected by the vaginal approach alone. In this case, one must then decide whether to perform an anterior suspension of the vagina and uterus or to choose some form of sacropexy (2). An anterior approach has the advantage of avoiding the uretrosigmoid anastomotic sites and, in addition, would place the suspended uterus between the weak anterior vagina and the direction of intra-abdominal pressure. I would recommend a Pfannenstiel incision with mobilization of an inferior strip of aponeurotic fascia 1 to 2 cm in width and as long as the incision (Fig. 40.1). These fascial strips could then be tunneled through the internal inguinal ring beside the ligament and retroperitoneally to the lower uterine segment and upper portion of the cervix. These should be sutured under tension anteriorly with interrupted nonabsorbable sutures so as to elevate and bring forward the cervix and uterus (Fig. 40.2). Excess anterior vaginal tissue should be excised approximately in the midline, or this portion of the operation could be performed by a vaginal approach. Anterior suspension of the uterus could be accomplished in a variety of ways. If the round ligaments are normal in size and not at-

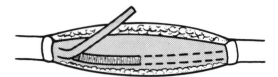

Figure 40.1: A Pfannenstiel incision has been made and a strip of aponeurotic fascia 1.5 cm wide and 8 cm long has been mobilized.

tenuated (as is often the case in patients with exstrophy), a modified Gilliam suspension should be performed (Fig. 40.2). If the round ligaments are attenuated, a separate fascial strip from the upper portion of the aponeurotic fascia can be used to suspend the fundus of the uterus anteriorly or one can suture the fundus directly to the anterior abdominal wall. Of the above methods of suspending the fundus of the uterus, the modified Gilliam suspension would be the least likely to be disrupted by pregnancy as the round ligaments will stretch when the uterus enlarges.

The second option for suspension of the genitalia involves some type of sacropexy (2, 4). This operation is performed by suturing a strip of nonabsorbable material to the posterior vagina and lower uterine segment. The supporting strip is then tunneled retroperitoneally on the right side of the rectum and sutured to the periosteum of the sacrum. A variety of

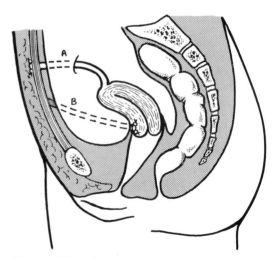

Figure 40.2. A modified Gilliam suspension has been performed to support the fundus of the uterus (A) and aponeurotic fascial strips have been utilized to support the lower uterine segment (B).

synthetic mesh materials as well as fascial strips can be utilized to suspend the genitalia. The advantage of this type of suspension is that the normal axis of the vagina is maintained and the resulting suspension is very durable. Two major disadvantages in this patient would be the danger of disrupting the uretrosigmoid anastomoses and the absence of the uterus anteriorly which would predispose the patient to recurrence of the anterior vaginal prolapse secondary to the force of intra-abdominal vaginal pressure. In addition, the fixation of the uterus posteriorly might result in compromise of the urinary diversion when the uterus enlarged in pregnancy.

When all options are considered, the best procedures are vaginal hysterectomy and sacrospinous ligament suspension in the patient who does not desire future childbearing, and anterior abdominal suspension in those patient who desire to retain childbearing capacity. In any case, a relaxing perineoplasty should be per-formed if necessary to retain or improve coital function. Should the patient become pregnant, cesarean section at term is the preferable method of delivery to avoid disruption of the surgical repair.

References

1. Damm PN: Geburt bei spaltbecken. *Zentralb f Gynak* 61:440, 1937.
2. Hendee AE, Berry CM: Abdominal sacropexy for vaginal vault prolapse. *Clin Obstet Gynecol* 24:1217, 1982.
3. Jeffs RD: Exstrophy and cloacal exstrophy. In Whitehead ED, Leiter E (eds): *Current Operative Urology*, Philadelphia, Harper and Row, 1984.
4. Käser O, Iklé FA, Hirsch HA: *Atlas of Gynecological Surgery*, 2nd ed. New York, Thieme-Stratton, 1985.
5. Overstreet EW, Hinman P Jr: Some gynecologic aspects of bladder exstrophy. *West J Surg* 64:131, 1956.
6. Randall CL, Nichols DH: Surgical treatment of vaginal inversion. *Obstet Gynecol* 38:327, 1971.
7. Winter CC, Goodwin WE: Malformation of the urinary bladder. In Karafin L, Kindall AR (eds): *Urology*, Hagerstown, MD, Harper and Row, 1974.

CHAPTER **41**

Posterior Colporrhaphy—
Lost Needle

ROBERT F. PORGES, M.D.

CASE ABSTRACT

A posterior colporrhaphy and perineorrhaphy were being accomplished following vaginal hysterectomy and anterior colporrhaphy upon a married 52-year-old multipara. The technique being used included "levator" stitches intended to bring the medial bellies of the pubococcygei together between the vagina and the rectum. As a deep levator stitch was placed, an audible "snap" was heard, and it was discovered that the swedged-on needle had been broken at its midpoint, and the missing needle segment was no longer visible. Although the fractured end of the missing segment could be initially felt but not visualized, additional palpation pushed it deeper within the substance of the muscles to a point where it could no longer be palpated.

DISCUSSION

Every effort must be made to retrieve the end of the broken needle, the length of which can easily be determined by comparison with a similar needle to the one having been passed.

Anatomy

In Figure 41.1, the relationship of the medial border of the levator muscle to the rectum is shown clearly. The posterior aspect of the medial border of the levator muscle hugs the wall of the rectum several centimeters above the anal spincter. The levator muscle and the vagina intersect obliquely, rather than perpendicularly, resulting in a more distal intersection between the anterior wall of the vagina and the levator muscle.

The rationale for the placement of sutures into the levator muscle is to bring the muscle bundles anterior to the rectum, thereby reducing the dimensions of the genital hiatus both anteroposteriorly and laterally. Usually one does not see as much of the muscle within the operative field as is shown in Figure 41.1. In those elderly women who stand to gain the most from posterior repair, the fibers of the levator muscle often will be attenuated and set far laterally, resulting in a very wide genital hiatus.

Technique of Posterior Colporrhaphy

While individual surgical preferences may vary, following triangular denudation of the distal portion of the posterior wall of the vagina and portion of the perineum (Fig. 41.2) the pelvic urogenital diaphragm is incised on each side to provide access to the levator muscle. The levator muscle may be identified by its tone and the direction of the muscle fibers which span in an anteroposterior direction and may be palpated readily from the inferior border of the pubic ramus medially to the arcus tendineus more posteriorly. Some surgeons grasp the levator muscle with an Allis clamp, pulling it into the operative field, making it more accessible for placement of the suture. The disadvantage of the Allis clamp is that it traumatizes the delicate muscle fibers and often results in some bleeding from the border of the muscle. Other surgeons dig the needle directly into the depth of the muscle and pull the muscle medially and more superficially into the operative field. It is just exactly this maneuver that may cause the needle to snap if the traction on the muscle is not exactly along the course of the curve of the needle. One or two, seldom three, sutures are usually sufficient for the levator muscle.

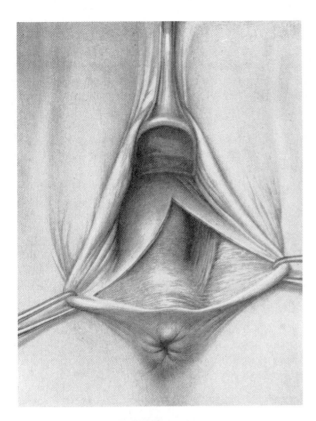

Figure 41.1. The relationship of the medial border of the levator muscle to the levator is shown. Reproduced with permission from Halban J: *Gynakologische Operationslehre*. Vienna, Urban & Schwarzenberg, 1932.

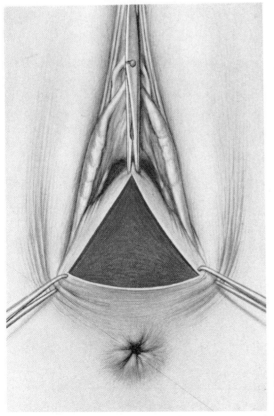

Figure 41.2. Triangular denudation of the distal posterior vaginal wall and postition of the perineum. Reproduced with permission from Halban J: *Gynäkologische Operationlehre*. Vienna, Urban & Schwarzenberg, 1932.

Prevention. Use a large, fairly thick needle with swedged-on 0 Dexon or an equivalent suture. Instead of pulling the bulk of the muscle medially with the needle, push the index finger against the rectal wall medial to the levator muscle so that the needle will be passed into a free space, only deeper in the operative field. Always pass the needle in a path corresponding to its own curve. Do not invent a new curve for the needle with your own wrist. The cervix is another area in gynecologic surgery where if the needle is not passed exactly in its own curve, it may snap.

How To Find The Needle. Normally, the needle-holder will grasp the needle at the three-quarter:one-quarter junction so that if the needle does break it will be likely to do so halfway between the needle tip and the needle holder, leaving a substantial length of needle fragment within the tissues.

Many operating rooms have some form of metal detector, and ophthalmologists occasionally use powerful magnets to retrieve metal from the eye. If these instruments are available they may be found useful. The most practical way to retrieve the needle is to probe for it with a tonsil clamp, using the digit of the other hand in back of the levator muscle as a baffle.

Occasionally, a clue to the location of the needle may be obtained by placing a finger into the rectum. If this fails then sutures should be placed above and below the site of needle passage for traction and hemostasis. The portion of the muscle between these sutures may even be excised. In unusual circumstances, a Schuchart incision may provide better access to the levator muscle directly and assist in the retrieval of the broken needle.

Selected Readings

Halban J: *Gynäkologische Operationslehre*. Vienna, Urban & Schwarzenberg, 1932.

CHAPTER **42**

Mass in the Lateral Wall of the Vagina

WINFRED L. WISER, M.D.

CASE ABSTRACT

A 16-year-old nulligravid patient who had been regularly menstruating for 3 years was troubled by increasing dysmennorrhea and a persistent intermenstrual dark bloody discharge. Although the uterus appeared to be of normal size, pelvic examination was somewhat difficult to perform. It was determined that there was a mass distending the full lateral wall of the left side of the vagina. The mass measured approximately 3 cm in diameter and appeared to be cystic, although the mass was tense. Careful examination revealed a pin-hole size opening in the lateral vaginal wall about 3 cm cranial to the hymenal ring, and pressure on the mass expressed some dark mahogany discharge through the opening.

DISCUSSION

There are a few cases of lateral vaginal wall masses. A differential diagnosis must include:

1. Obstructed hemivagina
2. Mesonephric, paramesonephric and urogenital sinus cysts
3. Leiomyoma
4. Vaginal adenosis
5. Vaginal hematoma
6. Advanced vaginal malignancy

The patient described above demonstrates the diagnostic dilemma of the lateral vaginal mass. Her history and physical findings are highly suggestive of failure of lateral fusion and central canalization of müllerian ducts which results in a double uterus, a patent vagina, and an obstructed hemivagina. If this diagnosis is correct, she will likely have ipsilateral absence of the kidney (Fig. 42.1).

Mesonephric cysts are found along the route of the Gartner's ducts. Paramesonephric cysts occur at any point in the vaginal wall; urogenital sinus cysts arise in the vestibule. These embryonic cysts are seldom symptomatic.

Leiomyomas most frequently occur in the anterior wall of the vagina but may be found along the lateral vaginal wall. They may extend cephalad into the hollow of the sacrum and vary in consistency from firm to semicystic. The predominant symptom is the sensation of partial vaginal obstruction.

The woman with a traumatic vaginal hematoma will give a history of recent trauma or vaginal delivery.

Lateral vaginal fusion defects are associated most frequently with a uterus didelphys. However, they may be associated with a bicornuate or septate uterus. The hemivagina may be completely or partially obstructed. The point of obstruction may vary from low in the vagina to near the corpus of the uterus (Fig. 42.2). With incomplete obstruction, a fistula may occur at any point in the vaginal septum or there may be lateral communication with the double uterus usually at the cervix.

Symptoms and physical findings correlate with the degree of obstruction (i.e., complete or incomplete obstruction), the location of the obstruction, and the presence or absence of a communicating fistula.

Symptoms in women with complete obstruction are progressive, severe dysmenorrhea with intermittent episodes of intermenstrual, lower

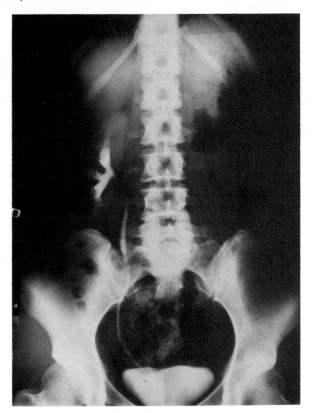

Figure 42.1. IVP—unilateral absence of kidney and collecting system.

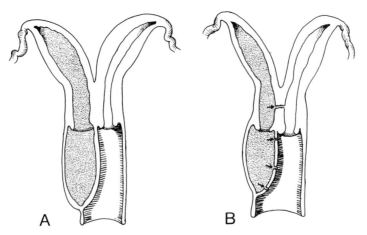

Figure 42.2. *A.* Double uterus, double vagina with complete obstruction, hematocolpos, hematometria on one side. *B.* Double uterus, double vagina with incomplete obstruction of hemivagina.

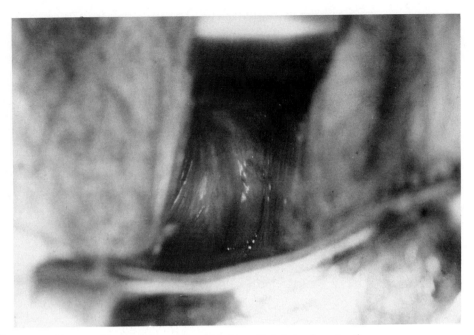

Figure 42.3. Obstructed hemivagina on the right side with bulging hematocolpos.

abdominal aching pain: this pain usually begins 1 to 2 years following menarche. These women have a normal menarche, regular menstrual cycles, and occasional premenstrual spotting. They always present with a bulging lateral mass (Fig. 42.3). Women who have incomplete vaginal obstruction present with lower abdominal pain and moderate-to-severe dysmenorrhea. In addition, they have an intermittent, foul-smelling, mucopurulent discharge, and a history of polymenorrhea with irregular staining between menses. An ill-defined or recurring mass may be found on physical examination. A pelvic abscess in the obstructed vagina may be the presenting sign in some women but it is more common in those women with a very small connecting fistula where a previous attempt at dilatation of the fistula has been made.

The diagnosis of this problem requires a high degree of suspicion. Palpation of a cystic mass in the lateral vaginal wall, a tender pelvic mass, and/or visualization of old blood coming from the lateral vaginal wall should increase suspicion of an obstructed hemivagina. A hysterosalpingogram is helpful if there is a lateral communication at the level of the cervix. In the completely obstructed hemivagina, a hysteros-

alpingogram may be useful to define what appears to be a normal unicornuate uterus on the side opposite the mass. An intravenous pyelogram (IVP) revealing ipsilateral absence of the kidney increases the likelihood of diagnosis. Aspiration of old blood from the mass in complete obstruction completes the diagnosis.

Treatment is simple. A large window is made between the two vaginas by excising a portion of the thick-walled septum. Because the septum is thick, the surgeon may be somewhat apprehensive in making the initial entry into the blind pouch. When the obstruction is complete, manifested by a bulging mass, an incision can be easily made over the mass. Placing a needle into the hematocolpos is helpful in establishing the optimal site of the incision. When a fistula is present between the two vaginal canals, a small probe with a hook can be passed through the fistula and traction applied toward the midline. An incision can then be made in the septum with relative ease (Fig. 42.4). The mucosa of the blind vaginal pouch is velvety smooth and glistening in appearance. The vaginal cavity and uterus should not be irrigated since irrigation increases the chance of pelvic infection. Once a window—which is large

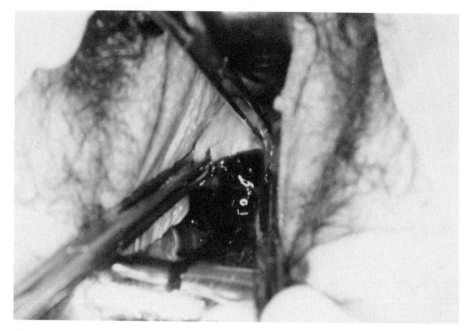

Figure 42.4. Incision through wall of obstructed hemivagina. Old blood from hematocolpos.

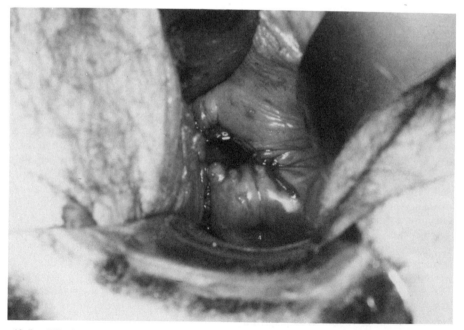

Figure 42.5. Window completed between obstructed vagina and normal vagina.

enough to prevent stricture—has been made, interrupted hemostatic sutures of 3-0 chromic catgut are placed in its circumference (Fig. 42.5).

The most common error in management of the obstructed hemivagina is failure to make the correct diagnosis before initiating a treatment regimen. The patient is frequently subjected to an abdominal exploration. The surgeon finds a double uterus with one side enlarged with a hematometria. The mass below the uterus extends to the pelvic floor. The hematometria should not be drained through the uterine fundus. The abdomen should be closed and a vaginal window made from below.

In the completely obstructed hemivagina, the epithelium is always composed of cuboidal cells, whereas the incomplete obstructed canal will be lined with squamous cells. When the canal is lined with cuboidal cells, a period of 2 to 3 years may be required for the metaplastic process to produce a squamous cell lining. Therefore, following creation of a vaginal window, these patients are likely to have a profuse, waterlike discharge for months, until a squamous epithelium has replaced the cuboidal epithelium.

Reproduction, following treatment of nonneglected cases, appears to be approximately the same as that in women with the equivalent uterine deformity but without an obstructed vagina. Pelvic endometriosis may result if the obstruction is not recognized and treated early. The incidence of endometriosis, however, is more common in the duplicated uterus without vaginal obstruction.

Selected Readings

Jones HW Jr: Reproductive impairment and malformed uterus. *Fertil Steril* 36:137, 1981.

Jones HW Jr, Wheeless CR: Salvage of the reproductive potential of women with anomalous development of the mullerian ducts: 1868-1968-2068. *Am J Obstet Gynecol* 104:348, 1968.

Rock JA, Jones HW Jr: The double uterus associated with an obstructed hemivagina and ipsilateral renal agenesis. *Am J Obstet Gynecol* 138:339, 1980.

Yoder IC, Pfister RC: Unilateral hematocolpos and ipsilateral renal agenesis: report of two cases and review of the literature. *AJR* 127:303, 1976.

CHAPTER 43

Wolffian Duct Cyst at the Vaginal Vault

JOHN A. ROCK, M.D.
RICARDO AZZIZ, M.D.

CASE ABSTRACT

A 3-cm cyst on the right side of the vaginal vault of a 23-year-old patient had become a source of dyspareunia. The cyst with its lining was surgically excised by sharp dissection. Because of some troublesome oozing at the base of the cavity from which the cyst had been removed, several figures-of-eight sutures using O chromic were placed, effectively controlling the bleeding. On the morning of the second postoperative day, the patient called complaining of severe backache. By that afternoon, the pain appeared to be concentrated in the right costovertebral angle. The patient felt anorexic and nauseated. The following morning the abdomen was distended with minimal bowel sounds. The temperature rose to 38.7 degrees C. A urinalysis revealed 1+ hematuria, with occasional WBCs and bacteria. The blood WBC count was 12,300 per ml, with a left shift, and the hematocrit was 36.

DISCUSSION

The differential should include unilateral ureteral obstruction with superimposed pylonephritis, simple pylonephritis, or acute appendicitis. The findings on physical examination will be similar in all three diagnoses. With appendicitis, there may be a greater tenderness to palpation and rebound over McBurney's point, although this is not always true with a retrocecal appendix. A urinalysis will be negative in 90% of surgical injuries to the ureter. On the other hand, it may reveal hematuria secondary to bladder manipulation and catherization.

A ureteral obstruction is usually secondary to ligation, or excessive kinking from a suture in the periureteral tissue. Ureteral edema and inflammation can cause an incomplete occlusion to progess to a complete obstruction. A stitch placed through the ureter will commonly not result in obstruction, but occasionally a fistula.

An intravenous pyelogram (IVP) should be performed as soon as a ureteral obstruction is suspected. With a complete occlusion, the kidney will continue to excrete urine for some time, albeit at a decreased rate. The ureter will distend, although water is continuously reabsorbed from it. Since iodinated contrast media is heavier than urine, the most dependent portions of the obstruction will be opacified first. Higher doses of media and delayed films, up to 24 hours in the event of nonvisualization, should be employed. Approximately 10 days after a complete ureteral obstruction, the kidney ceases to filtrate enough contrast material to produce a urogram. In these cases, a tubular nephrogram may still be seen. If the IVP is not helpful, a sonogram usually reveals the dilated and tortuous obstructed ureter. Injection of iodinated contrast dye through either the percutaneously (antegrade pylography) or cystoscopically (retrograde pylography) placed ureteral stents also aid in the locating the precise site of obstruction.

Management

Once a ureteral obstruction is diagnosed the operator must: (a) assess renal function, ipsi and contalaterally, (b) treat any infectious process, (c) drain the affected kidney, and (d) repair the obstruction.

Due to the presence of high iodine concentrations in contrast materials assessing kidney function, a tubular nephrogram does not necessarily correlate with a good parenchymal function, alternatively, a radionucleotide scan provides important prognostic information relating to renal function. Experimental evidence in dogs indicates that irreversible vascular damage to the kidneys occurs 30 to 40 days after ureteral ligation. Nevertheless, there are isolated reports in humans of full renal recovery up to 12 weeks after occlusion. In the present case one should expect good kidney function if the obstruction is relieved. The serum creatinine, blood urea, nitrogen, and electrolytes should be carefully followed.

Concurrent pyelonephritis places the patient at risk for septic shock and aggravates her renal damage. In addition, a surgical repair of the ureter becomes more difficult and prone to failure. Either a second generation cephalosporin (e.g., Cefamandol) or a broad spectrum semisynthetic penicillin (e.g., Piperacillin) provides an appropriate spectrum of activity, with minimal side-effects. Of these antibiotics, 70% is excreted into the urine unchanged. Nevertheless, the dosage requires adjustment for decreasing renal clearance as measured by serum creatinine. Patients with unilateral obstruction will usually have a normal creatinine clearance, if the unaffected kidney is healthy. Final antibiotic decisions should await the appropriate culture and sensitivity studies. Drainage of the kidney aids dramatically in resolving infection.

The alternatives for drainage and treatment of the obstruction include: (a) deligation only; (b) ureteral or nephrostomy stent placement, with or without deligation, and including the possibility of a later repair; (c) early surgical intervention.

A cystoscopically placed ureteral stent (size 5 or 6 French, Silastic) permits drainage of the infected urine, provided it passes into the renal calyces beyond the obstruction. In a small number of patients, the ureteral occlusion will spontaneously resolve without sequelae, as the misguided suture dissolves. The stent should be left in place for a minimum of 10 to 14 days, securing it to a transurethral Foley catheter. In the majority of cases in which the offending suture remains in situ a ureteral stricture subsequently occurs. This is independent of the type of suture or stenting. A later surgical repair or transureteral calibration is required in this event. Unfortunately, due to the associated edema and inflammation of the bladder mucosa, visualization of the ureteral stent is sometimes impossible. Attempts at cannulation of the obstructed ureter should be performed judiciously since ureteral perforation, in these circumstances, can create a retroperitoneal urinoma and abcess.

If the ureter cannot be cannulized beyond the obstruction, a percutaneous nephrostomy should be performed under sonographic guidance. Under no circumstances should the kidney remain obstructed. Drainage should be continued for 6 weeks to 3 months. The patient unfortunately will carry with her a constant reminder of the complication. As before, the ureteral occlusion will sometimes resolve spontaneously with residual stricture.

In view of the high incidence of ureteral strictures when the stitch is left in place, a deligation should be attempted. In dogs, if the suture is removed within the first week of obstruction, the majority of cases resolve without sequelae. With removal between 7 and 14 days, there is full recovery in 50% of the cases. If the deligation occurs after 2 weeks of occlusion, most ureters demonstrate a persistent mild to moderate pyelocaliectasis. In the present case, attempts at deligation should be performed transvaginally. Removing the sutures 48 hours after surgery will usually not disrupt the hemostasis achieved. Unfortunately, the area will be difficult to expose and the tissues very friable. Care should be taken not to cause further damage to the ureter. Concomitant stenting of the ureter produces the best results.

In any case, follow-up IVP studies should be performed at regular intervals since strictures or fistulas have been observed to develop up to a year later. If a fistula develops, or a stricture is unresponsive to transureteral dilatation, a surgical repair of the ureter is required. This should be performed at no earlier than 6 weeks, preferably at 3 months. In the present case, with an occlusion so near to the ureteral-vesical junction, the preferred method of repair is a ureteroneocystotomy with or without a flap procedure.

Various surgeons now favor an early aggressive surgical approach if the obstruction is recognized within 72 hours. In these cases, the damaged portion of the ureter is resected. Since our patient presents with acute pylonephritis, such an approach would not be advisable.

Prevention

As the ureter passes underneath the uterine artery, through the cardinal ligament, it curves caudally, anteriorly, and medially forming the so-called "knee." The portion of ureter beyond the uterine artery is on an average 1.9 cm long, most of which is intravesicular in nature. The "knee" is located 0.8 to 2.5 cm lateral to the cervix, 1.2 cm cranial to the lateral vaginal vault, and 1.8 cm medial to the ischial spine. As the ureter enters the base of the bladder, it lies approximately 1 cm above the anterior vaginal fornix.

In this patient, the anatomy has been distorted by a Wolffian duct cyst present in the vaginal vault. Gartner duct cysts are dilatations of Wolffian remnants comprised of a single layer of cuboidal or columnar cells, with a thin smooth-muscle coat. The cysts may be multiple and lie lateral to the uterus within the broad ligament, extending downward and anteriorly between the bladder, cervix, and vagina. They appear in the lateral vaginal vaults as usually asymptomatic submucosal cysts.

In removing these cysts, the operator must keep in mind that Gartner duct cysts, unless very superficial, are extremely difficult to excise completely. Their close proximity to the cervical/vaginal branches of the uterine and vesical arteries, as well as their extension deep into the parametria creates a situation where hemostasis can be difficult to control. A partial resection with marsupialization to the vaginal mucosa will usually be sufficient to alleviate any symptoms. The only bleeding will arise from the cut edges of the vaginal mucosa, which may be controlled with a continuous running-locking suture including only the mucosa and underlying fascia.

A cyst at the base of the broad ligament and upper vaginal vault will displace the ureter medially toward the cervix. Furthermore, since the operator also exerts downward and lateral traction on the cervix, the ureter is displaced even further medially and downward into the vaginal canal, where it can be readily ligated by a misplaced suture. The surgeon operating in the vaginal vault should keep in mind the pertinent anatomy and the distortions in order to minimize the risk of a ureteral injury.

Selected Readings

Bright TC, Pers PC: Ureteral injuries secondary to operative procedures. *Urology* 9:22, 1977.

Carlton ED, Russell S, Guthrie AG: The initial management of ureteral injuries: A report of 78 cases. *J Urol* 105:335, 1971.

Hoch WH, Kursh ED, Persky L: Early, aggressive management of intraoperative ureteral injuries. *J Urol* 114:530, 1975.

Kunz J: Urological complications of gynecological surgery and radiotherapy. In Keller PJ, (ed): *Contributions to Gynecology and Obstetrics*, Vol II. New York, Karger AG, 1984.

Raney AM: Ureteral trauma: Effects of ureteral ligation with and without deligation - experimental studies and case reports. *J Urol* 119:326, 1978.

Reisman DD, Kamkolz JH, Kantor HI: Early deligation of ureter. *J Urol* 78:363, 1957.

Smith AD: Percutaneous nephrostomy tubes and ureteral stents. In Kaye KW, (ed): *Outpatient Urologic Surgery*, Philadelphia, Lea & Febiger, 1985, pp. 131-144.

Spruce HM, Boone T: Surgical injuries to the ureter. *JAMA* 176:1070, 1961.

CHAPTER **44**

Retroperitoneal Postoperative Hemorrhage

R. CLAY BURCHELL, M.D.

CASE ABSTRACT

A vaginal hysterectomy and repair had been accomplished on a 38-year-old para 7. The patient was not anemic at the onset of surgery, and blood loss was estimated at 500 cc during the operative procedure. The vagina was lightly packed at the conclusion of surgery.

On the first postoperative day the patient was reasonably comfortable but somewhat restless. The blood pressure was recorded as 100/70 and the pulse rate 110, at rest. A routine hemoglobin and hematocrit were reported as 8 gm and 24%, respectively. Palpation of the abdomen disclosed some lower abdominal tenderness but without discrete masses. Bowel sounds were active, and the patient was not particularly nauseated.

DISCUSSION

The abstract presents a typical history of a patient with severe postoperative hemorrhage after vaginal surgery. Unfortunately, this complication occurs more commonly than it should and is often unrecognized. When there is severe internal hemorrhage, particularly if it is retroperitoneal, adequate treatment may not be instituted and a significant number of patients have died without effective therapy.

Obviously, the first problem in the history presented is to make a diagnosis. The blood counts should be repeated, but, in my experience, a marked reduction in hematocrit and hemoglobin postoperatively always means blood loss which must be explained. There is virtually never any benefit in praying, denying, or hoping that something is amiss with the laboratory determinations. What is amiss is that there has been unrecognized operative or postoperative hemorrhage and the patient needs treatment.

In this situation it is unlikely that all the bleeding occurred at operation and was unrecognized. It is common to underestimate the operative bleeding by some factor (even half), but in this patient there is an unexplained loss of 3 or more units of blood. Thus, the most likely diagnosis is postoperative hemorrhage and this is probably retroperitoneal since the gastrointestinal tract does not seem to be disturbed.

A rapid pulse either at rest or upon having the patient sit up suddenly would help to confirm the diagnosis. Absence of shifting dullness with abdominal and flank percussion would tend to support retroperitoneal rather than intraperitoneal hemorrhage. With a large retroperitoneal hemorrhage, hematomas may have dissected laterally and anteriorly so that there may be flank dullness, but this will not shift when the patient is moved. At times, hematomas have extended superiorly to the diaphragm and interfered with diaphragmatic excursion. Ultrasound examination might demonstrate a retroperationeal mass and support the diagnosis.

From the abstract one could assume that the active bleeding had stopped as there should be a marked change in vital signs in 24 hours with continued hemorrhage of this severity; the change in blood count shows that the bleeding has been severe. Assuming that the active bleeding has stopped, there are basically two options for subsequent care.

One option is to transfuse the patient, use all supportive measures as necessary based upon the clinical course, and attempt to avoid operation. The other option is to operate immediately after transfusion, evacuate the hematoma, and insure hemostasis. There are pros and cons with each option.

A useful approach to the decision-making process is to consider the worst and best outcomes with each option and subsequently balance the conflicting forces. The significant danger with not operating is that the hematoma may become infected. An infected retroperitoneal hematoma is a most serious complication of pelvic surgery and, at best, results in prolonged morbidity; at worst, death ensues. A large hematoma is difficult to drain without operating transabdominally, and there is the certainty of total peritoneal infection with a celiotomy. A common sequela of an infected retroperitoneal hematoma is septic pelvic thrombophlebitis because the great veins of the pelvis and abdomen are surrounded by the abscess. If thrombophlebitis ensues and an anticoagulant-antibiotic regimen is not effective, the vena cava must be ligated or death is virtually certain.

On the other hand, with the best possible outcome for the nonoperative course, the bleeding may not recur, the hematoma may not become infected, and there may be very little subsequent morbidity. In time, the hematoma will resorb without permanent sequelae. The key question is based on the risk of the hematoma becoming infected.

The other approach is to operate when the patient is in good condition. This approach necessitates a major operation, evacuation of a large hematoma, and probably dissection of a large retroperitoneal area. The operation demands anatomic familiarity with the operative area, and not all gynecologists will feel comfortable with the operation. This, however, should not preclude the operative option from being considered. The advantages to the operative approach are that any pelvic bleeding can be stopped with certainty and the hematoma can be evacuated so that there will not be a large culture media for abscess formation. Even if the retroperitoneal space does become infected, a large abscess should not form and antibiotics should be effective. Again, one is balancing the odds of an infected hematoma against the morbidity of a major operation to prevent a disaster that may not occur.

There are several other considerations that may assist in making the decision. Prior to the days of antibiotics, it was known that a postoperative patient could be reoperated within 24 to 36 hours without serious danger of infection. If the abdomen were reopened after the first day and within a week, peritonitis was virtually certain. Although antibiotics enable the surgeon to operate when necessary, this old rule of thumb is of some help. When postoperative hemorrhage is discovered within the first day, there are significant advantages to operating. If the hemorrhage is discovered after several days, there may be advantages to waiting unless there are any signs of infection. When an abscess develops, it must be drained. In addition, if a patient with a hematoma is several days postoperative and there is no sign of infection, it may provide some security that an infection will not ensue.

In the patient presented, with the internal bleeding discovered on the first postoperative day, the best treatment would be early operation with evacuation of the clots. It is also important that any bleeding points be ligated. A very effective procedure is bilateral internal iliac artery ligation. This operation will prevent the necessity of religating all the pedicles and has been found effective in second operation for postoperative hemorrhage. Since iliac ligation has no effect on the hemodynamics of ovarian artery flow, the ovarian arteries should be surveyed and religated if they are a source of bleeding. In my personal experience, there have been several deaths when patients were observed, but no serious morbidity from early operation.

In a situation of this type, there is naturally a good deal of retrospective critique. Is hemorrhage inevitable in some patients, or should it always be preventable? What steps can be taken to prevent postoperative bleeding? Suffice it to say that the surgeon is always subject to some self-censure when there is a serious complication, even if the objective view is that it could not have been prevented.

In a series reporting the clinical use of internal iliac ligation, we found that the procedure was utilized for postoperative hemorrhage twice as often after vaginal as after abdominal hysterectomy (4). There are several reasons why postoperative hemorrhage is more common after vaginal than abdominal procedures. The operator has only one good opportunity to ligate vessels with the vaginal operation—the first time the pedicle is sutured. If tags are not left on the pedicle, it retracts upward; if tags are present, there is likelihood of traction causing bleeding. A total survey of the field at the end of the operation is not available with vaginal hysterectomy. The procedure must be done correctly at each step.

An additional factor is that many gynecologic surgeons are not thoroughly familiar with tissue planes in the vaginal approach and thus are unable to stay out of trouble. One of the commonest mistakes is to circumcise the cervix too low, with the result that the vaginal cuff is too small for the subsequent operation. Pedicles are poorly ligated from inadequate exposure, and hemorrhage is likely.

Postoperative hemorrhage of significance is virtually always arterial in origin. Small veins tend to cease bleeding because there is no pulse pressure to prevent clotting. A small artery, however, will continue to bleed for hours and often will not stop spontaneously. The prevention of postoperative hemorrhage is based upon understanding the arterial anatomy, careful suturing of pedicles the *first time*, and gentle handling of tissues so that, once placed, pedicle sutures are not dislodged or loosened. Postoperative hemorrhage should be rare and might always be preventable in a theoretical sense for a specific patient. Unfortunately, statistics do catch up, and any surgeon will have a small incidence of postoperative hemorrhage.

When this complication occurs, a good clinician will not deny the change in vital signs hoping that there is no hemorrhage but will make a prompt diagnosis and institute early treatment. There are more options for therapy before than after the patient has gone into shock.

Internal iliac artery ligation certainly has a place in the treatment of pelvic hemorrhage. Understanding how and why the operation results in hemostasis will enable the surgeon to decide when to utilize the procedure. Understanding is hampered by a number of misconceptions about the pelvic blood supply and internal iliac ligation, and these should be corrected.

First, the blood supply to the human female pelvis is unbelievably abundant. After ligation of the main arteries (internal iliac), there is no deprivation of blood supply. There is an interlacing network of collateral anastomosis which functions immediately. Since the collateral network is already present, the concept that collateral channels develop over a period of time after ischemia is untrue for the human female pelvis. The second major point is that iliac ligation always promotes clotting, even though it may not always, by itself, stop the bleeding. As the blood flows through the small-diameter anastomosis after internal iliac ligation, the high arterial pulse pressure is "damped out" so that clots are not dislodged from vessels once they form.

Bilateral ligation affects the pulse pressure in the entire pelvis. Unilateral ligation has primarily a unilateral effect, so that ligation of one vessel will suffice if the bleeding is arising from a unilateral source. When the bleeding site is unknown or in the middle of the pelvis, both vessels should be ligated. Understanding the physiology of iliac ligation leads to several other obvious conclusions (1, 2). The operation will be effective with hemorrhage from uterine atony and certainly should be employed prior to a decision to perform cesarean hysterectomy with patients who desire more children. With uterine atony the ovarian arteries should also be ligated as they supply large amounts of blood to the upper portion of the fundus. The uterine blood supply is sufficient to support a term pregnancy after ligation of all four vessels—both internal iliac and both ovarian arteries (6).

The operation is technically simple and not difficult for the experienced gynecologic surgeon to learn. Nevertheless, it is too infrequently used and some women have unnecessary hysterectomy simply because it is not in the surgeon's armamentarium at the crucial time. All gynecologists should not only be competent but confident of their competency to perform internal iliac ligation when indicated.

The ability to perform the operation only requires a knowledge of the retroperitoneal anatomy and the patience to dissect carefully. The actual ligation of the vessel is unimportant in the learning process. Anatomy of the iliac vessels and of the ureter should be learned from fresh dissection by any gynceologist in training if he or she is to be capable of preventing accidents in subsequent practice.

When iliac ligation alone does not stop the

bleeding, pelvic packing will be an additional help. The so-called "umbrella pack" has been found to be particularly useful because, with this ingenious concept of Logothetopulos as adopted from Mikulicz, positive pressure of any desired amount can be applied to pelvic bleeding sites (3, 5, 7, 8). Obviously, in the most critical situations there two hemostatic agents to reinforce each other, and together they should control any pelvic bleeding.

References

1. Burchell RC: Arterial physiology of the human female pelvis. *Obstet Gynecol* 31:855, 1968.
2. Burchell RC: Physiology of internal iliac artery liga-tion. *J Obstet Gynaecol Br Commonw* 75:642, 1968.
3. Burchell RC: The umbrella pack to control pelvic hem-orrhage. *Conn Med* 32:734, 1968.
4. Burchell RC, Mengert WF: Internal iliac artery liga-tion: A series of 200 patients. *Int J Gynecol Obstet* 7:85, 1969.
5. Logothetopulos K: Eine absolut sichere Blutstillungs methode bei vaginalen und abdominalen gynakolo-gischen operationen. *Zentralbl Gynaekol* 50:3202, 1926.
6. Mengert WF, Burchell RC, Blumstein RW, et al: Preg-nancy after bilateral ligation of the internal iliac and ovarian arteries. *Obstet Gynecol* 34:664, 1969.
7. Mikulicz J: Ueber die Anwendung der Antisepsis bei Laporatomieen, mit besonderer Rucksicht auf die Drainage der Peritoneal hohle. *Arch Klin Chir* 26:111, 1881.
8. Parente JT, Dlugi H, Weingold AB: Pelvic hemostasis: A new technique and pack. *Obstet Gynecol* 19:218, 1962.

CHAPTER 45

Bleeding 3 Hours Following Vaginal Hysterectomy

GEORGE W. MITCHELL, JR., M.D.
FREDDY M. MASSEY, M.D.

CASE ABSTRACT

A vaginal hysterectomy and repair had been performed on a 42-year-old woman because of troublesome menorrhagia unrelieved by previous curettage, with mildly symptomatic cystocele and rectocele. Although the surgery proceeded swiftly, the blood loss throughout the procedure was greater than usual and, at the conclusion of the procedure, a Foley catheter was placed in the bladder and a pack placed in the vagina. Three hours from the conclusion of the operation the surgeon was notified that the postoperative vaginal bleeding was persistent and excessive, the packing was saturated with blood, which was slowly soaking some sanitary napkins that had been placed.

DISCUSSION

A small amount of bleeding may be expected after every vaginal hysterectomy and repair, and the nursing service on the surgical floor must be alerted to this fact in order to avoid unnecessary calls. The decision to intervene depends upon both quantitative and qualitative factors. Usually a sponge or light pack has been placed in the vagina immediately following the conclusion of the surgical procedure, and this sponge is ordinarily saturated with a serosanguineous discharge, which may be profuse enough to soil the perineal pad and the immediately adjacent bedclothes. If the discharge is red rather than serosanguineous and if it is definatively progressive, so that the spot outside the packing continues to increase in size, there is a strong likelihood that the bleeding will not stop spontaneously, and a look at the operative site is indicated. More objective confirmation of blood loss can be obtained by the postoperative hematocrit, which should be routinely ascertained when the patient is in the recovery room, or shortly thereafter, and should be repeated when there is any suspicion that bleeding persists. The time factor is also important, in that most small bleeding points which would be likely to be sealed by clotting should

be dry within an hour of the operation. Persistence of bleeding 3 hours after the operation strongly suggests that hemostasis has not been secured. A patient who has bled excessively during the procedure should be kept under particularly close observation postoperatively because of the possibility that normal clotting will not have taken place.

Gynecologists often tend to forget that abnormal uterine bleeding may not be a manifestation of uterine disease or simple uterine dysfunction. A history of menorrhagia unrelieved by conservative treatment should serve as an indication for a good bleeding history and complete preoperative blood studies, including bleeding time, to rule out a bleeding tendency; if abnormal values are found, a consultation with the hematology service is essential. Often such a consulatation will permit elective surgery to go forward but will recommend that such adjuncts as platelet transfusions or fresh frozen plasma be immediately available.

Intraoperative control of bleeding is of the utmost importance in vaginal, as in other types of surgery. Some surgeons believe erroneously that bleeding from the broad tissue planes that have been opened is to be expected and that this bleeding can be left uncontrolled until the conclusion of the operation, when it may be eliminated by closing the vaginal mucosa, and packing. In addition to careful ligature, preferably double ligature, of the major vascular pedicles, small bleeding points of the vaginal mucosa and the bladder and rectal muscle should be clamped and either tied or coagulated. Many surgeons find it simpler and quicker to use the electrocoagulation unit to seal these small vessels. Abnormal bleeding during the operation suggests the possibility of a bleeding diathesis, as previously noted, or the possibility that the wrong tissue planes have been dissected.

At the conclusion of the operation, the uterosacral, cardinal, and ovarian ligaments which had been previously ligated should be carefully inspected for further bleeding. This is most easily done by leaving the second suture on each of these ligaments long and using that suture for traction to pull the stump back into the field. The uterine vessels, which should not be directly placed on traction, will usually be exposed by this maneuver. When the vaginal mucosa has been closed over the cystocele and rectocele repair, there should be a short delay before packing to make certain there is no persistent bleeding. If there is, it is essential to reopen the vaginal mucosa at this time and search for the source of the bleeding. Not infrequently, this will be far superior and lateral to the vesical neck, where the rich venous plexuses of the urogenital diaphragm may have been ruptured during the dissection. This area is difficult to expose, but it is necessary to place one or two mattress of figure-of-8 catgut sutures in the area to bring this bleeding under control.

There are varying opinions about whether to close the vaginal mucosa completely following vaginal hysterectomy and repair, to leave the cuff open, to insert a small drain, or to place the dissected area and the peritoneum immediately above the vaginal cuff under constant drainage. Each has its own supporters, but if the operative field is dry, the vaginal cuff can safely be closed without drainage. If there is some concern about hemostasis and some slight drainage persists, it is well to leave the vaginal cuff open. Drains are seldom necessary and, postoperatively, if left in too long, may constitute a hazard because of the introduction of infection.

The amount of packing to be placed in the vagina after surgery is also the subject of some debate. Common sense dictates that, if very heavy packing of the type associated with radium applications must be inserted, the surgeon does not feel very secure about hemostasis. This type of packing is most uncomfortable to the patient and may cause damage to the bladder or rectum or gangrene of the vaginal flaps. A loose packing of gauze soaked with some medication, such as iodoform, to reduce unpleasant odor is introduced to assist with hemostasis, obliterate dead space, and prevent the soiling of bedclothes and linen, which can be objectionable to the patient and her family. Such a pack should never be left in longer than 24 hours.

When the call comes from the floor that a patient is bleeding progressively and/or the hematocrit is falling after vaginal hysterectomy and repair, the surgeon must order the patient to the examining room where, with the patient in lithotomy position and in a good light, he can remove the first pack and carefully inspect the operative site. If the bleeding is not excessive and seems to be coming from the vaginal closure anteriorly or posteriorly, one or two superficial sutures at the bleeding site may serve to control it. Otherwise, heavier packing is indicated. This should be done using gauze rolls 2 to 3 inches in width and a long dressing forceps. At the time of this examination, the patient should also be examined for the possibility of intraperitoneal bleeding. The signs one ordinarily associates with this may be masked by the effect of recent surgery, and the hematocrit is the best check of the situation. A culdocentesis may be attempted if the issue remains in doubt. The secondary pack should not be left in longer than 24 hours, even if it is effective, and should again be removed in the treatment room under good conditions for another examination. If the secondary pack is unsuccessful and the bleeding continues, other steps are necessary.

If, at the time of first examination, removal of the pack reveals large clots, if the bleeding is excessive, or if the location of the bleeding seems to be at the vaginal apex, it is unlikely that a secondary pack will prove effective. The surgeon has a choice of trying this, of course, so long as the patient's general condition remains stable, but he should be thinking about re-exploration in the operating room.

When transferred to the operating room, the patient should be given general anesthesia and again inspected vaginally. Any obvious bleeding points may be ligated at this time, but brisk bleeding strongly suggests the likelihood that a large vessel has escaped its ligature. This is particularly true if the bleeding is arterial. At this point, the vagina should be packed to make its identification easier suprapubically, and an abdominal incision, either vertical or transverse, made through the peritoneum. Good exposure of the pelvic floor is often difficult to obtain because of the presence of hematomas and the disruption of tissues by surgery. Both ovarian pedicles should be identified and, if necessary, religated and an attempt made to localize the uterine artery and vein. If this is impossible, consideration must be given to ligating the uterine artery and vein on either side, at their origin from the hypogastric vessels. If the clotting has progressed to the lateral pelvic walls, making identification of these vessels difficult, it may be necessary to ligate the hypogastric artery close to its origin from the common iliac. Under these serious circumstances, ligation of both arteries is indicated, even if the bleeding seems to be from only one side. If bleeding is coming from an unsecured ovarian artery, it should be ligated. How rapidly the surgeon must proceed from simple nonoperative bleeding to hypogastric artery ligation depends, of course, upon the magnitude of the bleeding and the patient's general condition. Serious complications require serious measures.

CHAPTER 46

Unanticipated Spontaneous Vaginal Hemorrhage Following Straining at Stool on Tenth Postoperative Day

DAVID H. NICHOLS, M.D.

CASE ABSTRACTS

A vaginal hysterectomy with repair and bilateral salpingo-oophorectomy had been performed on a 42-year-old patient because of troublesome, persistent menometrorrhagia and some mild degree of genital prolapse. The postoperative convalescence was smooth and unremarkable. But on the tenth postoperative day (3 days after discharge from the hospital), the patient called her surgeon to report that, following some straining at stool, the postoperative vaginal bleeding, which had almost stopped, had suddenly increased and was now flowing so freely that it ran down her leg and she was unable to contain it.

DISCUSSION

This is an uncommon but potentially serious problem, and the source of her bleeding may be either venous or arterial, most likely the latter. The major vessels from which hemorrhage can arise in the patient described are a uterine artery, a vaginal artery, or an ovarian artery. Another source of bleeding is from spontaneous transvaginal evacuation of an old postoperative hematoma. The character of the blood is significant in identifying the etiology. Bright red blood which readily clots is generally of arterial origin and may occur from either "scab" disruption secondary to prematurely increased physical activity, prematurely timed coitus, or consequent to increased intra-abdominal pressure from straining at stool. A profusion of dark unclotted blood suggests evacuation of a hematoma which, although dramatic by its volume, is usually self-limited.

Sanguinal purulent discharge may indicate spontaneous evacuation of an infected hematoma or of an abscess cavity. In the latter instance there will generally have been antecedent fever, and if there was coincident fresh bleeding it may have resulted from premature absorption of a vascular pedicle ligature or an erosion by the abscess into a nearby blood vessel. An additional source of hematoma might be that which is secondary to a previously undiagnosed blood dyscrasia or coagulopathy, but in most instances there will be a history of a previous bleeding tendency and ease of bruising.

For the complication described in the abstract, the vagina should be examined in either the office, the hospital emergency room, or the hospital operating room depending upon the amount of hemorrhage, either with or without anesthesia. An examination must be accompanied by an examination light from an adequate source. The immediate treatment depends upon what is found at the examination:

A bleeding artery should be clamped and ligated. At the site of the colporrhaphy, this will generally be a branch of the vaginal artery; at the vault of the vagina, it may be either uterine or ovarian.

If a specific site of bleeding cannot be identified, microfibrillar collagen (Avitene) may be applied (carefully avoiding any region near the ureter, lest it initiate periureteral fibrosis with future obstruction!) and the vagina packed for 24 to 48 hours. A transurethral Foley catheter may or may not be necessary, depending upon the extent of vaginal distention from the packing. At the end of 24 to 48 hours, the pack is gently removed and the patient observed for an additional 24 hours.

A complete blood count, hematocrit, and bleeding and clotting time determination are made and appropriately treated if abnormal.

Ascorbic acid (vitamin C) 500 mg two or three times daily may be administered and stool softeners and laxatives prescribed to eliminate straining at stool in the immediate future.

Intramuscular administration of the adrenochromes (Adrenosem) may be helpful in temporarily increasing blood coagulability.

The patient should remain at rest until a new clot has formed and has begun to be organized at the site of the bleeding. The protocol for postoperative convalescence is then restarted.

If the above measures are not successful, bilateral hypogastric artery ligation may be performed through either a transperitoneal or extraperitoneal exposure. If this procedure does not promptly stop the hemorrhage and the services of a skilled radiologist are available, selective embolization through a vascular catheter may be employed.

The prevention of delayed postoperative hemorrhage begins with a careful preoperative work-up to diagnose and treat any possible coagulopathy. Postoperative care should include a comparison of the postsurgical with the preoperative hemoglobin and hematocrit, and instructions to the patient on going home should include: adequate rest, the prescription of stool softeners and laxatives to avoid straining at stool, the avoidance of excessive exertion, and postoperative prohibition of coitus for 4 to 6 weeks.

Adequate hemostasis at surgery is essential, and postoperative supplementation by vitamin C may be desirable, especially if the patient is a smoker, to diminish the effect of nicotine-induced oxidation of ascorbic acid.

Careful examination of the patient described above disclosed some "scab disruption" in the vault of the vagina, the cause uncertain but possibly from some straining at stool or from unreported coitus. There was generalized ooze with no single site of bleeding. A vaginal pack was inserted and the patient placed on bed rest. The packing was removed 24 hours later, and the patient was observed for an additional 24 hours, then ambulated and sent home with prescriptions for vitamin C and stool softeners. The remainder of the convalescence was uneventful.

CHAPTER 47

Accidental Cystotomy During Vaginal Hysterectomy

RICHARD F. MATTINGLY, M.D.

CASE ABSTRACT

A vaginal hysterectomy and repair were being performed on a 35-year-old multipara because of recurrent dysfunctional uterine bleeding (unrelieved by repeated curettage and hormonal therapy) and some pelvic floor relaxation. The uterus was in first degree prolapse, with a modest cystocele and recotcele. Traction to the cervix brought the latter down to the vaginal outlet.

A posterior colpotomy was made without difficulty, but a problem was encountered in finding the anterior peritoneal fold. The more the operator dissected in this area, the less his visibility, and the more troublesome the bleeding became. Suddenly there was a free flow of clear fluid, and it was evident the dissection had encroached upon and lacerated the bladder.

DISCUSSION

The close anatomic relationships of the bladder, uterus, and upper vagina cause the bladder to be the most vulnerable and frequently injured organ of the lower urinary tract during pelvic surgery. The bladder and lower genital tract are so intimately approximated in their embryologic development that they have been characterized as the "uroreproductive unit." Pathologic, microbiologic, and physiologic alterations of one organ may alter the normal function of the other. It is understandable, therefore, that bladder injury may occur during dissection and the cervix and lower uterine segment. Although accurate data are difficult to obtain, bladder injury occurs in approximately 0.5% to 1.0% of all major pelvic surgery. Vaginal hysterectomy is associated with a much lower incidence of bladder injury as compared to abdominal hysterectomy, a ratio of approximately 1 to 6, respectively. This is due to the fact that there is little deformity of

the uterus, and intrapelvic pathology is usually absent when vaginal hysterectomy is selected as the operative procedure of choice. However, careful dissection of the bladder base from the cervix and lower uterine segment and identification and opening the anterior peritoneal fold during a vaginal hysterectomy are recognized to be the most difficult technical steps of this operation. Bladder injury during attempted entry into the peritoneal cavity is far more frequent than injury to the terminal ureter or rectum.

Factors Related To Bladder Injury

Previous pelvic surgery is the most frequent cause of alterations of the pelvic anatomy that predispose to bladder injury during vaginal hysterectomy. For this reason, previous operative procedures, such as cesarean section, myomectomy, or any procedure which could produce advancement of the bladder peritoneum on the anterior wall of the uterine fundus, render a patient at risk for potential bladder injury. When these preceding conditions exist, a vaginal hysterectomy has a greater potential of bladder injury than when the procedure is done by the abdominal route. Many skilled surgeons do not consider these prior pelvic operations to be totally contradictory to the performance of a vaginal hysterectomy. Yet, only extensive surgical experience can surmount the adhesive scars and advancement of the bladder base from a previous low cervical cesarean section. In such cases, the surgeon would be well advised to make certain that the patient has been informed of this small, but important, risk of bladder injury during vaginal hysterectomy.

Uterine enlargement due to small myomata or adenomyosis may also cause distortion of the anterior cul-de-sac and bladder base. Occult pelvic endometriosis may also involve the bladder peritoneum, produce coincidental bleeding, and make entry into the peritoneal cavity hazardous. Previously, bladder advancement was a common technique used for uterine suspension which, if known preoperatively, would be a serious contraindication to vaginal hysterectomy. However, this type of uterine suspension is no longer utilized and only rarely will a gynecologist be confronted by an elderly patient in whom this historic procedure was performed many decades previously.

Operator experience must be included as one of the important risk factors associated with bladder injury at the time of vaginal hysterectomy. It is an admitted fact that the partially obscured dissection beneath the bladder base in search of an elusive peritoneal fold is one of the most difficult portions of this operative procedure. Extensive operative experience is required for the surgeon to feel totally secure and technically precise in the dissection of this troublesome area. While many operative series fail to document operator experience to be a significant factor in the frequency of bladder injury, the best example of this statement is the individual gynecologic surgeon who can recall vividly the period in his operative career when he had the greatest difficulty with this operation. There can be little doubt that as technical experience increases, dissection of the fascial plane between the bladder and lower uterine segment is done with greater ease and facility while inadvertent injury to the bladder wall becomes a very infrequent and unusual surgical event.

Several intraoperative factors influence the ease with which the anterior bladder peritoneum is demonstrated during a vaginal hysterectomy. The current practice of the submucosal and interstitial infiltration of the vaginal fornices and bladder base with a dilute solution of Neo-Synephrine (1:200,000) in order to decrease troublesome bleeding has produced a dual effect when used for a vaginal hysterectomy. While this technique does create the desired response of vasoconstriction and decreased capillary oozing, it also produces marked distortion of the normal tissue planes. As a consequence, identification of the layer of fibroareolar tissue that separates bladder base and cervix, frequently called the pubovesicocervical fascia, is easily lost. Many surgeons use blunt dissection too early in the separation of the bladder from the cervix and uterus. This approach may develop an incorrect tissue plane which, if too vigorous an attempt is made to separate tissue bluntly, can cause a tear through the muscular wall of the bladder base. The key sign of this surgical misadventure is the appearance of an extensive amount of bleeding from the operative field which is well beyond that seen in the most vascular portions of the hysterectomy. It is important at this moment during the operation to discontinue the blunt or sharp dissection and to take stock of the source of the bleeding problem. The mere application of more vasoconstricting solution (Neo-Synephrine) to the operative field will do little to identify anatomic landmarks. These landmarks must be accurately visualized, or the continuity of the bladder wall must be documented. This can be done by instilling the bladder with 200 cc of sterile saline or milk and observing for evidence of bladder leakage.

An additional factor that has created more clinical confusion than it has proven to be a scientific fact concerns the degree of pelvic vascularity. The patient's use of oral contraceptive agents is the particular issue at point. Historically, when large amounts of estrogen and progestogen were used as contraceptive agents, the pelvic vasculature was frequently compared to that of a pseudopregnancy state. However, the current use of low-dose or minidose amounts of contraceptive steroids does not increase the vascularity of the pelvic viscera when given to menstruating females. Because of a greater risk of an inadvertent, early pregnancy if a contraceptive agent had been omitted, we advise our patients to continue to use a mini-dose oral contraceptive until the time of surgery and have observed no diffence in bleeding complications from this procedure.

Operative Technique

Our technique for a vaginal hysterectomy is basically one that has been modified from the Heaney procedure, originally described in 1942. As demonstrated in Figure 47.1A, the submucosa of the vaginal fornices is infiltrated with 10 cc of a dilute solution of Neo-Synephrine (1:200,000) to produce vasoconstriction of small capillaries and to reduce bleeding from the vaginal mucosa to a minimum. Use of a larger amount of fluid interstitially can produce distortion of tissue planes between the cervix and bladder. A semiannular incision is made initially in the anterior fornix, just above the portio of the cervix and below the attachment of the bladder (Fig. 47.1B). Although we do not find it necessary in most cases, a uterine sound or Kelly hemostatic forceps may be passed through the urethra and into the bladder to demonstrate how low the bladder base is attached to the cervix. This step in the identification of the bladder wall can be of considerable assistance in an elderly patient with an elongated cervix who has a large, redundant cystocele and in whom tissue planes may be difficult to define due to atrophic change. As shown in Figure 47.1C, *sharp scissor dissection* is used to initiate the release of the bladder wall from the cervix. This important step should not be bypassed for the more rapid method of blunt finger dissection (Fig. 47.1D). It is our experience that this initial sharp dissection provides easy access to the loose fibroareolar tissue plane that separates the bladder from the cervix and lower uterine segment. Too frequently, the impatient surgeon attempts to separate the bladder from the uterus bluntly without first having excised and released these dense areas of adherence, which are always present in the midline. This is one of the most frequent causes of bleeding from the wall of the adherent bladder which, if great pressure is vigorously applied, may cause a tear in the bladder musculature or frank disruption of the full thickness of the bladder wall. Failure to free the adherent bladder base may also produce a false tissue plane which may lead to dissection into the wall of the bladder or into the vascular wall of the cervix and lower uterine segment. Once the anatomy of the bladder base and uterine wall has become obscured and the surgeon encounters increased bleeding with each effort to dissect blindly beneath the bladder, he should promptly cease the dissection, clearly identify the continuity of the bladder wall, and ligate the sources of bleeding. When the tissue plane has erroneously involved the anterior wall of the cervix and uterus or the posterior wall of the bladder, the all too familiar gush of blood upon withdrawal of the dissecting finger or thumb from the operative field is good evidence that dissection has occurred in the wrong surgical plane. Most commonly, the surgeon will err in the direction of the uterus rather than the bladder, as he is painfully aware of the possible complications from bladder trauma.

In many instances, the operative field is too obscured with bleeding to make an accurate visual determination of the boundaries of the bladder wall. When the operator has reached this point of surgical frustration, the following steps have proven to be exceedingly helpful:

1. Obtain adequate but gentle exposure of the surgical field.
2. Avoid trauma to the bladder wall by firm pressure from an angulated, narrow bladder retractor.
3. Carefully identify all bleeding vessels and control each with individual suture ligature (do not use cautery).
4. Distend the bladder with 200 cc of sterile saline or sterile milk.
5. Follow the wall of the bladder from the vaginal margin to the apex of the surgical field. The wall of the bladder should be carefully inspected to determine if there is a defect in the muscularis or mucosa from which there may be significant bleeding.
6. In the rare event that an occult entry into the bladder lumen has occurred, this will be demonstrated best by the use of sterile milk, which will show the leakage of a whitish fluid from the bladder wall.

Once the bleeding sites have been controlled and the integrity of the bladder wall has be clearly demonstrated, the surgeon should now look carefully for the pearly white border of the peritoneal fold (Fig. 47.1E). The bladder peritoneum should be conclusively differentiated from the bladder wall (the latter can be easily recognized by distension with fluid). The plica of the peritoneum should then be incised

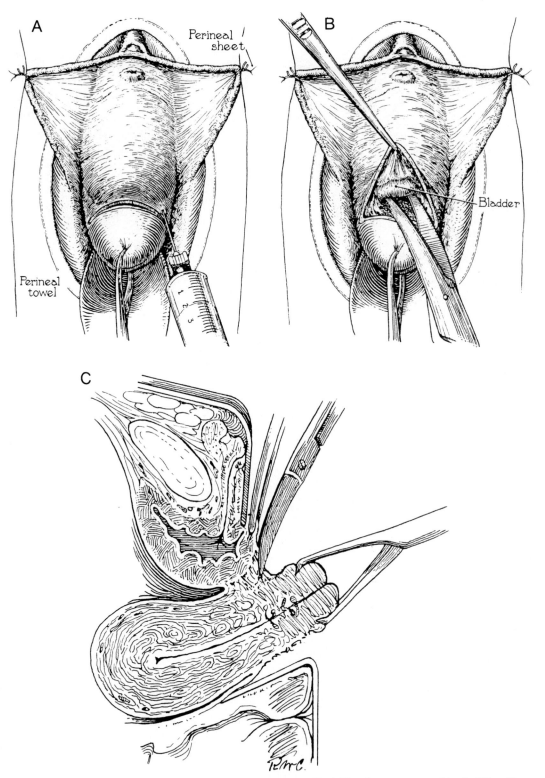

Figure 47.1. Heaney technique for vaginal hysterectomy. *A*. The labia minora are sutured back. Dilute Neosynephrine or normal saline is injected. The incision is made. *B*. The bladder is separated from the uterus with sharp dissection. *C*. Lateral view of dissection of bladder base from cervix and lower uterine segment. Note that the scissors are directed toward the uterus.

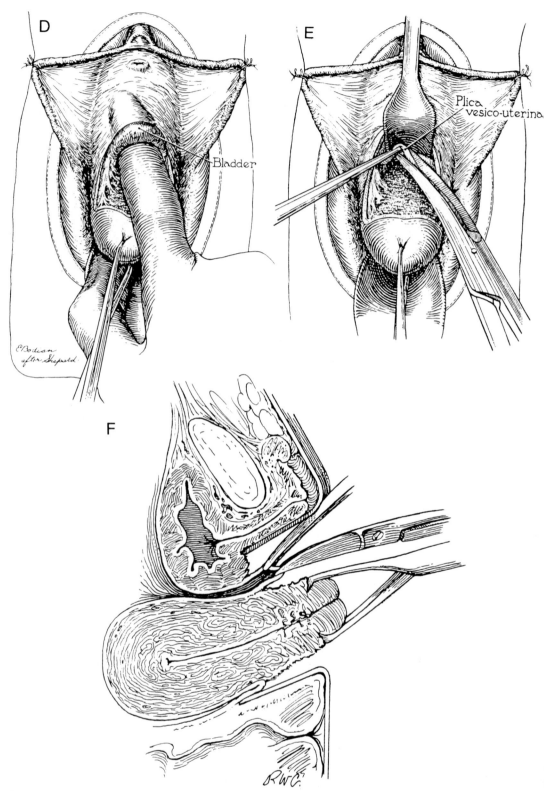

Figure 47.1. (cont.) *D*. The bladder is separated to the plica of bladder peritoneum by blunt finger dissection. *E*. The bladder peritoneum is incised. *F*. Lateral view showing identification and opening of anterior peritoneal reflection. Reprinted with permission from Mattingly RF, Thompson JD: *TeLinde's Operative Gynecology*, 6th ed., Philadelphia, JB Lippincott, 1985.

(Fig. 47.1*F*), the pelvis explored (Fig. 47.1*G*).

If excessive delay is encountered in attempting to identify the anterior peritoneum, as can frequently occur with a cervical or lower uterine segment myoma, excessive puttering may cause further damage and bleeding. In such an event, it is preferable to discontinue this surgical approach and, instead, enter the posterior cul-de-sac. Following entry into the peritoneal cavity, the index and middle fingers of one hand can be inserted through the cul-de-sac of Douglas, passed over the uterine fundus, and used to distend the boundaries of the anterior peritoneal fold which can be safely incised (Fig. 47.2). In most instances, the operator will find the previous dissection between the bladder and uterus to be well advanced beyond the normal peritoneal fold and that the pearly white appearance of the undersurface of the peritoneum

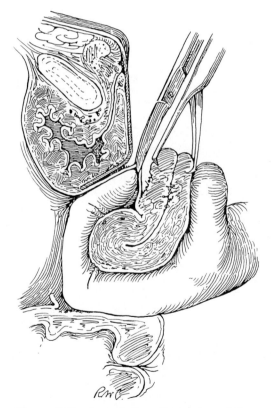

Figure 47.2. Lateral view of posterior cul-de-sac approach for identification and incision of bladder peritoneum between index and middle fingers. Reprinted with permission from Mattingly RF, Thompson JD: *TeLinde's Operative Gynecology,* 6th ed. Philadelphia, JB Lippincott, 1985.

has been obscured by dissection in an improper tissue plane. Entry into the anterior peritoneal space secondarily, after initial entry into the cul-de-sac of Douglas, creates no difficulty for the proper execution of the vaginal hysterectomy. Although we do not favor this secondary method of anterior entry, as we find this approach to be a more cumbersome and obscured technique, there are many gynecologists who routinely enter the peritoneal cavity by this method.

Should inadvertent entry into the bladder occur during this segment of the operation, this can usually be identified all too clearly by the sudden gush of clear or blood-tinged fluid that follows the scissor incision of the fold of tissue that was thought to be the anterior peritoneum. This may also occur following vigorous, blunt finger dissection of the bladder base from the uterine wall.

To have this complication occur and to fail to recognize the bladder injury could prove to be a more serious medical-legal liability. The problem of failure to identify a small, unsuspected defect in the bladder at the completion of the anterior cul-de-sac dissection can be overcome with the instillation of sterile water or saline which has been lightly tinged with methylene blue or indigo-carmine dye. While we cannot discount the value of this prophylactic and innocuous procedure, we have reserved this type of bladder study for those cases where there has been even the slightest concern about possible injury to the bladder wall.

Surgical Repair of Bladder Laceration

It must be clearly understood that the surgical injury to the bladder during a vaginal hysterectomy will occur almost exclusively in an area of the bladder base that is *above and separate from* the trigone and lower ureters. These anatomic facts are important in undertaking the surgical repair of the bladder defect. The student of pelvic anatomy will quickly recall that the female urethra measures approximately 4 cm from its origin at the vaginal introitus. The urethrovesical junction is located at or near the junction of the middle and upper third of the anterior vaginal wall. The trigone and ureteral orifices are contiguous with the upper one-third of the vagina and anterior fornix, as can be easily demonstrated by the insertion of ureteral catheters. The remainder of the bladder base rests intimately on the cervix and lower portion of the lower uterine segment

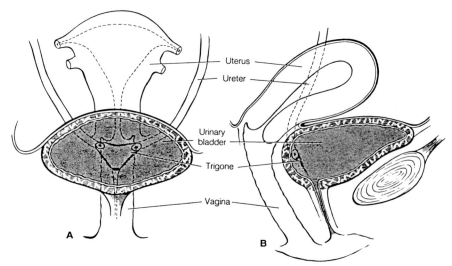

Figure 47.3. *A.* Anterior view of the normal anatomy of the ureter and bladder. The terminal end of the ureter passes medially from the lateral pelvic wall and crosses over the anterior fornix, where it enters the trigone of the bladder, which rests on the upper one-third of the anterior vaginal wall. *B.* Sagittal view of anatomical relationship of ureter and bladder base. Note that the ureter enters the trigone in the area of the upper one-third of the vagina. Reprinted with permission from Mattingly RF, Thompson JD: *TeLinde's Operative Gynecology,* 6th ed. Philadelphia, JB Lippincott, 1985.

(Fig. 47.3). Injury to the bladder during the dissection of the tissue plane that separates the cervix and lower uterine segment from the bladder base will involve only that portion of the bladder wall that is above the trigone. For this reason, it is usually unnecessary to inspect the bladder by water cystoscopy prior to repair of the bladder defect. Only if the bladder injury has occurred in the upper third of the vagina during the anterior colporrhaphy, just beyond the urethrovesical junction, should water cystoscopy be performed. Bladder inspection by water cystoscopy will demonstrate the site of injury in relationship to the trigone.

Once the bladder opening has been identified, the lateral boundaries of the bladder wall should be marked by traction sutures. It is our experience that immediate repair of the bladder defect is advisable rather than deferring the repair until completion of the hysterectomy. Occasionally, the bladder defect is so close to the anterior peritoneal fold that exposure of the site of injury is made easier if the peritoneal cavity is opened prior to the repair. The immediate bladder repair avoids loss of identification of the anatomic landmarks and the extent of the bladder injury. Therefore, it is preferable to repair the bladder wall when the injured area has

been clearly outlined and prior to loss of the anatomic boundaries of the bladder defect.

Technically, the bladder wall is closed in three layers (Fig. 47.4). A continuous suture of fine 000, delayed-absorbable suture material is used for the inititial layer of closure. Ideally, this suture should be placed in the submucosa and should invert the bladder mucosa to provide a more dependable watertight bladder seal and to avoid a foreign body reaction in the bladder mucosa. Practically speaking, this is difficult to achieve; therefore, it is far preferable to pass the suture directly through the mucosa and submucosa to ensure complete closure of the bladder defect. A locking suture is known to be more hemostatic but should not be used on the bladder base to avoid ischemic necrosis and segmental separation of the mucosa. The initial suture line should be placed without undue traction on the delicate and fragile bladder mucosa. It is important that the repair in the bladder base be watertight. Therefore, the integrity of the initial suture layer should be tested with the instillation of sterile milk or chromagen-tinged sterile water or saline. If there are sites of obvious leakage from the mucosal margins, these areas should be reinforced with interrupted, inverting horizontal mattress sutures,

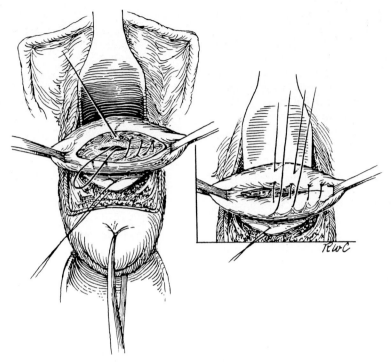

Figure 47.4.   Closure of accidental laceration of bladder in two layers; continuous 3-0 chromic or delayed absorbable suture includes bladder mucosa and intermuscularis in first layer; interrupted inverting 2-0 sutures in muscularis form the second layer. Free margin of bladder peritoneum held with suture may be advanced over the suture line for addtional support to watertight closure. Reprinted with permission from Mattingly RF, Thompson JD: *TeLinde's Operative Gynecology,* 6th ed. Philadelphia, JB Lippincott, 1985.

placed in the same plane as the bladder defect. A second layer of interrrupted 000 delayed absorbable sutures is placed in the muscularis to support and invert the initial suture line. Finally, adjacent paravesical fascia should be approximated as a third layer, using interrupted, 00 sutures. Should a fascial layer prove to be difficult to identify, an additional supporting layer of sutures in the muscularis can be used, or alternatively, the bladder peritoneum can be drawn beneath the bladder base and used as a final supporting layer to the bladder defect. The repaired bladder base should be thoroughly inspected for residual bleeding, which must be meticulously controlled before the operation is complete.

After the bladder wall has been repaired, the vaginal hysterectomy is completed as per usual. In the event that preoperative assessment of the vagina indicated the need for an anterior colporrhaphy with plication of the vesical sphincter for the correction of stress urinary incontinence, this procedure should be performed, disregarding the previous repair to the bladder wall. Obviously, the bladder base should not be traumatized during the anterior colporrhaphy, but the same technique for the cystocele repair should be utilized with careful attention directed to the bladder base to avoid any further injury to the operative site of the previous bladder repair.

Postoperative Care   Bladder drainage may be achieved by means of a urethral or a suprapubic catheter. It has been our practice to use a suprapubic catheter to avoid trauma to the repaired bladder mucosa from a large balloon of a urethral retention catheter. Regardless of the choice of bladder drainage, it is critical to the proper healing of the bladder wall that the bladder remain empty and the bladder wall undistended for a period of 7 days. If this can be assured by the use of a urethral catheter, this should be the drainage method of choice. If there has been clinical experience with the use of the suprabubic catheter, this is the method which we find to be preferable.

The benefit of prophylactic antibiotics to avoid interstitial infection and to ensure primary bladder healing has not been documented adequately to date. In the premenopausal patient, the use of perioperative antibiotics with broad-spectrum Gram-positive and Gram-negative antimicrobial effectiveness has been shown to decrease the incidence of infectious morbidity in women undergoing vaginal hysterectomy. If preoperative antibiotic use has been initiated, whereby a therapeutic tissue level of the antibiotic has been achieved during the operative procedure, we would recommend no more than a 24-hour antibiotic treatment because of the bladder injury. If preoperative antibiotics had not been initiated prior to the identification of the bladder injury, we would consider the short-term use of prophylactic antibiotics to be valuable when initiated promptly with the repair of the bladder wall. Unfortunately, there are no data available, based on a randomized, prospective, double blind study that would prove the clinical value of this latter method of prophylactic antibiotic use with bladder injury. It is highly probable that meticulous surgical technique and accurate reapproximation of the bladder wall are far more critical to assure proper tissue healing than is the therapeutic use of prophylactic antibiotic agents. While unsupported by any scientific evidence, we have maintained the patient at bed rest for 24 hours during the initial postoperative period to ensure adequate seal of the bladder mucosa. Thereafter, ambulation of the patient should be no different than for a patient without bladder injury. As is known to every pelvic surgeon, the success or failure of primary healing of a repaired bladder is dependent on the surgical technique and anatomic closure of the bladder wall at the time of the injury. If the bladder remains undistended at all times, the degree of ambulation of the patient should have little effect on tissue healing.

The suprapubic catheter is clamped on the seventh postoperative day. This may be done as an outpatient if the patient's condition permits an earlier hospital discharge. The patient is carefully observed so that bladder distention does not occur. If the patient is unable to void in the presence of bladder symptoms, the suprapubic catheter is opened and the bladder is completely drained, regardless of the period of time of catheter closure. Thirty minutes later, the suprapubic catheter is closed again in similiar time sequence, leaving the catheter closed for 3- to 4-hour periods if the patient has initiated voiding. The patient must be catheterized accordingly, per urethra, if a urethral catheter has been used to drain the bladder. Only when the residual urine volume is less than 100 cc is the catherization discontinued or the suprapubic catheter removed. Before doing so, a urine culture is obtained and the urine sediment is examined for microscopic evidence of bladder infection, which, when present, is treated with appropriate oral antibiotics.

Although bladder injury is a more common complication of an abdominal rather than a vaginal hysterectomy, injury to the bladder base per vagina is the more serious of the two types of bladder complications. Failure of healing of the repaired bladder based can lead to a troublesome vesicovaginal fistula. When bladder injury occurs in the dome of the bladder at the time of abdominal hysterectomy, there is rarely any sequela if the bladder wall is closed in any fashion. Only in the dependent portion of the bladder base is it essential that the repaired bladder defect be watertight with the avoidance of the smallest sinus tract in the repaired bladder wall. Should such an intramural defect occur, it is possible that it may lead to a residual vesicovaginal fistula. Therefore, while injury to the bladder base occurs less frequently than injury to the bladder dome, the bladder base is at higher risk for the subsequent development of a vesicovaginal fistula, due to continued presence of urine on the suture line and the antomic factors that influence tissue healing.

Selected Readings

Everett HS, Mattingly RF: Urinary tract injuries resulting from pelvic surgery. *Am J Obstet Gynecol* 71:502,1956.

Heaney NS: Techniques of vaginal hysterectomy. *Surg Clin North Am* 22:73,1942.

Jaszczak SE, Evans TN: Intrafascial abdominal and vaginal hysterectomy: A reappraisal. *Obstet Gynecol* 59:435,1982.

Mattingly RF, Borkowf HI: Lower urinary tract injuries in pregnancy. In: Barber HK, Graber EA (eds): *Surgical Disease in Pregnancy*, Philadelphia, WB Saunders, 1974.

Mattingly RF, Moore DE, Clark DO: Bacteriologic study of suprapubic bladder drainage. *Am J Obstet Gynecol* 114:732,1972.

Mattingly RF, Thompson JD: *TeLinde's Operative Gynecology*, 6th ed., Philadelphia, JB Lippincott, 1985.

Williams TJ: Urologic injuries. In: Wynn RM (ed): *Obstetrics and Gynecology*, Annual 1975, vol. 4. New York, Appleton-Century-Crofts, 1975, pp. 347-368.

CHAPTER **48**

Urine Leakage Through Vagina After Vaginal Hysterectomy and Anterior Colporrhaphy

RICHARD E. SYMMONDS, M.D.

CASE ABSTRACT

A vaginal hysterectomy and anterior colporrhaphy had been performed on a 37-year-old multiparous patient with symptomatic genital prolapse. On the third postoperative day, the Foley catheter was removed and the patient was found to be leaking urine through the vagina.

DISCUSSION

Regardless of the surgeon's experience and ability, an occasional bladder perforation will occur with vaginal hysterectomy and anterior colporrhaphy; if fistula formation is to be prevented, the bladder injury must be recognized and repaired. The recognized injury that is repaired immediately will almost never lead to fistula formation. Leaving a retention catheter in the bladder for 7 to 10 days after all difficult vaginal hysterectomies that may have been traumatic to the bladder provides additional "insurance," for instance, with a vaginal hysterectomy that is done after a low cervical cesarean section or a previous anterior uterovaginal surgery of another type, some bladder "demuscularization" may occur without actual perforation. In such patients, prolonged catheter decompression of the bladder may obviate the development of a fistula.

With a patient leaking urine 3 days after vaginal hysterectomy and anterior colporrhaphy, the bladder distention associated with a cystoscopic evaluation should be avoided and a more simple effort should be made to determine the nature of the fistula. With the insertion of a tampon in the vagina and the instillation of methylene blue into the bladder, leakage of urine (rather than peritoneal fluid) often can be confirmed by the presence of dye on the vaginal tampon; this finding suggests that a vesicovaginal fistula is present. If, after a time, the methylene blue has failed to stain the vaginal tampon, another tampon is inserted, followed by the intravenous administration of indigo carmine. If this dye stains the vaginal tampon, whereas the methylene blue in the bladder had failed to do so, the patient can be considered as having ureterovaginal fistula.

With confirmation of a vesicovaginal fistula by the dye test, cystoscopic evaluation need not be done merely to determine the size or location of the fistula. It is much too soon to consider surgical intervention to correct the fistula; generally, cystoscopic overdistention of the bladder will not be beneficial and could be detrimental. A large-caliber transurethral catheter should be inserted to maintain bladder drainage and decompression; on occasion, even fistulas of rather large size can heal spontaneously. This is true, in particular, for the high fistula that is leaking urine through the vaginal vault by a relatively long and perhaps circuitous tract where fibrotic obliteration of the tract (rather than epithelialization) can occur. During catheterization, the patient can be up and about and even dismissed from the hospital; rest in bed or assuming the prone position usually does not promote healing of the fistula. If the fistulous tract fails to heal with catheter drainage within 4 to 6 weeks, it is unlikely to do so.

If the patient continues to leak urine after the catheter has been removed, the catheter should be left out to allow the irritation and infection that has occurred from prolonged catheterization to subside. Any consideration of surgical correction of the fistula should be deferred for approximately 3 months. During this time, the suture material from the hysterectomy should have been absorbed or expelled, edema and infection will have subsided, and the tissues will become soft, pliable, and "workable." The use of cortisone does not significantly speed up this process. The first surgical effort to correct the fistula has the best possibility of success; thus, one should be certain that the tissues are in absolutely optimal condition before repair is attempted.

When the "two-dye test" has reliably excluded the presence of a vesicovaginal fistula and suggests that the urinary leakage is from a ureterovaginal fistula, cystoscopic investigation of its location should be promptly done. An effort should be made to insert a ureteral catheter well above the level of the ureterovaginal fistula; when this can be accomplished and the catheter has been left in place for 2 to 3 weeks, approximately 30% of the fistulas subsequently will heal spontaneously. The fortunate patient who obtains spontaneous healing of the ureterovaginal fistula must be observed most carefully by the use of excretory urography after intervals of 3, 6, and 12 months to be sure that a stricture of the ureter does not occur. A delayed stricture of the ureter can severely impair or even totally destroy renal function; such a stricture can be occult and completely "silent" clinically.

Occasionally, a ureteral catheter cannot be inserted because of its kinking or distortion at the level of the fistula; in this instance, additional action is not urgent, provided the kidney is not being jeopardized by high-grade obstruction and infection. If the kidney is being drained well by the fistula and there is no infection, one can procrastinate and allow the patient sufficient time to recover from the operation. After 10 to 15 days, another effort can be made to insert a ureteral catheter; on occasion, due to the subsidence of edema, suture relaxation or dissolution, or other changes, a ureteral catheter can be inserted, and this may promote spontaneous healing of the fistula.

The situation becomes urgent when the patient has significant pyeloureterectasis, poor drainage, and upper urinary tract infection;

permanent impairment of function or even loss of the kidney can result. Depending on the patient's condition, the surgeon must consider either a prompt nephrostomy or an abdominal approach to repair the ureterovaginal fistula. When the patient is critically ill and toxic, a nephrostomy (open or percutaneous) is the safer approach.

If 3 days after vaginal hysterectomy and repair the patient has no evidence of vault infection and is in reasonably good condition, immediate repair of a ureterovaginal fistula frequently is the treatment of choice. This soon after a vaginal hysterectomy there may be relatively little edema or tissue reaction to the surgery involving the higher pelvic portion of the ureter and the broad ligament; abdominal exploration and a ureteroneocystostomy frequently can be accomplished utilizing relatively normal tissues. This is in decided contrast to the quality of the tissues that usually will be found in the patient in whom a ureterovaginal fistula has developed several days after total abdominal hysterectomy for conditions such as endometriosis, pelvic inflammatory disease, and malignancy. Any consideration of accomplishing an immediate repair of a ureteral injury after abdominal hysterectomy for such problems is to be definitely deplored.

When the condition of the patient has indicated the need for a temporizing nephrostomy, definitive repair of the ureterovaginal fistula should be deferred for 2 or 3 months. Depending on the degree of urinary extravasation and infection that has occurred, an earlier approach may reveal significant edema, inflammatory reaction, and suture material that can make the dissection difficult and the repair less than satisfactory.

In summary, bladder-ureteral injuries must be recognized and repaired at surgery. When doubt exists at the time of surgery, the instillation of dye (or milk) into the bladder may disclose an otherwise unrecognizable perforation. Even when an actual bladder perforation has not occurred, prolonged catheterization after operation is advisable whenever the surgeon considers the degree of bladder trauma to be unusual and excessive.

Once the fistula has occurred, the surgeon should not be coerced into early surgical intervention by the anxious patient and her family. In a series of 600 patients referred to us with fistulas, more than half had had an unsuccessful fistula repair. The most prevalent cause of the unsuccessful repairs appeared to have been premature surgical efforts to correct the fistula. The initial repair should be deferred until the tissues are in optimal condition.

Selected Readings

O'Connor VJ Jr, Sokol JK, Bulkley GJ, et al: Suprapubic closure of vesicovaginal fistula. *J Urol* 109:51, 1973.

Symmonds RE: Prevention and management of genitourinary fistula. *J Cont Educ Obstet Gynecol* 21:13, 1979.

Symmonds RE: Ureteral injuries associated with gynecologic surgery: Prevention and management. *Clin Obstet Gynecol* 19:623, 1976.

Symmonds RE, Hill LM: Loss of the urethra: A report on 50 patients. *Am J Obstet Gynecol* 130:130, 1978.

CHAPTER 49

Vesicovaginal Fistula Following Total Abdominal Hysterectomy

JOHN D. THOMPSON, M.D.

CASE ABSTRACT

Because of chronic, annoying, dysfunctional uterine bleeding, unresponsive to hormonal manipulation and dilatation and curettage (D & C), an abdominal hysterectomy was performed on a 36-year-old woman whose two children had both been delivered previously by low cervical cesarean section.

Because of considerable adherence between the posterior surface of the bladder and cervix at the site of the cesarean section scar, considerable difficulty was encountered establishing a bladder flap. Much oozing from the posterior surface of the bladder was controlled by interrupted mattress stitches of 3-0 chromic catgut.

Although the urine was blood tinged, the Foley catheter was removed the morning of the second postoperative day. On the eighth postoperative day, the patient noted partial urinary incontinence and was totally incontinent on the ninth postoperative day. No diagnostic studies were performed, and the patient was sent home with an indwelling transurethral Foley catheter connected to a leg bag. Urine was leaking through the vagina 8 weeks later, whenever the catheter was clamped.

DISCUSSION

When a major complication is encountered in the surgical treatment of gynecologic disease, a careful review of the patient's clinical history and physical findings will be done to determine if the operation was indicated in the first place. From the clinical history given, it does seem that this patient did need the operation, although information about the amount of bleeding, the presence or absence of anemia, the number of D & Cs performed, etc., is not given. After it is determined that the operation was indicated, one may then ask if the operation was performed correctly, and here there may be some reason to question the judgment of choosing the abdominal rather than the vaginal approach in this patient. Certainly, in the absence of pelvic pathology (such as tumors or indurated tissue), a vaginal hysterectomy can usually be performed with ease even though the patient has had no previous vaginal deliveries.

In the author's opinion, the vaginal approach is preferable when hysterectomy is indicated in a patient who has had previous low cervical cesarean section(s). The dissection of the bladder from the lower uterine segment is easier when done vaginally, especially since it is always possible to put an instrument in the bladder through the urethra to help locate the proper plane of dissection. If there are no contraindications to vaginal hysterectomy, then a history of previous low cervical cesarean section should be an indication rather than a contraindication to the vaginal approach.

Vesicovaginal fistulas are sometimes caused by gynecologic malignancies, but gynecologic surgery for benign disease (as in this case) is the most common etiology, accounting for approximately 75% in this country. Obstetric causes of vesicovaginal fistulas are extremely rare in the United States but are common in some developing nations. Although there are several points that should be emphasized in the primary prevention of vesicovaginal fistulas, the most important point is careful and correct technique of gynecologic operations. Steps in abdominal hysterectomy to reduce the incidence of bladder injury include identification of the proper plane between the bladder and the cervix, sharp dissection rather than pushing with a sponge stick or a sponge-covered index finger, intrafascial technique of removal of the cervix when operating for benign uterine disease, adequate mobilization of the bladder inferiorly and laterally, and care in clamping and suturing the vaginal cuff. When performing vaginal hysterectomy, sharp dissection should be used to identify the proper plane between the bladder and the lower uterine segment; traction, countertraction, and adequate exposure are essential; abandon a difficult dissection anterior to the cervix and complete the dissection posterior to the cervix first; if necessary, identify the anterior peritoneum by placing a finger through the posterior cul-de-sac; and identify the limits of the bladder by placing an instrument in the bladder through the urethra. If it is anticipated that the hysterectomy will be technically difficult to perform vaginally, it should be done abdominally.

Damage to the bladder muscle should be reinforced with a 4-0 Vicryl sutures, and the edge of the peritoneum that covers the bladder should be sutured to the anterior edge of the vaginal cuff. This latter technique is extremely helpful in preventing postoperative vesicovaginal fistulas (Fig. 49.1). If cystostomy has actually occurred, careful approximation of the bladder mucosa with a 4-0 Vicryl should then be reinforced by at least two layers of interrupted vertical mattress 4-0 Vicryl sutures placed in the bladder muscle. Again, the peritoneal edge behind the bladder should be sutured to the anterior margin of the vaginal cuff. In both circumstances, an indwelling transurethral Foley catheter should be left in place for 1 to 2 weeks depending on the extent of the injury and the security of the repair. Above all, injuries to the bladder should be discovered and repaired before the operation is completed.

Now, returning to the case history, it is noted that the patient became partially incontinent of urine on the eighth postoperative day and totally incontinent on the ninth day. This is about the time in the postoperative period when most vesicovaginal fistulas resulting from damage with subsequent ischemia and necrosis of the

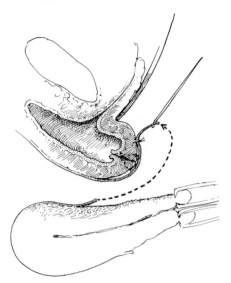

Figure 49.1. An anterior peritoneal flap is tacked in place over the operative repair providing the security of an additional fresh tissue layer. Reprinted with permission from Nichols DH, Randall CL: *Vaginal Surgery,* 2nd ed. Baltimore, Williams & Wilkins, 1983.

bladder wall will develop. However, it is also stated that "no diagnostic studies were performed." This is a critical error. It is absolutely necessary to know whether the incontinence is the result of injury to the bladder or injury to the ureter(s). This patient could have a unilateral ureterovaginal fistula, bilateral ureterovaginal fistulas, a vesicovaginal fistula, or a vesicovaginal fistula in combination with a unilateral or bilateral ureterovaginal fistula. Although certain historical points are helpful in making the diagnosis, special diagnostic procedures are necessary to locate and determine the extent of the injury exactly. These include transurethral instillation of dye into the bladder, intravenous injection of indigo carmine, intravenous pyelography, and cystoscopy with retrograde pyelography. Not all of these studies will be needed in each patient. But certainly a patient with a vesicovaginal fistula will at least need an intravenous pyelogram (IVP) in order to be certain that the ureters are normal. Eventually, cystoscopy will also be needed to locate the fistula, to determine if there is only one or possibly more than one, and to locate the margins of the fistula in relation to the ureteral orifices. These items of information are essential in proper performance of vesicovaginal fistula repair.

It was formerly taught that one must wait at least 6 months after the operation of injury before attempting a vesicovaginal fistula repair. This teaching was based on the idea that this much time was required for the tissues to become sufficiently healthy to hold sutures and to heal. Recent experience indicates that most simple postoperative vesicovaginal fistulas may be repaired successfully without delay. Certainly, this is the opinion of the author. More complicated fistulas may require a waiting period for the tissues to improve, but this is rarely in excess of 3 months.

After a fistula is diagnosed, one can offer the patient the option of wearing or not wearing an indwelling transurethral bladder catheter. Some patients will have so much discomfort from the catheter that they will prefer instead to wear rubber pants and/or disposable diapers until a repair can be done. A careful preoperative evaluation is carried out with particular reference to the proximity of the ureteral orifices to the fistula margin, the presence of more than one fistula, ureteral stenosis, urinary tract infection, and the degree of induration of the tissues. If the fistula has developed in a patient with a gynecologic malignancy, biopsy of the margins of the fistula may be indicated. Preoperative steroids are of questionable value and are no longer used by the author.

Several points in the operative technique should be discussed. The transvaginal approach is preferred for simple fistulas. When dealing with more complicated fistulas (large, postirradiation, postradical pelvic surgery, multiple, or close to the ureteral orifices), a multiple approach technique including transvaginal, transabdominal, and transvesical may be needed. If the fistula margin is close to the ureteral orifices, placement of ureteral catheters to facilitate dissection and avoid ureteral injury is helpful.

When doing a transvaginal repair, one needs good exposure of fistula margins. Occasionally, a Schuchardt incision will be needed if the vaginal introitus is tight. If it is needed, it should be done without hesitation. A wide and thorough dissection and mobilization of the bladder base is carried out with preservation of all muscle and connective tissue possible on the bladder site rather than the vaginal flap. Indurated tissue is removed, and bleeding vessels are secured (Figs. 49.2 - 49.5). The track of the fistula is excised completely and in such a way

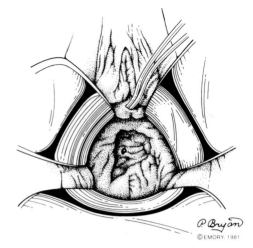

Figure 49.2.   The vesicovaginal fistula is shown.

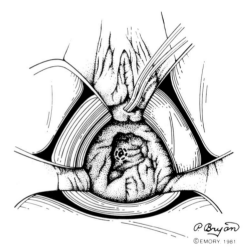

Figure 49.3.   The vesicovaginal fistula is outline by the *broken line*.

as to allow exact identification of the fresh edge of the bladder mucosa (Fig. 49.6). The choice of sutures is important. The author's present preference is for 3-0 Vicryl sutures throughout the repair. The first layer of interrupted vertical mattress sutures includes the bladder mucosa and adjacent bladder muscle (Fig. 49.7). The bladder side of the fistula must be closed securely. The adequacy of the closure is tested by instilling 200 to 300 cc of a weak solution of methylene blue into the bladder through the catheter. If there is any point of leakage, reinforcement is required. This first layer closing the bladder mucosa must be watertight (Fig.

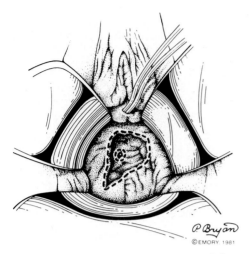

Figure 49.4.   The lateral limits of proposed dissection are shown by the *outer broken line*. Ureteral catheters may be placed if the fistula margins are close to the ureteral orifices. For patients with a simple, fresh posthysterectomy vesicovaginal fistula, indurated tissue must be removed.

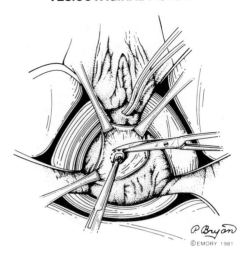

Figure 49.6.   The track of the fistula is excised completely and in such a way as to allow exact identification of the fresh edge of the bladder mucosa.

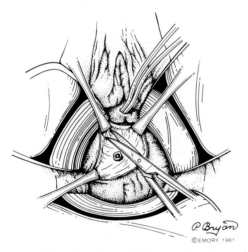

Figure 49.5.   A wide and thorough dissection and mobilization of the bladder base is carried out with preservation of all muscle and connective tissue on the bladder.

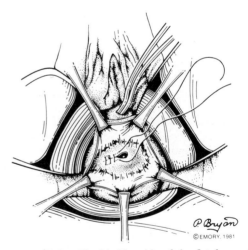

Figure 49.7.   The bladder side of the fistula must be closed securely. The first layer should be watertight. Reinforcement of any point of leakage is required.

49.8). Following this, several (two or three) horizontal mattress sutures of 3-0 Vicryl are placed in such a way that tissue is approximated "broad surface to broad surface without tension." Further dissection and mobilization must be carried out if there is tension. Omental or bulbocavernosus fat flaps may be used to reinforce the repair, but these are not needed in repair of simple fistulas. Finally, the excess vaginal mucosa is trimmed away, and the vaginal edges are approximated horizontally with sutures (Fig. 49.9). At the end of the repair, 5 cc of indigo carmine are injected intravenously. The bladder is emptied, and 200 cc of clear sterile saline are instilled. A cystoscope is inserted to watch for efflux of dye from the ureteral orifices.

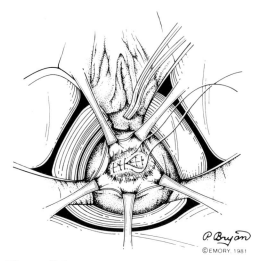

Figure 49.8. Several horizontal layers of interrupted vertical mattress sutures of 3-0 Vicryl are placed in such a way that tissue is approximated "broad surface to broad surface without tension."

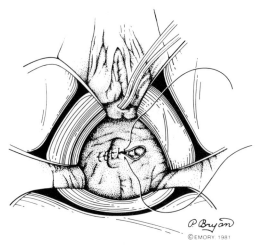

Figure 49.9. Excess vaginal mucosa is trimmed away, and the vaginal edges are approximated horizontally with sutures.

Vesicovaginal Fistula

Postoperatively, adequate bladder drainage must be provided. Although a suprapubic cystostomy may be needed for complicated fistulas, a transurethral Foley catheter can be used for simple fistulas easily and securely repaired. Usually, the catheter is left in place about 10 days. However, this time may be shorter or longer depending on the size of the fistula and the security of the closure. If a patient has had a proper repair of a very small fistula, she may be discharged on the third day after operation without a catheter. Early ambulation is allowed in patients with simple fistulas. Maintenance of an adequate urine output is more important in preventing urinary tract infection than the use of urinary antiseptics.

It should be understood that this discussion has been written with the above case presented in mind. Very special operative techniques and postoperative care will be needed for complicated fistulas. Even urinary diversion above the bladder will be indicated for a few patients. However, urinary diversion should be reserved for patients with "impossible" fistulas or vesicovaginal fistulas associated with severe bilateral ureteral obstruction. Of course, this is an entirely different problem when compared to the patient with a small postoperative vesicovaginal fistula who generally can be successfully managed by a simple transvaginal repair soon after the fistula is diagnosed.

Selected Readings

Collins CG, Collins JH, Harrison BR, et al: Early repair of vesicovaginal fistula. *Am J Obstet Gynecol* 3:524, 1971.

Fearl CL, Keizur LW: Optimum time interval from occurrence to repair of vesicovaginal fistula. *Am J Obstet Gynecol* 104:205, 1968.

Mattingly RF, Thompson JD: *TeLinde's Operative Gynecology*, 6th Ed. Philadelphia, JB Lippincott, 1985, chap. 27.

Moir JC: Vesicovaginal fistulae as seen in Britain. *J. Obstet Gynaecol Br Commonw* 80:598, 1973.

Nichols DH, Randall CL: *Vaginal Surgery*, 2nd ed. Baltimore, Williams & Wilkins, 1983.

Persky L, Herman G, Geurrier K: Non-delay in vesicovaginal fistula repair. *Urology* 13:273, 1979.

Ridley JH: Surgery for vaginal fistulae. In Ridley JH (ed): *Gynecologic Surgery: Errors, Safeguards, and Salvage*, 2nd ed. Baltimore, Williams & Wilkins, 1981.

Robertson JR: Vesicovaginal fistula: The gynecologist's responsibility. *Obstet Gynecol* 42:611, 1973.

CHAPTER 50
Unrecognized Clamping of Ureter at Hysterectomy

RICHARD E. SYMMONDS, M.D.

CASE ABSTRACT

A difficult abdominal hysterectomy, complicated by endometriosis and fibroids, had just been completed on a 37-year-old patient. After removal of the uterus and control of bleeding from deep within the pelvis, it was found that a Kelly hemostatic clamp had inadvertently placed on a ureter and that the hemostat had been there for at least 30 minutes by the time the condition was discovered.

DISCUSSION

The continuing high incidence of ureteral injury with total abdominal hysterectomy (0.5% to 2%) is deplorable. Such injury can be almost completely avoided by the simple preliminary measure of demanding routine identification of the ureters above the level of disease as the initial step in every abdominal hysterectomy. The ureter then can be dissected down and displaced out of the diseased area, and injury can be either avoided or at least recognized. Regardless of experience or ability, any surgeon can injure the ureter during its dissection from the diseased area, but the injury should be recognized and immediately repaired to obviate a fistula. The insertion of ureteral catheters is not necessary for ureteral identification and may merely increase trauma to the ureter during its dissection, as noted by Shingleton. Surgeons who do not have sufficient knowledge of the pelvic anatomy to practice routine and constant identification of the ureter should not operate in the pelvis. Once the injury has occurred, as with a clamp placed across the ureter for at least 30 minutes, the method of repair will be governed by (a) the location and severity of the injury (high or low on the ureter), (b) the nature of the disease process for which the hysterectomy was accomplished (infected, malignant), (c) the condition of the patient (critical, short-term prognosis), and (d) the training and experience of the operator. The

surgeon who has little experience and knowledge regarding the proper management of ureteral injuries should obtain prompt consultation with someone knowledgeable in this area.

The clamp or ligature placed across (or around) the ureter should be promptly removed; generally, if removed within a few seconds of the time it was placed, tissue damage will be minimal and no repair is required. A ureteral catheter can be inserted to splint the area if desired. Insertion can be accomplished most expeditiously by doing a simple anterior cystotomy, sliding the ureteral catheter up the ureter, and passing its lower end down through the urethra, where it can be tied to the urethral retention catheter; both catheters are left in place for approximately 10 days.

When the clamp has been placed across the ureter and allowed to remain in place for 30 minutes or longer, the damage to tissue if untreated will lead to subsequent necrosis and to either a ureteral sticture or fistula formation. While simple trauma to the ureteral sheath or an incision in the ureter can be repaired with a few interrupted 4-0 chromic catgut sutures, this type of crush injury will require resection.

The location of the clamping injury is not stated in the present case; however, the ureter is frequently clamped or ligated at the pelvic brim level along with the infundibulopelvic ligament and ovarian vessels. At this high level, the repair is best accomplished by an end-to-end ureteroureterostomy. Both ends of a small ureter may need to be slightly spatulated in order to allow one to accomplish an accurate, somewhat oblique anastomosis. Excessive suture material should be avoided; perhaps no more than four to six interrupted sutures should be used. Each suture should include the ureteral sheath as well as full thickness of the ureteral wall. Opinion is divided regarding the necessity of inserting a ureteral catheter for splinting; however, the author prefers to splint a ureteroureterostomy, inserting a ureteral catheter as noted above. There is no difference of opinion regarding the need to provide some form of extraperitoneal drainage down to the level of the anastomosis. A suction drain of the Hemovac type can be inserted through the abdominal wall retroperitoneally down to but not actually touching the anastomosis.

More frequently, the clamp will have been placed across the ureter at the level of the uterosacral ligament, uterine artery, or lateral vaginal angle. After resection of the damaged section of ureter, the continuity of the urinary tract can be best and most accurately restored by accomplishing a simple end-to-side ureteroneocystostomy; this is particularly true when the injury has occurred in a deep, perhaps obese and sanguineous pelvis, where an end-to-end ureteroureterostomy may be difficult to accomplish. By doing an anterior cystotomy and inserting a finger in the bladder to "tent-up" the most accessible portion of the bladder, the surgeon can quickly accomplish an end-to-side (mucosa-to-mucosa) anastomosis between the end of the ureter and the side wall of the bladder. Any tension on the anastomosis must be avoided by mobilizing the bladder and displacing it upward toward the pelvic brim. Similarly, the upper segment of the ureter can be additionally mobilized or a "bladder-hitch" can be accomplished to relieve tension on the anastomosis. A bladder-hitch requires that the bladder be displaced upward and attached with interrupted absorbable sutures to the fascia of the iliopsoas muscle just lateral to the iliac artery bifurcation.

Generally, the urologist will advise (and accomplish) an antireflux type of ureteroneocystostomy (Politano-Leadbetter). The relatively inexperienced surgeon, when repairing a ureteral injury, probably should accomplish the more simple end-to-side anastomosis without an antireflux mechanism, because this will carry a lesser risk of producing subsequent obstructive problems.

Splinting a ureteroneocystostomy with a ureteral catheter is not necessary; however, the bladder should be drained with a transurethral catheter for 10 days. Again, some type of extraperitoneal suction drainage should be inserted down to but not touching the area of the ureteroneocystostomy.

When the ureteral injury has occurred in a patient whose condition is precarious or when the surgeon is not "comfortable" with ureteral surgery and immediate urologic consultation is not available, a temporizing method of managing the ureteral injury is advisable. A small Silastic catheter is brought out through an extraperitoneal stab wound in the abdominal wall—a "catheter ureterostomy." At least this will not do any additional harm, and it will protect the kidney until the patient's general condition has improved or until an experienced surgeon is available to accomplish a definitive repair. Similarly, with ureteral injury in a patient with a short-term prognosis (carcinomatosis, for instance), rather than a complex operation to repair or replace the ureter, the proximal end of the ureter can be merely ligated; this will produce prompt renal nonfunction and, in the absence of upper urinary tract infection, no significant clinical symptoms. If this is to be accomplished, it is absolutely essential to know that the patient has good renal function on the other side.

With the total abdominal hysterectomy technique, the admonition has always been to clamp parallel or close to the cervix and intrafascially in order to avoid ureteral injury. The passage of time has indicated that this has not been adequate either to prevent ureteral injuries or to promote their recognition. With endometriosis (as in the case presentation), with pelvic inflammatory disease, and with large uterine and broad ligament tumors, clamping close to the cervix or intrafascially may be impossible; similarly, with various types of uterine malignancy, intrafascial clamping is undersirable. Until it is taught and practiced that the routine identification of ureters, bladder base, and rectum represents an essential early step in the total abdominal hysterectomy technique, a high incidence of unrecognized injuries and fistula formation will continue with this operation.

Selected Readings

Higgins CC: Ureteral injuries during surgery: A review of 87 cases. *JAMA* 199:82, 1967.

Lee RA, Symmonds RE: Ureterovaginal fistula *Am J Obstet Gynecol* 109:1032, 1971.

Solomons E, Levin EJ, Bauman J, et al: A pyelographic study of ureteric injuries sustained during hysterectomy for benign conditions. *Surg Gynecol Obstet* 111:41, 1960.

Symmonds RE: Ureteral injuries associated with gynecologic surgery: Prevention and managemnt. *Clin Obstet Gynecol* 19:623, 1976.

Talbert LM, Palumbo L, Shingleton H, et al: Urologic complications of radical hysterectomy for carcinoma of the cervix. *South Med J* 58:11, 1965.

Chapter 51

Crushed Ureter with Transabdominal Hysterectomy

CLAYTON T. BEECHAM, M.D.

CASE ABSTRACT

An abdominal hysterectomy necessitated by an uncommonly large fibroid—extending from the base of the broad ligament to the umbilicus—presented a number of problems at surgery. Both corpus and cervix uteri were essentially all tumor. Exposure of parametrial and broad ligament structures was difficult. As the tumor and uterus were lifted from the operative site, a hysterectomy clamp was seen to include both uterine artery and ureter. The latter had been crushed within the clamp for at least 1/2 hour. This misapplication was about 2 cm from the ureterovesical junction where the uterine artery crosses the ureter.

DISCUSSION

The Problem

Obviously, the ureter has been injured; what is the extent of the injury?

1. Has the ureter been severed like the uterine artery

2. Is the ureter simply injured by the crushing but otherwise intact?

Approach to Problem

Immediately, the uterine artery must be traced laterally from the clamp, isolated, and doubly ligated. Once the artery is secure, the crushing hysterectomy clamp is removed. Prior to removal, ureteral dilation will have been noted. After removal, if the ureter has been severed, the cut ends will be visible and there will be urine dripping or spurting from the lumen. Dilation will disappear quickly; the gynecologist should proceed at once with a ureteroneocystotomy.

If the surgeon has been fortunate, when he removes the hysterectomy clamp, he will find the ureter intact but the walls adherent to each other (from the crush). Untreated, this will lead to the formation of a ureterovaginal fistula in about 7 days. However, if such a ureter is kept open and draining into the bladder, it will not slough and form a fistula.

Solution to the Problem.

1. **Treatment of the Lesser Injury— Crushing.** The surgical objective is to open the ureteral canal where it has been crushed and then splint the lumen from the kidney to the bladder. This is done by opening the dome of the bladder in order to look directly down on the ureteral orifices in the trigone and, then, introducing a #5 ureteral catheter up to the point of injury. Gentle upward pressure on the catheter, while squeezing the crushed ureter, will allow it to pass through the point of injury up to the kidney pelvis. While holding it in place with upward pressure, the distal end can be passed down along the indwelling Foley catheter (in the urethra) to the meatus.

Closure of the cystotomy should be two layered using plain catgut. Do not place a drain in the retroperitoneal space since it may further traumatize the already injured ureter. After vascular oozing from the cut vaginal edges has been controlled by a continuous suture, leave the vaginal apex open but peritonealized. This will provide adequate drainage for serum and/or urine should there be a leak.

The ureter, with its upper tract catheter in place, will dilate almost immediately; kidney function will not be impaired. *An unobstructed ureter will heal* and does so rapidly.

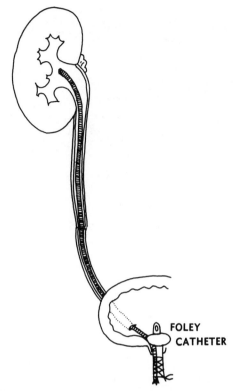

Figure 51.1. A 5 ureteral catheter in place from kidney pelvis into bladder and stabilized exteriorly by a firm tie to a Foley catheter.

After abdominal closure, tie the splinting ureteral catheter to the Foley so as to hold it in position from the kidney down (Fig. 51.1). Do not isolate the ureteral catheter for collection of urine because there will be little drainage—most of the output will pass into the bladder.

Postoperative rules are essential if the compromised ureter is to heal and function normally. Ureteral peristalsis and dilatation tend to push the upper tract catheter down into the bladder; such danger is minimized by keeping the patient in bed for 2 weeks. She must not be allowed head elevation beyond that provided by one pillow. Her back must be straight. However, the patient must be encouraged to move from side to side keeping her legs active. Such patients must *not* be allowed to sit up. Prophylactic anticoagulants and urinary antiseptics, of course, must be maintained.

On the seventh postoperative day, radioopaque material is injected into the upper urinary tract catheter; x-rays will reveal slight hy-

dronephrosis and hydroureter, but there will not be any evidence of leakage at the site of injury.

On the 14th postoperative day, the patient may ambulate after both catheters have been removed. Films taken 3 months after primary surgery will demonstrate normal function and no evidence of a compromised ureter.

2. Treatment of Partial or Complete Ureteral Severance. Ureterovaginal fistulas follow uncorrected injuries. Should a ureter be angulated by a suture which incorporated its wall or be partially or totally cut, as it must be in this case, a fistula will result.

The treatment of choice is immediate ureteroneocystostomy: the ureter, above and below the injury or severance, must be dissected free from its retroperitoneal bed. If the ureter is cut, it should be transected immediately above the injury where the tissue is healthy. The bladder dome is opened sufficiently to allow a clear working space in the trigone. A 2-cm stab incision is made into the trigone near the ureterovesical orifice on the injured side, and, the ureteral catheter is brought into the bladder cavity (Figs. 51.2 and 51.3). At the same time the ureteral cut end, with 00 chromic catgut in each flap of its Y, is brought through its stab incision. The Y flaps are sutured into the full thickness of the bladder wall (Fig. 51.4).

Coiled up ureteral catheter (in the bladder cavity) can then be worked down alongside the Foley catheter. At the close of surgery, the upper tract catheter is then anchored just under the bulb (Fig. 51.5). Care is necessary in order that traction is not applied to the ureteral catheter as it is being tied to the Foley; its tip must remain in the kidney pelvis. The bladder is closed with two layers of plain 0 catgut.

Postoperative care is identical to that described for crushing injuries.

Testing for Ureteral Patency

If one is not certain damage to a ureter has accrued, as encountered in cases of advanced endometriosis and pelvic inflammatory disease, a specific test should be made. These diseases, when long-standing, disfigure the base of the broad ligament, and, in doing so, their dense adhesions obscure the ureter. Dissecting the ureter from this bed is often accompanied by bleeding over a wide retroperitoneal area. Control of the vascular ooze is, at times, difficult. If there is any uncertainty about ureteral

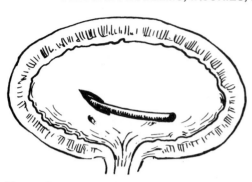

Figure 51.2. Ureteral catheter brought into the bladder through a stab wound near the ureteral orifice on the affected side.

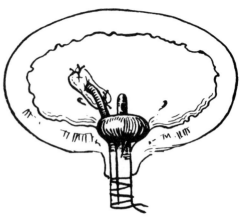

Figure 51.5. Ureteral catheter anchored snuggly to the indwelling Foley catheter.

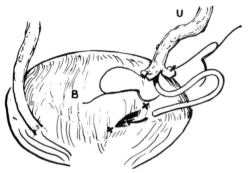

Figure 51.3. Ureteral catheter and cut ureter (*u*) with its Y on 00 chromic catgut sutures brought through the bladder (*B*) stab wound.

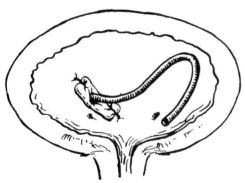

Figure 51.4. Y flaps of ureter sutured into bladder mucosa and muscle.

damage (when the pelvis is ready to be peritonealized) the bladder dome should be opened so the ureteral orifices can be observed while indigo carmine is injected intravenously. If dye is not excreted, an upper urinary tract catheter should be passed. An obstruction or kink will be easily diagnosed, and, if found, regardless of vascular oozing, the ureter must be dissected out. Corrective action, as mentioned above, can then be instituted.

Avoiding Ureteral Injury

Gynecologic surgeons must have a passion for safeguarding the ureter and be alert to the nuances of pelvic vascular structures. In its simplest form, prophylaxis against ureteral injury involves routine hysterectomy (Fig. 51.6).

Traction on a uterine cornual clamp will stretch not only the broad ligament but the ureter as well. Opening the anterior leaf of the broad ligament will usually bring the ureter into view. It is surrounded by loose, avascular fibroconnective tissue. Exposed, the ureter is gently pushed laterally and downward with the finger—*not gauze*—moving it away from the cervix. Doing this while maintaining traction not only safeguards the ureter but delineates the uterine artery more clearly.

Problems with this step in a hysterectomy occur with endometriosis and long-standing inflammatory disease. These diseases often disfigure the area to a point where ureter and uterine artery are not easily distinguishable. Also,

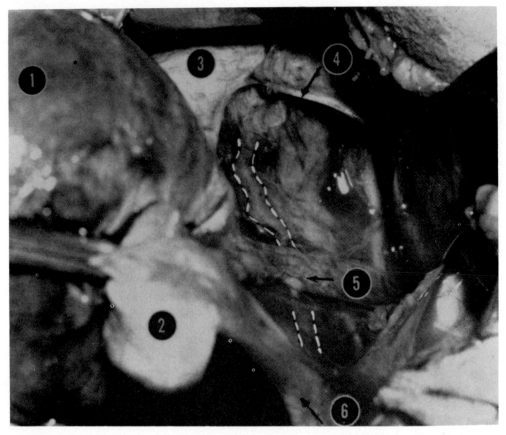

Figure 51.6. *1,* hysterectomy; uterus with fibroid under traction by cornual clamp; *2,* right ovary; *3,* bladder peritoneum; *4,* cut edge of anterior broad ligament peritoneum showing a normal avascular space. The parametrium or transverse cervical ligament, containing the uterine artery is under tension from the traction (*5*); *6,* the infundibulopelvic ligament. The course of the ureter is noted by the *dotted white lines.*

broad ligament or cervical myomas may be large enough to obstruct the surgeon's view and make dissection extremely difficult.

An option, if such problems are anticipated, is to introduce ureteral catheters prior to surgery. Such placement dilates the ureters and makes them easy to feel.

Endometriosis, Stages 2, 3, and 4, involves the posterior leaf of the broad ligament, the uterosacral ligaments, and the posterior cul-de-sac. It is then that the ureters tend to be drawn toward the cervix, thereby making them prone to injury. If ureters are buried in extensive disease and attempts to uncover them are complicated by bleeding, it is wise to pick up the ureter at the pelvic brim—open the posterior peritoneum and dissect it down to the mass of endometriosis. In the course of this dissection,

the uterine artery should be isolated laterally and doubly ligated.

However, in cases of Stage 3 and 4 endometriosis with their cul-de-sacs full of disease, there is another helpful step: After the bladder has been dissected off the cervix, a stab incision is made into the anterior vaginal fornix. Through this vaginal opening a tenaculum is placed on the *posterior cervical lip,* and with firm traction the cervix is pulled away from the cul-de-sac endometriosis. The maneuver tends to move the ureter laterally while defining more clearly the uterine artery and its branches. Next, the posterior vaginal fornix is incised (under tension), and the cervix will come away with minimal bleeding or disturbance to the endometriosis.

Should there be any question about the integrity of the ureter at the completion of dissection, a cystotomy should be done so direct observation of indigo carmine excretion is possible. This is the simplest way to insure an intact upper urinary tract with normal function.

Selected Readings

Beecham CT: Technique of correcting low ureteral injuries. *Clin Obstet Gynecol* 5:549, 1962.

Beecham CT: Classification of endometriosis. *Obstet Gynecol* 28:437, 1966.

Beecham CT, Bates JS: Retroperitoneal endometriosis with ureteral obstruction. *Obstet Gynecol* 34:242, 1969.

Conger KB, Beecham CT, Horrax TM: Ureteral injury in pelvic surgery: Current thought on incidence, pathogenesis, prophylaxis and treatment. *Obstet Gynecol* 3:343, 1954.

CHAPTER 52
Transvaginal Ureteral Transection with Vaginal Hysterectomy and Anterior Colporraphy

JOHN D. THOMPSON, M.D.

CASE ABSTRACT

During the course of a vaginal hysterectomy and rather difficult repair upon a 55-year-old postmenopausal multipara, a loss of urine was evident during the dissection preceding the repair of a very large cystocele.

Although at first a bladder laceration was suspected, instillation of methylene blue through a transurethral catheter was unrewarding. Subsequent intravenous administration of indigo carmine demonstrated obvious leakage, and it was evident that the ureter had been severed near the vesicoureteral junction.

DISCUSSION

Dr. Thomas Green of Boston was fond of saying, "The venial sin is injury to the ureter; the mortal sin is failure of recognition." In the case described above, the urethral injury was promptly recognized. Prompt recognition, preferably at the operation of injury, and prompt repair will provide better results with fewer kidneys lost.

Ureteral injury occurs in approximately 0.25% of gynecologic operations. About two-thirds of these will occur during abdominal procedures and one-third during vaginal procedures. There is a suggestion that the incidence of injury is increasing. Because injury to the ureter can have devestating effects on kidney function, can cause serious illness in the patient, and is a leading cause of malpractice suits against pelvic surgeons, prevention of ureteral injury must be a matter of serious concern. When doing a vaginal hysterectomy, a properly developed vesicocervical space and a retractor placed under the bladder will help elevate the ureter out of harm's way. The ureter can sometimes be palpated in the bladder pillars, which helps in accurate placement of clamps. The bladder pillars should be clamped as separate structures

adjacent to the cervix. This maneuver will allow the ureters to be elevated even more. Only small bites should be taken in paracervical tissue and parametrial tissue adjacent to the cervix. Again, strong traction on the cervix laterally to the side away from the placement of clamps and retraction of the bladder upward will help protect the ureters. Double clamps should not be used when clamping and ligating the cardinal ligaments and uterine vessels. The width of double clamps causes the lateral clamp to be placed too close to the ureter. Blind clamping and mass ligatures to control bleeding should be avoided. And, the gynecologist should be especially "ureter conscious" when doing an anterior colporrhaphy, posterior culdeplasty, and partial vaginectomy (Fig. 52.1). Hofmeister found the sutures are placed as close as 0.9 cm away from the ureter when doing an anterior colporrhaphy. Just why the ureter is not injured more often during the anterior colporrhaphy is a mystery. Ureters are especially susceptible to injury during the posterior culdeplasty technique of McCall. Care should be taken that no culdeplasty suture is placed on the lateral pelvic side wall higher than the uterosacral ligament. If a partial vaginectomy is done with the vaginal hysterectomy (usually for

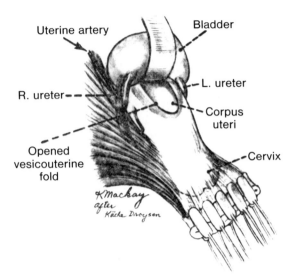

Figure 52.1. This illustration shows relationships between the bladder, ureter, uterus, and uterine artery. Notice the traction on the cervix downward exaggerates the knee of the ureter. This illustration includes partial vaginectomy. Tissues must be separated as close as possible from the vagina, cervix, and uterus in order to avoid injury to the ureter.

carcinoma-in-situ extended to adjacent vaginal fornices), the risk of ureteral injury, in our experience, is increased 23 times to almost 1%. Therefore, this operation requires extreme caution, remembering to release the vaginal cuff completely from the underlying paravaginal tissue before beginning to clamp the bladder pillars and cardinal ligaments. One must also remember that in vaginal surgery, traction is applied to the cervix in a downward direction. As the uterus descends, the ureters are pulled into the operative field by the uterine vessels, and the so-called "knee" of the ureter is exaggerated (Fig. 52.2).

Prompt recognition of all ureteral injuries from vaginal surgery will be possible if routine cytoscopy is carried out at the end of every vaginal hysterectomy and/or anterior colporrhaphy. Before discontinuing the anesthesia, the anesthetist is asked to inject 5 cc of indigo carmine intravenously, the bladder is emptied or urine and refilled with approximately 200 cc of clear sterile saline, and a cystoscope (or other suitable endoscope) is inserted through the urethra. If indigo carmine is seen effluxing from both ureteral orifices, it may be assumed that ureteral injury has not occurred. This procedure generally adds about 5 minutes to the operating time. It can yield valuable information about the patient and give a gynecologist a great sense of comfort.

When ureteral injury is discovered intraoperatively during a vaginal procedure, repair may be done transvaginally or transabdominally.

When a simple transection of the ureter close to the vesicoureteral junction is present, the author's preference is for transvaginal ureteroneocystostomy. There are advantages to a transvaginal approach. For example, the ureter should be reimplanted into the bladder as close

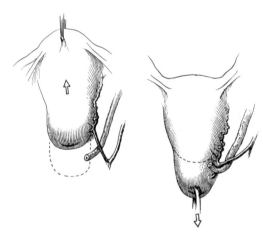

Figure 52.2. The relationship of the ureter to the uterine artery during hysterectomy. The *dotted line* represents a usual position of the uterus. In the drawing on the *left*, the relationship between the uterine artery and the ureter is shown when upward traction is applied to the uterine fundus as in abdominal hysterectomy. The drawing on the *right* demonstrates the change in this relationship when downward traction is applied as during vaginal hysterectomy. Reprinted with permission from Nichols DH, Randall CL: *Vaginal Surgery*, ed. 2. Baltimore, Williams & Wilkins, 1983.

to the bladder base as possible. When doing the ureteroneocystostomy transvaginally, the bladder base is the only part of the bladder available for reimplantation. The best site can be identified by placing an instrument into the bladder. A small incision is made through the bladder muscle and mucosa. The reimplantation must be done without tension on the suture line. This is an extremely important point in achieving a successful result. If necessary, the ureter can be carefully dissected free of its attachments superiorly in order to provide a tension-free anastomosis. The author's preference is for the use of a small-caliber plastic indwelling catheter as a stent. The stent is inserted through the urethra into the bladder, out through cystostomy incision, and then passed up the ureter to the kidney (Fig. 52.3). The damaged end of the ureter is excised. The ureteral lumen is enlarged. Two sutures of 4-0 Vicryl are placed on each side of the end of the ureter and then placed through the bladder mucosa and muscularis from the inside to the outside (Fig. 52.4). When these sutures are tied, the ureter will be drawn into the bladder. The sutures should be placed and tied in such a way that the ureter is not twisted. The anastomosis is reinforced with sutures that approximate the muscularis of the bladder and perivesical fat over the lower ureter. This will strengthen and protect the site of reimplantation and will also decrease the possibility of reflux. A bulbocavernosus fat flap may also be used to protect the reimplantation site, but this is usually not nec-

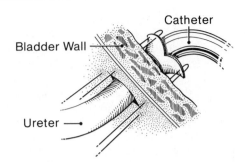

Figure 52.4. Two sutures of 4-0 Vicryl are placed each side of the end of the spatulated ureter and sewn through the bladder mucosa and muscularis. When tied, the ureter will be drawn into the bladder as shown.

essary. These tissues must not cause obstruction by compressing the ureter too tightly. A continuous locked suture is placed in the vaginal edge for hemostasis. The vaginal vault is lightly packed and left open. The ureteral stent is tied tightly at the external urethral meatus to an indwelling Foley catheter in the bladder. Each is connected to a collection bottle. The vaginal pack is removed in approximately 24 hours.

The ureteral stent is irrigated to maintain patency. It is allowed to remain in place for 10 to 14 days before removal. An intravenous pyelogram (IVP) is done before discharge and at any subsequent time the patient's symptoms suggest ureteral obstruction. Otherwise, an IVP and voiding cystourethrogram (VCUG) should be done about 2 to 3 months postoperatively.

If routine cystoscopy at the completion of vaginal hysterectomy with or without repair should reveal absence of efflux of dye from one ureter, then an attempt should be made to pass a catheter up that ureter. If an obstruction is demonstrated, the ureteral catheter should be left in place while the ureter is dissected free to locate the obstruction. Usually, a suture will be found. If a suture is found adjacent to the ureter so that it is sharply bent, the suture may be removed and the catheter can be passed beyond the obstruction. If a suture is found around or through the ureter, deligation should be performed. Then, the damaged ureteral tissue should be removed and a ureteroureterostomy performed utilizing a stent. About four 6-0 Vicryl sutures will be sufficient to accomplish the anastomosis. Simple deligation should not be relied on if the suture has been tied around the

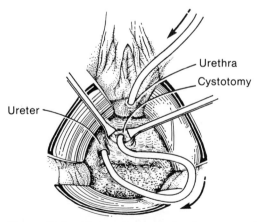

Figure 52.3. The urethral stent has been inserted through the urethra into the bladder, out the cystotomy incision, and passed up the ureter.

ureter or passed through the ureter and tied.

There are circumstances under which one should abandon or not attempt transvaginal repair. If, for some unusual reason, the ureteroneocystostomy cannot be done without tension, then the transvaginal approach should be abandoned in favor of an abdominal technique that will allow the anastomosis to be done without tension. If one is dealing with indurated or irradiated tissue, dissection to locate and free the ureter and repair the damage may be difficult. Certainly, the author is aware of no circumstances under which it would be proper to solve a ureteral injury problem by simply tying off the ureter vaginally without attempting a repair. It would also not be proper to wait for several weeks before attempting repair. A stenosis of the ureteral lumen at the site of injury with obstruction and impairment of kidney function will occur within a short time. This can usually be avoided if a proper repair is done promptly.

Selected Readings

Everett SH, Mattingly RF: Urinary tract injuries resulting from pelvic surgery. *Am J Obstet Gynecol* 71:502, 1956.

Flynn JT, Tiptaft RC, Woodhouse CR, et al: The early and aggressive repair of iatrogenic ureteric injuries. *Br J Urol* 51:454, 1979.

Fry DE, Milholen L, Harbrecht PJ: Iatrogenic ureteral injury: Options in management. *Arch Surg* 118:454,1983.

Hofmeister FJ: Pelvic anatomy of the ureter in relation to surgery performed through the vagina. *Clin Obstet Gynecol* 25:821, 1982.

Kaye KW, Goldberg ME: Applied anatomy of the kidney and ureter. *Urol Clin North Am* 9:3, 1982.

Mattingly RF, Thompson JD: *TeLinda's Operative Gynecology,* 6th ed. Philadelphia, JB Lippincott, 1985, Chap. 14.

Nichols DH, Randall CL: *Vaginal Surgery,* ed. 2. Baltimore, Williams & Wilkins, 1983.

Symmonds RE: Current concepts in gynecologic surgery. *Clin Obstet Gynecol* 19:619, 1976.

Thompson JD, Benigno BB: Vaginal repair of ureteral injuries. *Am J Obstet Gynecol* 3:601, 1971.

Van Nagell JR Jr, Roddick JR Jr: Vaginal hysterectomy, the ureter and excretory urography. *Obstet Gynecol* 39:784, 1972.

CHAPTER 53

Unilateral Postoperative Ureteral Obstruction

DAVID H. NICHOLS, M.D.

CASE ABSTRACT

A vaginal hysterectomy and repair were performed on a 43-year-old multipara to relieve a symptomatic genital prolapse. Each elongated uterosacral ligament was shortened about 1 inch and attached to the vaginal vault early in the operation. Following the hysterectomy, the ligaments were brought together in the midline by still another polyglycolic acid (Dexon) stitch placed beneath the vagina and posterior to the site of peritoneal closure. On the morning of the second postoperative day, the patient complained of pain in the right flank, and tenderness was demonstrated in the right costovertebral angle. The patient experienced emesis. Bowel sounds were present though hypoactive. The patient was afebrile. An infusion intravenous pyelogram was performed immediately, which demonstrated a normal collecting system on the left side, but appearance of the dye was delayed 10 minutes on the patient's right side where a mild hydronephrosis and hydroureter with obstruction 3 to 4 cm from the ureterovesical junction were evident (Fig. 53.1). There were no positive findings on abdominal palpation.

DISCUSSION

Unilateral costovertebral tenderness in an afebrile postoperative patient is indicative of ureteral obstruction until proven otherwise. In the above instance, the obstruction was probably produced by ureteral kinking from the final but misdirected uterosacral ligament suture. Presence of the radiopaque dye in a dilated ureter suggests incomplete obstruction, as some urinary fluid flow is necessary to convey the dye into the ureter. Pain appearing on the second postoperative day instead of the first suggests obstruction due to postsurgical edema and kinking of the ureter as from periureteral suture placement, rather than occlusion by a suture placed through or around the ureter. The absence of chills and fever speaks against a pyelonephritis.

Postoperative ureteral obstruction may be either "silent" or symptomatic and, if unrelieved, may result in ureterovaginal fistula, pyelonephritis, or destruction of the kidney. With ultimate absorption of the suture the obstruction may undergo spontaneous resolution. Renal atrophy or fistula formation is more common with complete obstruction, while ascending bacteria from an incomplete obstruction may result in acute pyelonephritis.

In the author's view, the costovertebral angles of every pelvic surgical patient should be palpated the evening of the day of surgery and any *unilateral* accentuation of pain promptly investigated. A diagnosis of possible postoperative ureteral obstruction should be confirmed or excluded by infusion pyelography as soon as it is suspected. If early in the postoperative period, the usual gastrointestinal preparation may be waived and a single intravenous injection of contrast material given; to be followed by 5-, 10-, and 20-minute radiographs, interpreted immediately. If the diagnosis of obstruction is confirmed, it should be promptly relieved by passage of a splinting ureteral catheter or, failing this, deligation or ureteroneocystotomy, or percutaneous nephrostomy (4, 5) 2 or 3 days later if a catheter still cannot be passed. If a catheter cannot be

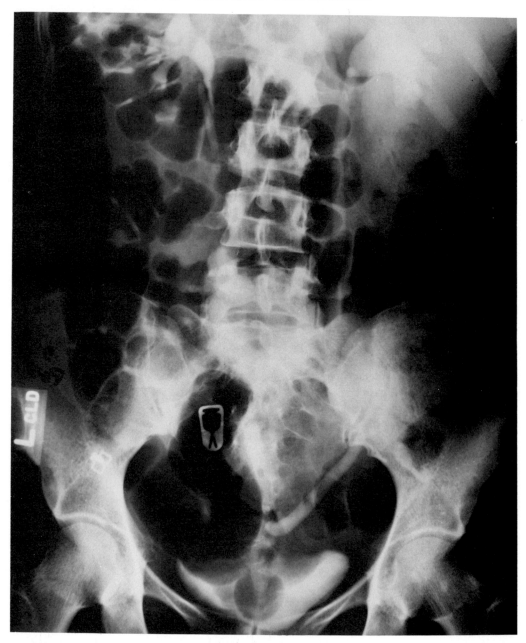

Figure 53.1. Postoperative infusion intravenous pyelogram (IVP) showing dilation of right ureter with medial displacement and obstruction near the vault of the vagina.

passed initially, the ureter is more likely occluded than kinked, with more ominous prognosis. Delay only risks compounding the problem by increasing local edema and the possibility of upper urinary infection, further lessening the chance of successful subsequent passage of a splinting ureteral catheter.

The simplest treatment is prompt cystoscopic placement of a splinting ureteral catheter. The 25-cm 6F pigtail (1–3) stent is a good size and choice for the average adult female (Maynard JF: personal communication), although a range of sizes from which to choose should be available. It should be left in place until there has been adequate time for suture absorption. The length of time depends upon the type of suture material that was used in the primary procedure—in the range of 2 weeks for catgut and 1 to 2 months for polyglycolic acid type suture. The pigtail catheter is a plastic "with a memory" having a coil at each end. Using a stilette, it is placed with one end inserted into the renal pelvis and the other into the bladder. The catheter has multiple perforations through its wall to insure adequate drainage. When the estimated time of suture absorption has been reached, and excretory urography shows no evidence of obstructive uropathy, the catheter may be easily removed through an operating cystoscope by an endoscopic forceps in the hands of an experienced cystoscopist.

In the patient described in the abstract, a pigtail catheter was placed endoscopically the day the obstruction was diagnosed, relieving the obstruction. The patient was discharged on the eighth postoperative day, and the catheter was removed uneventfully through the cystoscope in an ambulatory facility several weeks later. The subsequent follow-up intravenous pyelogram was normal.

References

1. Hepperlen TW, Mardis HK, Kammandel H: Self-retained internal ureteral stents: A new approach. *J Urol* 119:731, 1978.
2. Hepperlen TW, Mardis HK, Kammandel H: The pigtail ureteral stent in the cancer patient. *J Urol* 121:17, 1979.
3. Mardis HK, Hepperlen TW, Kammandel H: Double pigtail ureteral stent. *Urology* 14:23, 1979.
4. Mazer MJ: Permanent percutaneous antegrade ureteral stent placement without transureteral assistance. *Urology* 14:413, 1979.
5. Rutner AB, Fucilla I: Percutaneous pigtail nephrostomy. *Urology* 14:337, 1979.

CHAPTER **54**

Stitch Penetration of Bladder at Vaginal Hysterectomy and Repair

GEORGE W. MITCHELL, JR., M.D.
FREDDY M. MASSEY, M.D.

CASE ABSTRACT

A 70-year-old para 2 with symptomatic second degree prolapse received a vaginal hysterectomy and repair. Although the urine was clear at the conclusion of the surgical procedure, it was bloody on the first postoperative day. There was no flank pain, examination of the costovertebral angles was negative, and the patient was afebrile. Cystoscopy failed to demonstrate obvious laceration, showing only considerable edema of the base of the bladder. Although an intravenous pyelogram (IVP) was negative, the hematuria persisted.

DISCUSSION

Following a vaginal hysterectomy, with or without repair, it is customary to insert either a suprapubic or urethral catheter and to observe whether or not the urine that has accumulated during the procedure is clear. If the urine is examined microscopically, it will invariably show red blood cells, since this operation always causes some trauma to the bladder wall. When the urine is pink, it is probable that no serious injury has occurred, but, depending upon what has transpired during the operation, the surgeon may wish to reassure himself by cystoscopy or by filling the bladder through the catheter to make sure that is is competent. Microscopic hematuria ordinarily persists for several days, but grossly bloody urinary drainage immediately following surgery, or occurring secondarily, is a sure sign that something is amiss, and investigation without delay is essential.

Hematuria occurring as a result of pyelonephritis is most unusual unless there has been partial occlusion of one of the ureters, and even then it is unlikely before the third of fourth postoperative day. In its full-blown form, pyelonephritis is associated with flank pain, chills, fever, anorexia, and general malaise, and a urine culture will be positive unless the ureter has been completely occluded. In the case under discussion, none of the classic signs and symptoms was present, and, because of the sequence of events, it was logical to conclude that the hematuria occurring on the first postoperative day was the result of direct injury to the bladder, with an outside possibility of some previously unsuspected occult intrinsic lesion in the bladder.

An IVP is the most appropriate test of ureteral patency and renal function in the postoperative phase, and this should be done prior to cystoscopy so that during the latter procedure the condition of the ureters is known and appropriate steps to determine the location and degree of injury to the ureters may be taken. The condition of the bladder should be checked with a cystoscopic instrument having a lens set at an angle of 30 to 45 degrees so that the recesses of the organ may be easily seen. The urethra should be checked with a panendoscope, with the water or carbon dioxide running constantly to give the necessary distension. Rinsing the bladder several times may be necessary to evaluate clots and achieve adequate visualization. Clots tend to adhere to damaged areas or to stitches that have been placed through the bladder wall to the mucosal side, and they must be displaced with jets of water or a clot evacuator so that the extent of the damage can be accurately evaluated.

Few surgeons use nonabsorbable suture material for vaginal hysterectomy and repair, but some continue to place silk sutures at the urethrovesical neck, in accordance with the Kelly tradition. Nonabsorbable suture material is more commonly used for suprapubic suspension of the vesical neck, as in the Marshall-Marchetti-Krantz operation, or the Burch modification. When nonabsorbable sutures have been used and a stitch penetrates the bladder or urethra, it should show up well at cystoscopy because of its color. Such a stitch can sometimes be cut transvesically or transurethrally, and, with a little luck, it may retract out of the lumen, especially if a suprapubic suspension has been done. Failing that, an attempt should be made to pull the suture out after cutting it, and if this is also unsuccessful, a retroperitoneal suprapubic cystostomy may be necessary to remove the offending ligature. Leaving such a foreign body in situ causes intractable cystitis and eventual stone formation.

Absorbable suture materials, such as catgut or those made with polyglycolic acid, which have penetrated the bladder wall are more difficult to identify. Fine catgut sutures in the range from 2-0 to 3-0, with a life expectancy of 14 to 21 days, can probably be left in situ, unless they encompass enough tissue to produce significant necrosis. Such sutures may cause the symptoms of bladder infection but usually will not remain in the lumen long enough to give rise to late side-effects, such as stone formation. Heavier catgut suture material of the kind ordinarily used for ligation of the major vascular pedicles during vaginal hysterectomy or polyglycolic acid sutures should be cut and an attempt made to remove them as in the case of nonabsorbable suture material, the implication being that the heavier suture has been used for heavy duty and, in addition to its longer life potential, probably incorporates a larger amount of necrotic tissue.

A laceration of the bladder should be repaired intraoperatively as soon as it is diagnosed, the only problem being that the surgeon must be certain that no portion of the ureter is included in the repair. Closure should be in two layers, with continuous fine plain or chromic catgut encompassing the submucosa and the inner muscular layer, and continuous chromic catgut or polyglycolic acid suture in the outer muscular layer in the same plane. Injuries of this kind most commonly occur when the bladder is being mobilized from the anterior surface of the cervical isthmus. When this dissection is accomplished only with difficulty, the competency of the bladder should be tested at once by the transurethral introduction of some easily identified fluid like sterile milk, which does not stain the operative field, or methylene blue.

When a surgical laceration escapes detection and is discovered postoperatively by cystoscopy, there are two possible courses of action. The majority of minor lacerations will close spontaneously if the bladder is kept on constant drainage, and bleeding will usually stop. The indwelling catheter should be irrigated at least twice daily, or at any time when the flow of urine slows or stops, because of the possibility of its being plugged with blood clots. To avoid distention, no more than 30 to 50 cc of irrigating fluid should be injected. A hanging bottle of saline connected to a two-way catheter, forming a closed system, is best for this purpose. The indwelling catheter should remain for at least 2 weeks to allow good healing. If a small amount of bleeding continues but no fistula develops, the lacerated area can be superficially fulgurated cystoscopically. This method is occasionally used by urologists for the closure of tiny vesicovaginal fistulas. Larger lacerations that sometimes occur during morcellation to remove a larger uterus vaginally are usually discovered during surgery but, if not, should be repaired postoperatively by a suprapubic transvesical approach.

Whenever doubt exists about the possibility of bladder injury during surgery, continuous urinary drainage should be instituted and continued for longer than the usual 5 days. There is no harm in explaining to the patient that this is a safety precaution, necessary because unexpected problems were encountered during surgery.

CHAPTER **55**

Bladder Management at Postpartum Hysterectomy

R. CLAY BURCHELL, M.D.

CASE ABSTRACT

A para 5 at term was admitted in precipitate labor and birth ensued 1 hour later. Moderate vaginal bleeding began postpartum and continued, despite massage of the uterus, oxytocics, and normal blood-clotting studies. In view of the diagnosis of uterine atony and the patient's parity, the decision was made after 2 hours to perform hysterectomy. At this time, the estimated postpartum blood loss was 600 to 800 cc.

When the bladder peritoneum was opened after the upper pedicles were ligated, it was considered virtually impossible to separate the bladder from the lower uterine segment because of large varices (1 cm in diameter) on the bladder and the uterus.

DISCUSSION

This patient presents a dilemma for the operating surgeon. She obviously needs a hysterectomy and the operation is partially completed. A total hysterectomy, the most desirable procedure, appears to be difficult, dangerous, or impossible to perform. This is a recurrent problem with cesarean or postpartum hysterectomy. There is often a marked dilation of veins on the lower uterine segment and on the bladder, particularly with multiparous patients. If these veins are torn, massive bleeding will result, yet it seems almost impossible to separate the tissues without tearing the veins.

Every obstetrician has noted the distention of veins on the anterior portion of the lower uterine segment at cesarean section. If these veins are observed carefully it will be noted that there is less distention following birth of the baby. In a study, it was found that venous pressure varied between 30 and 3 cm of water (Burchell, unpublished data). High pressures between 18 and 30 cm. of water were observed before birth and pressures usually fell to approximately 3 cm of water after delivery.

Nevertheless, there is a good surgical solution if the operator possesses the required *knowledge* and *skill*. The specific operative ability required is based on the utilization of sharp dissection and a knowledge of bladder anatomy (4). This operative ability is not ordinarily required in obstetrics and gynecology so that it may not have been previously developed. Sharp dissection is best learned at an operation on a nonpregnant patient when there is no emergency. Detailed knowledge of the anatomy in this area is also necessary. The tissue layers between the cavity of the bladder and the cavity of the uterus are: bladder mucosa, bladder muscularis, arteries and veins, endopelvic fascia, arteries and veins of the uterus, either uterine myometrium or cervical stroma depending upon the specific area, and finally the endometrium or the endocervical glands (Fig. 55.1A).

The endopelvic fascia (vesicouterine or vesicocervical in this area) is always interspersed between veins of bladder and uterus, providing a potential cleavage plane. This fascia appears as a loose areolar tissue condensed in some areas so as to essentially form ligaments (5, 6). This tissue is easily dissected by blunt dissection in the nonpregnant patient.

All tissues are more friable in pregnancy so that if large veins are present they will tear more easily than the fascia will separate. Hence, blunt dissection in the pregnant patient is likely to

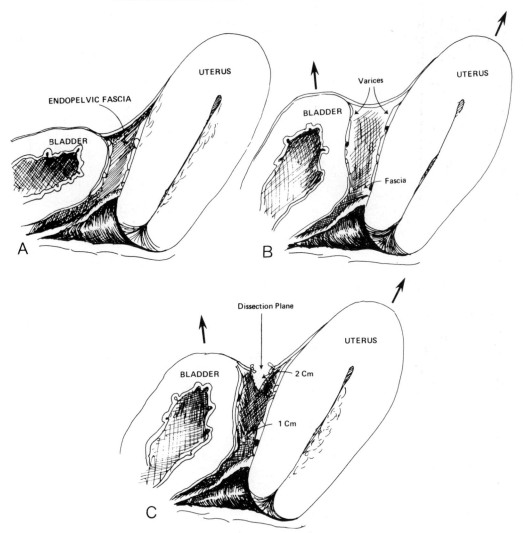

Figure 55.1. *A.* The endopelvic fascia is interspersed between the veins on the surface of the bladder and uterus. *B.* Traction on the bladder and uterus in tangential directions places the peritoneum on stretch so it can be sharply dissected. *C.* The fascial plane is wider (2 cm) and less dense near the fundus than close to the cervix (1 cm). There is always a bloodless cleavage plane for sharp dissection.

produce a cleavage plane through the venous plexus rather than in the natural fascial plane. Obviously this results in massive hemorrhage!

Dissection

For sharp dissection, traction is placed on the uterus in the direction of the patient's head. Traction is placed on the bladder at a 45 degree angle so that the vesicouterine peritoneum and fascia are placed on stretch and hence easily visualized (Fig. 55.1*B*). It is mandatory to grasp the bladder walls in order to complete

this step. The main cause of injury and failure with sharp dissection is the operator's reluctance to grasp the bladder with an instrument that will not slip (toothed forceps, for example). With traction on both uterus and bladder, the endopelvic fascia will extend for a distance of approximately 2 cm between the organs (Fig. 55.1*C*). It is technically easy to sharply incise the fascial tissue with scissors by cutting *halfway* between the two organs. Even if there are large varices present, the operator can incise *halfway* between bladder and uterine veins, completing virtually bloodless dissection.

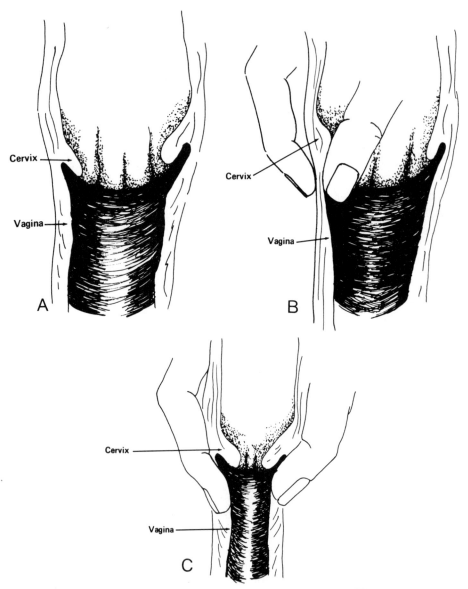

Figure 55.2. *A*. The cervix is always thicker than the vaginal wall. *B*. The cervix can be palpated with one finger inside and one finger outside the vagina. *C*. The cervix can also be palpated with both fingers outside the vagina.

As the dissection proceeds, the width of the fascial plane will diminish and the tissue will become more condensed. In the area of the internal os of the cervix, the distance between bladder and cervix is less than 1 cm and the fascial tissue is condensed into the so-called vesicocervical ligament. Nevertheless, there is always a space for bloodless sharp dissection if the operator has sufficient skill.

To remove the entire cervix (sometimes a problem with cesarean or postpartum hysterectomy) the dissection is carried to a point inferior to the cervix. Even a totally effaced cervix can be identified by either one of two methods. Both depend upon the fact that the cervix is always thicker than the vaginal wall (Fig. 55.2*A*). In one method the operator places a thumb in the vagina and a forefinger outside the vagina at a level below the cervix. If the fingers are approximated with some pressure and moved superiorly, an obstruction will be felt when the cervix is reached, no matter how well effaced it is (Fig. 55.2*B*). The other method is to place thumb and forefingers on the outside of the vagina anteriorly and posteriorly and repeat the same process (Fig. 55.2*C*).

Other Considerations

There are several other considerations with cesarean or postpartum hysterectomy. Sometimes there is marked vaginal bleeding from the vaginal cuff. This is seldom encountered in the nonpregnant patient. Bleeding can be controlled by placing ring clamps on the cuff. They are highly desirable in this situation because they compress a fairly large area, are gentle to tissues, and will not tear through. Clamps with teeth on them should not be used to control hemorrhage with friable tissues as they will only increase the hemorrhage by tearing the tissue. In cases where the bleeding is particularly severe, the vaginal cuff can be immediately sutured as it is incised. These sutures can be fairly broad, extending 1 cm or more, but one should take great pains to insure that there is no space between the individual figure-of-eight sutures.

Another consideration is whether a supracervical hysterectomy should ever be done. There is no doubt that the removal of the uterus, leaving the cervix intact, does avoid some of the difficulties with dissection of the bladder and may be necessary in rare instances. However, there are cogent reasons why the cervix should be removed. If the cervix remains there is danger of infection and subsequent pathology. If the operator has the surgical skill to remove the cervix, it can be done with very little difficulty.

Another consideration is the desirability of intraoperative internal iliac artery ligation. Iliac ligation is possible, sometimes desirable, and, rarely, even necessary, with cesarean or postpartum hysterectomy (2). It should not be done prophylactically or *routinely* because to do so would be unnecessary and will not necessarily prevent massive venous bleeding. The collateral circulation is so abundant in the human female that there can be considerable bleeding, even after iliac ligation (1). However, if bleeding cannot be controlled by conventional means, iliac ligation may be lifesaving.

In summary, cesarean or postpartum hysterectomy is a formidable procedure because of the threat of hemorrhage and the apparent difficulty with bladder management. Bladder dissection is the most difficult aspect of the entire operation because it is the major source of hemorrhage. This difficulty is easily overcome if the operator possesses the prerequisite knowledge of bladder anatomy and the skill and courage to sharply dissect the bladder even with dilated veins. With this knowledge and skill (best learned previously when there is no emergency), the operating surgeon presented with the patient described in this abstract will never doubt his or her ability to proceed with the operation.

References

1. Burchell RC: Arterial physiology of the human female patient. *Obstet Gynecol* 31:855, 1968.
2. Burchell RC: Internal iliac artery ligation: A series of 200 patients. *Int J Obstet Gynecol* 7:85, 1969.
3. Burchell RC, Mengert WF: Etiology of premature separation of the normally implanted placenta. *Am J Obstet Gynecol* 104:795, 1969.
4. Nichols DH, Milley PS: Clinical anatomy of the vulva, vagina, lower pelvis and perineum in gynecology and obstetrics. In Sciarra (ed): *Gynecology and Obstetrics*, Vol. 1. Hagerstown, MD, Harper & Row, 1977, pp. 1–16.
5. Range RL, Woodburne RT: The gross and microscopic anatomy of the transverse cervical ligament. *Am J Obstet Gynecol* 90:460, 1964.
6. von Peham H, Amreich J: *Operative Gynecology*, Vol. 1. Philadelphia, JB Lippincott, 1934, pp. 166–197.

CHAPTER **56**

Large Myomata Uteri and Stress Urinary Incontinence

RICHARD F. MATTINGLY, M.D.

CASE ABSTRACT

Hysterectomy had been recommended to a 45-year-old patient with a large, symptomatic fibroid uterus-that extended halfway to the umbilicus. The patient was a heavy smoker with coexistent chronic bronchitis and severe and socially disturbing stress urinary incontinence. The diagnosis was confirmed on pelvic examination, at which time Some obvious rotational descent of the bladder neck was noted. A Marshall test was positive, and urodynamic studies showed no evidence of neurogenic bladder dysfunction.

DISCUSSION

Coexisting disease processes are common to the female reproductive tract. Since uterine myomata occur in 30% to 40% of the adult female population, one might expect to encounter many women who have this anatomic abnormality of the uterus and, at the same time, have protrusion of the bladder base and posterior urethra through a widened levator muscle hiatus and a weakened urogenital diaphragm. The clinical symptoms that accompany a myomatous uterus and a cystourethrocele include an increasing degree of pelvic pressure, abnormalities in the cyclicity and amount of menstrual flow, and the presence of socially disabling stress urinary incontinence. While the clinical manifestations of these two entities may occur separately and independent of one disease process or another, when both entities are progressively symptomatic, the treatment requires individualized consideration and coordination of the surgical approach. It is uncommon that a large myomatous uterus will compress the ureters at the pelvic brim, similiar to a gravid uterus, and produce partial ureteral obstruction. Such a complication is a compelling indication for hysterectomy. Similiarly, pain caused by a degenerating (carneous) myoma occurs rarely and should not be used as a common indication for surgery.

Anatomic Considerations

The relationship of the bladder base to the lower uterine segment is usually quite typical when dealing with an enlarged uterus caused by myomata. In the case of the enlarged uterus with multiple myomata, the reflection of the bladder peritoneum (anterior cul-de-sac) onto the lower uterine segment and the location of the bladder base and trigone adjacent to the cervix and anterior vaginal fornix remain unaltered. As a consequence, bladder symptoms of urinary frequency and urgency are uncommon in patients with a myomatous uterus. However, when the anterior wall of the uterine fundus is greatly distorted by the presence of these benign tumors, there can be pressure against the bladder that causes urinary frequency. Also, it should be emphasized that the presence of anatomic stress urinary incontinence has no etiologic relationship to the uterine enlargement due to leiomyomata. The anatomic changes in the levator ani muscles and urogenital diaphragm occur separately from the enlargement of the uterus from myomata.

The basic physiologic defects that occur in a patient with the combined problem of a large myomatous uterus and disabling stress urinary incontinence are usually unrelated one to the other. The rare instance in which a large subserous myoma protrudes beneath the base of the bladder is the exception to this rule. In such cases, the symptoms of gradually increasing urinary frequency and nocturia may be sufficiently troublesome to warrant hysterectomy because of bladder symptoms alone. However, stress urinary incontinence has its own etiologic factors that can usually be demonstrated as a result of a generalized relaxation of the pelvic diaphragm, which produces both a cystocele and a rectocele. These anatomic changes are components of a hernia in the musculofascial support of the pelvic floor. Based on a proper understanding of these pathophysiologic events, the surgical treatment of these two entities must be approached as separate clinical problems.

Clinical Symptoms

Although uncommon, some women who have a uterus which is greatly enlarged and distorted by the presence of multiple myomata may be entirely asymptomatic. In such cases, these tumors may be carefully examined, documented to be confined to the uterus, and followed conservatively. Only if these tumors enlarge rapidly or gradually produce the characteristic symptoms of this disease do they require surgical removal. Classically, the most common symptom that requires the surgical removal of a large myomatous uterus is related to abnormal uterine bleeding. Enlargement of the uterine cavity causes an increase in endometrial surface area and an increase in the amount of menstrual bleeding. The average menstrual egress of 50 to 75 cc per cycle may increase to more than 200 or 300 cc in association with a very large uterine cavity. In the rare instance (0.5%) of sarcomatous change in the uterine myoma, the bleeding pattern can be very abnormal or produce no symptoms at all. Currently, it is possible to document uterine size by ultrasound measurement with relative accuracy. This study can be repeated at 6-month to 1-year intervals and can provide reasonable assurance of tumor size, which is poorly documented by pelvic examination and bimanual examination of the uterus.

The pressure symptoms of myomata uteri occur late in the growth cycle of these tumors. While the adjacent bladder may be associated with pressure symptoms, as has been previously discussed, the rectosigmoid colon rarely undergoes sufficient external pressure from an enlarged uterus to produce symptoms of constipation. Only in the occasional patient with an enlarged, incarcerated myoma in the cul-de-sac will the rectosigmoid colon undergo partial compression sufficient to produce bowel symptoms. Since constipation is not a common symptom of this uterine abnormality, the patient should not be counseled to the effect that a hysterectomy will produce relief of this type of chronic bowel dysfunction.

Historically, we have held to the dictum that the upper urinary track is not altered by the presence of large uterine myomata. However, this position has been changed in recent years since assessment of the urinary track has been performed frequently as a preoperative procedure. Silent ureteral obstruction at the pelvic brim can occur but is an uncommon finding in association with large myomata. When present, it is the result of a more symmetrically enlarged uterus where the posterior uterine wall presses directly against the posterior aspect of the pelvic inlet and sacral promontory, similiar to the physiologic enlargement of the gravid uterus. Ureteral dilation alone provides sufficient indication for hysterectomy despite the fact that no other symptom may exist. When hydronephrosis persists for an extended period of time, progressive blunting and irreversible deformity of the pyelocalyceal junction may lead to permanent renal damage. In most instances, however, brief periods of external ureteral pressure and partial obstruction at the pelvic brim do not produce lasting urinary tract abnormalities following hysterectomy.

Pelvic pain is not a significant feature of a myomatous uterus. Only in the rare instance of localized interstitial hemorrhage, such as that which may occur in pregnancy (carneous degeneration), is the symptom of pelvic pain a clinical finding. It is particularly puzzling to find a large subserous myoma that has undergone parasitic attachment to the vascular omentum without an apparent pelvic symptom during complete separation from the uterine masculature. If a patient is seen with serious pelvic pain, the gynecologist would do well to consider the adnexa, rather than the uterus, as the primary source of this aggravating symptom.

One of the most distressing sequelae of advancing age in a female is the progressive loss of urinary control that results from relaxation of the musculofascial support of the pelvic diaphragm. While the symptoms of stress urinary incontinence may be infrequent initally, the problem becomes more troublesome with advancing age and increasing parity. The symptoms become disabling when the patient is required to wear a perineal pad for protection at all times. This sudden, precipitous loss of urine that is associated with intra-abdominal pressure changes, such as coughing, sneezing, laughing, and sudden changes in body position, may be confused with the symptoms of urinary frequency and urgency in the presence of a large myomatous uterus. Such cases may suggest the occurrence of both an anatomic and a neurogenic bladder dysfunction. These conflicting symptoms may be accurately assessed by both cystometric and urodynamic pressure studies of the bladder and urethra. Such studies are important in determining the appropriate surgical approach to these disease entities.

Diagnostic Studies

Not infrequently, the question is asked as to the indication for hysterectomy for an asymptomatic patient with myomata uteri, based on uterine size alone. Speaking frankly, there is no uniform answer to this question. However, there is general agreement among experienced clinicians that an asymptomatic, myomatous uterus should be removed when there has been sufficient enlargement to obscure the clinical evaluation of either adnexa. Regrettably, some surgeons have interpreted this axiom quite loosely and have removed uteri that contain very small tumors. Prior to performing a hysterectomy for small, asymptomatic myomata, it would be well for the gynecologist to balance the risks of the surgical mortality of a hysterectomy (0.1% to 0.2%) and the inadvertent injury to the urinary tract and bowel (1% to 2%) with the rare occurrence of sarcomatous degeneration of a myoma (0.5%). On balance, the combined mortality and serious complication rates of a hysterectomy in the 1980s far exceed the minimal risk of the patient dying from malignant degeneration of a myoma. However, when the risk of an ovarian malignancy enters into the consideration of pelvic surgery, the clinical risks are different. Since ovarian carcinoma is the most lethal of all gynecologic cancers, with less than 30% overall 5-year survival, due principally to late diagnosis, a more aggressive surgical approach is indicated when adnexal pathology cannot be clearly differentiated from uterine myomata.

Having determined that the patient has clear indications for an abdominal hysterectomy, what diagnosis criteria are important in the selection of a surgical procedure that will also correct the anatomic deformity of the pelvic diaphragm and will relieve the patient's symptoms of stress urinary incontinence? In making this clinical decision, it is essential to determine that one is dealing specifically with anatomic stress incontinence and not a neurogenic dysfunction of the bladder. This differential diagnosis is not always easy. A careful history is essential to make certain of the specific type of bladder dysfunction. Urinary urgency and urge incontinence are commonly associated with an irritating lesion somewhere in the urinary tract. Therefore, a complete urologic study should be made in such circumstances, including an intravenous pyelogram, water cystoscopy, and a cystometric study of the bladder contractile pattern. Depending on these findings, a urethral pressure profile and urodynamic studies may be useful if there is still uncertainty as to the precise cause of the incontinence.

The more simplistic method of diagnosing a relaxed vaginal outlet, including descensus of the bladder neck and posterior urethra, is by pelvic examination. With the bladder partially filled, one can easily demonstrate the instantaneous loss of urine with coughing and straining, both in the supine and in the erect position. By the simple technique of elevating the posterior urethra to a more normal retropubic position with pressure of the examining fingers on either side of the urethra, the stress incontinence should be controlled. It is important to emphasize the time sequence of the intra-abdominal pressure and the loss of urine from the urethra. In true anatomic stress incontinence, the urinary loss occurs immediately following the intra-abdominal pressure. If there is a delay in the loss of urine by approximately 10 to 20 seconds following the intra-abdominal pressure, the possibility of a neurogenic bladder must be considered. Clinically, the degree of posterior rotation of the urethra and bladder base can be identified by the relationship of the urethra to the axis of the symphysis pubis. By inserting a catheter into the urethra and bladder or by the placement of a sterile Q-tip into the bladder, one can determine the degree of displacement of the posterior urethra with the axis of the symphysis pubis. (Fig. 56.1). Although this is a very gross clinical test for determining

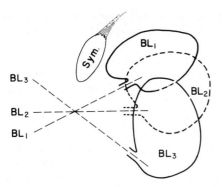

Figure 56.1. Relationship of urethra and bladder base to the axis of the symphysis pubis. BL_1 illustrates normal angle of inclination (10 to 30 degrees); BL_2 shows posterior rotation and straightening of urethrovesical angle (angle of inclination, 45 degrees); BL_3 demonstrates pronounced posterior rotation of urethrovesical junction associated with large cystocele. Reprinted with permission from Ridley JH: *Gynecologic Surgery: Errors, Safeguards and Salvage.* Baltimore, Williams & Wilkins, 1974.

the degree of herniation of the posterior urethra and bladder neck through the pelvic diaphragm, this has proven to be clinically applicable in many cases of stress urinary incontinence where more thorough diagnostic studies have not been required. More important, clinical evaluation of the degree of herniation of the bladder base (cystocele) and rectum (rectocele) is an important clinical determinant that must be made prior to selecting the appropriate operative procedure for the correction of stress urinary incontinence. When the symptoms of stress urinary incontinence are accompanied by the presence of a large cystourethrocele and rectocele, a vaginal colporrhaphy with correction of the cystocele and rectocele is always indicated, regardless of the nature of the abdominal disease. In such cases, it is necessary to perform an extensive vaginal repair of the bladder neck, bladder base, and anterior rectal wall prior to performing the abdominal procedure. In the event that there is only minimal relaxation of the anterior vaginal wall with only a small cystocele evident on pelvic examination, the combined abdominal hysterectomy and abdominal suspension of the urethra (Marshall-Marchetti-Krantz procedure) can be achieved by a combined procedure through an abdominal approach. Therefore, the degree of pelvic floor relaxation, as evidenced by the size of the cys-

tocele and rectocele, is the governing factor that determines whether a combined abdominal and perineal operative procedure will be required or whether the abdominal route can be used alone.

Choice of Operative Procedure

An abdominal hysterectomy is the preferable surgical treatment of a large myomatous uterus, while vaginal hysterectomy is an ideal surgical approach for the removal of a smaller myomatous uterus, no more than 10 weeks' gestational size. A larger uterus may prove to be a more hazardous surgical task by the vaginal route. The abdominal surgery may be tailored to the needs of the patient, including total hysterectomy, myomectomy, and conservation of one or both ovaries.

The choice of vaginal or abdominal correction of the clinical symptoms of disabling stress urinary incontinence should be made on the basis of the degree of relaxation of the pelvic diaphragm. If a large cystocele and/or rectocele is present, it is inappropriate for the gynecologist to assume that these anatomic deformities will be corrected by retropubic suspension of the posterior urethra. Any pelvic surgeon who has had operative experience with the Marshall-Marchetti-Krantz procedure will know that the suspension of the urethra to the posterior surface of the symphysis pubis does not correct a large cystocele. While the abdominal suspension of the urethra (Marshall-Marchetti-Krantz procedure) does increase intraurethral pressure and re-establish a more normal physiologic, retropubic, and intra-abdominal position of the posterior urethra and urethrovesical junction, this procedure does not correct the anatomic defect in the pelvic diaphragm, in particular, a cystocele. As a result, while incontinence may be corrected by retropubic urethral suspension, symptoms of pelvic pressure from a cystocele and/or rectocele will persist following the abdominal surgery alone. It is important that a vaginal repair of a large cystocele and rectocele be performed prior to performing a total abdominal hysterectomy for a large myomatous uteri. At that time, wide plication of the pubovesicocervical fascia and elevation of the urethrovesical junction to a retropubic position can be accomplished by an appropriate vaginal repair. Surgical correction of this anatomic defect is directed toward restoring the normal musculofascial support to the bladder neck and urethra. The Kelly urethral plication procedure that was originally described in 1913 remains one of the primary methods of vaginal repair of this condition. The successful repair of this hernia is dependent upon the thoroughness of the dissection and mobilization of the posterior urethra and the supporting fascia of the urogenital diaphragm. If wide dissection and plication of the pearly white fascia surrounding the bladder neck are achieved in a succession of vertical mattress sutures, elevation of the urethrovesical junction above the urogenital diaphragm from its dependent position can be easily achieved. Plication and reapproximation of the suburethral and subvesical fascia are essential for the effective repair of the cystocele as well as to replace the bladder neck within the confines of the true pelvis. High plication of the paraurethral fascia on each side of the urethrovesical junction to the strong pubourethral (subpubic) ligaments, using No. 1 delayed-ab-

sorbable suture, will provide assurance of long-standing urethral support (Fig. 56.2 A and B). A high rectocele repair that extends from the vaginal introitus to the apex of the vagina is essential if adequate support of the rectum and posterior vaginal wall with wide plication of the pararectal fascia and the medial borders of the levator ani muscle. The most common failing in the repair of a large rectocele is the inadequate dissection of the pararectal fascia, due to the extreme vascularity of the hemorrhoidal plexus in this portion of the pelvic anatomy. Meticulous ligation of these venous sinusoids and plication of the adjacent fascia will provide adequate control of the bleeding and will avoid subsequent hematoma formation.

In those cases where there is minimal relaxation of the vagina in conjunction with disabling stress incontinence, with only a small cystocele present, support to the urethra and the fascia of the anterior vaginal wall can be

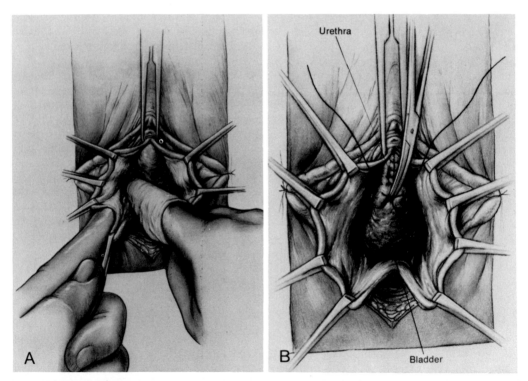

Figure 56.2.   *A.* Wide vaginal dissection of urethra, urethrovesical junction, and bladder base from anterior vaginal wall. *B.* Wide plication of margins of paraurethral and vesical fascia with elevation of urethrovesical junction. Delayed absorbable suture (No. 1 Vicryl) in fascia at bladder neck should be suspended to pubourethral (subpubic) ligaments on each side of urethra for assurance of high elevation of posterior urethra above pelvic floor. Reprinted with permission from Mattingly RF, Thompson JD: *TeLinde's Operative Gynecology,* 6th ed. Philadelphia, JB Lippincott, 1985.

achieved by an abdominal suspension of the uretha as described by Marshall, Marchetti, and Krantz. Many gynecologists and urologists propose that the support to the posterior urethra and urethrovesical junction is accomplished best by abdominal suspension of the urethra and paraurethral fascia to the symphysis pubis. However, a well-controlled, randomized, prospective study to support this contention has yet to be performed. Until such a study is available, one can only say with assurance that the long-term results of the Marshall-Marchetti-Krantz procedure are equally as effective as the Kelly vaginal plication procedure in controlling stress urinary incontinence. The distinct advantage of the Marshall-Marchetti-Krantz procedure in conjunction with an abdominal hysterectomy and closure of the peritoneal cavity, the retropubic space can be explored rapidly and through the same low midline abdominal incision. After mobilization of the urethra and paravesical fat, the fascia of the posterior urethra can be easily identified (Fig. 56.3). By placing a ''double bite'' of suture into the paraurethral fascia, using delayed-absorbable sutures of No. 1 Vicryl or Dexon, the urethra can be effectively suspended to the midline cartilage or the periosteum of the posterior symphysis. It is important to avoid hyperangulation when the posterior urethra is drawn to the posterior aspect of the symphysis pubis. The paraurethral fascia should be approximated to the median cartilage of the pubis at the same level as its normal retropubic position. This retropubic position is determined with one hand of the operator in the vagina while placing the paraurethral sutures under direct, palpable, anatomic control. Gentle pressure on either side of the posterior urethra by the operator's fingers will show the correct position for placement of the suture in the pubic cartilage. In this way, one simply elevates the urethra to its normal location in the true pelvis and avoids the hazard of producing neurogenic dysfunction of the bladder by excessive stretching and tension of the trigone. Two sutures are placed firmly into the fascia on either side of the urethra. The most important suture is the one placed near the urethrovesical junction. It is here that one needs to be particularly cautious to avoid the aggressive suturing and plication of the fascia near the urethrovesical junction which could entrap the terminal end of the pelvic ureter. An equally serious com-

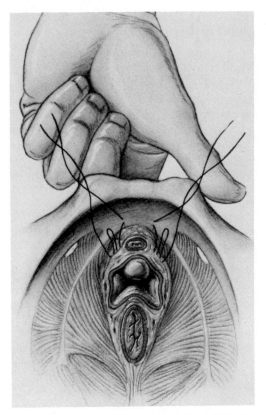

Figure 56.3. Cut-away view of the pelvic diaphragm, showing elevation of the urethra and paraurethral fascia by the surgeon's finger for accurate placement of ''double-bite'' sutures in fascia and adjacent periosteum or pubic cartilage. Reprinted with permission from Mattingly RF, Thompson JD: *TeLinde's Operative Gynecology,* 6th ed. Philadelphia, JB Lippincott, 1985.

plication is the hyperangulation of the urethrovesical junction by plicating the urethra too high on the symphysis pubis. We have seen cases in which both ureters were completely obstructed by this type of hyperangulation that required secondary surgical release. Although a third suture can be placed in the paraurethral fascia where convenient, it has been our concern that this may lead to an overcorrection of the normal urethral angle. If there is residual venous bleeding at the completion of the procedure from the paravesical plexus, the space of Retzius should be drained by a Penrose drain through a separate stab wound incision and *not* through the lower end of the midline incision. It is our preference to insert a suprapubic Silastic catheter through the dome of the bladder at the completion of this procedure, prior to closing the abdominal incision.

Abdominal Versus the Combined Abdominoperineal Procedure

The medical literature is replete with exaggerated predictions of the therapeutic benefits of one procedure or another, mainly vaginal repair or abdominal urethral suspension for the treatment of stress urinary incontinence. Frequently, the enthusiasm and clinical opinion of the investigator have replaced hard scientific data concerning the long-term surgical cure by one method or the other. Controlled, randomized, prospective studies of these two primary surgical techniques are needed to resolve this plaguing clinical problem. Without belaboring these highly controversial points, suffice it to say that the time-honored surgical approach to the correction of a hernia is to dissect out the margins of the hernial sac, plicate the attenuated musculofascial supports, and re-establish the normal anatomy at the site of the hernia. Whether this defect occurs in the thoracic diaphragm, the abdominal wall, the inguinal or femoral canal, or the pelvic floor, the basic surgical principles are always operative in the correction of this common anatomic problem. It is beyond the limits of good surgical principles to assume that the abdominal suspension of the urethra will correct a widened pelvic diaphragm that is associated with a large cystocele and rectocele. Therefore, one must approach each disease process and anatomic defect in accordance with the extent of the pathology and the anatomic abnormality that is involved. One can see the distinct benefit of the Marshall-Marchetti-Krantz procedure for patients with a minimal degree of pelvic floor relaxation. In such cases, the symptoms of stress urinary incontinence can be easily corrected by the abdominal suspension of the urethra. However, a large hernia of the pelvic diaphragm that has produced a prominent cystocele and rectocele must be corrected separately, per vaginam. Repair of the musculofascial support of the pelvic floor is always accomplished best by the vaginal route. Based on the proper execution of sound surgical techniques, one can assure the patient of comparable results of either the abdominal or the vaginal approach to the correction of or the vaginal approach to the correction of stress urinary incontinence. However, without proper understanding of the anatomic factors that are responsible for these defects, the mechanical approach to the correction of the musculofacial relaxation of the pelvic floor is likely to be unsuccessful.

Selected Readings

American Cancer Society: Cancer Facts and Figures, 1980. New York, 1981.

Bradley WE: The urologically oriented neurological examination. In Ostergard DR (ed): *Gynecologic Urology and Urodynamics: Theory and Practice*. Baltimore, Williams & Wilkins, 1980, pp. 444-554.

Crystle CD, Charme LS, Copeland WE: Q-tip test in stress urinary incontinence. *Obstet Gynecol* 38:313, 1971.

Curtis AH, Anson BJ, McVay CG: The anatomy of the pelvis and urogenital diaphragm in relation to urethrocele and cystocele. *Surg Gynecol Obstet* 68:161, 1939.

Green TH Jr: Urinary stress incontinence: Differential diagnosis, pathophysiology and management. *Am J Obstet Gynecol* 122:368, 1975.

Jeffcoate TNA, Roberts H: Observations on stress urinary incontinence. *Am J Obstet Gynecol* 64:721, 1952.

Jeffcoate TNA, Roberts H: The principles governing the treatment of stress incontinence of urine in the female. *Br J Urol* 37:633, 1965.

Kitzmiller JL, Manzer GA, Negel WA, et al: Chain cystourethrogram and stress incontinence. *Obstet Gynecol* 39:333, 1972.

Marshall VF, Marchetti AA, Krantz KE: The correction of stress urinary incontinence by simple vesicourethral suspension. *Surg Gynecol Obstet* 88:509, 1949.

Mattingly RF: *TeLinde's Operative Gynecology*, 5th ed. Philadelphia, JB Lippincott, 1977, pp. 531-572.

Morrow CP, Hart WR: The ovaries. In Romney S, Gray MJ, Little AB, Merrill JA, Quilligan EJ, Stander R (eds): *Gynecology and Obstetrics: The Health Care of Women*. ed. 2. New York, McGraw-Hill, 1981.

Ostergard DR: *Gynecologic Urology and Urodynamics: Theory and Practice*. Baltimore, Williams & Wilkins, 1980.

Richardson EH: A simplified technique for abdominal panhysterectomy. *Surg Gynecol Obstet* 48:248, 1929.

Stanton FL: Preoperative investigation and diagnosis. *Clin Obstet Gynecol* 21:705, 1978.

Tanagho EA: Colpocysto-urethropexy: The way we do it. *J Urol* 116:751, 1976.

Van Rooyen AJL, Liebenberg HC: A clinical approach to urinary incontinence in the female. *Obstet Gynecol* 53:1, 1979.

Zacharin RD: *Stress Incontinence of Urine*. Hagerstown, MD, Harper & Row, 1972.

CHAPTER **57**
Urinary Stress Incontinence in a Young Patient Who Wants More Children

W. GLENN HURT, M.D.

CASE ABSTRACT
Progressively socially disabling urinary stress incontinence is present in a 27-year-old, para 5, who has expressed a firm desire to have more children. Positive findings on pelvic examination include marked hypermobility of the urethra, a moderate-sized cystocele and rectocele, and a retroverted uterus in first degree prolapse.

DISCUSSION

The basic evaluation of all patients seen in consultation because of urinary incontinence begins with a general history and physical examination which are supplemented by an incisive urologic history (1), urologically oriented neurologic examination, and a detailed pelvic examination with special attention to the integrity of the pelvic support systems. Demonstration of incontinence is an essential part of the evaluation. A postvoid residual urine measurement is made to determine bladder efficiency, and the specimen is sent for urinalysis and/or culture to assure that there is no infection. The Q-tip test (2) is helpful in demonstrating proximal urethral mobility. Cystometry should be performed to estimate bladder volume and determine neurologic control of the micturition reflex. This basic evaluation may enable the clinician to make the diagnosis of urinary stress incontinence with added confidence. Findings during the basic evaluation may indicate the need for endoscopy, additional urodynamic testing, radiologic studies, and further consultation.

It is particularly helpful if the patient will come to her initial evaluation with a representative urinary diary and a listing of food intolerances, drug allergies, and current medications. Some physicians will furnish the patient with a gynecologic-urologic questionnaire to be completed at home and made a part of her history.

If the evaluation of this patient results in a final diagnosis of socially disabling pure urinary stress incontinence and if she has a firm desire to have more children, she should be counseled regarding what we know of the etiology and pathophysiology of this disorder and the advantage of a concerted effort to develop compensatory continence mechanisms through nonsurgical therapy until she completes childbearing, with full realization that surgery ultimately may offer the only real cure. Since vaginal delivery is thought to contribute to the development of urinary stress incontinence and since it is recognized that the first surgical attempt at correction of the disorder is the one most likely to succeed, I would outline my plan for the nonsurgical management of this patient's urinary stress incontinence and encourage her to complete childbearing as soon as is reasonable.

All patients with urinary incontinence need counseling regarding dietary indiscretions, especially if there is obesity and excessive fluid intake. Since some acid foods (i.e., tomatoes, strawberries, etc.) and those containing caffeine (i.e., coffee, tea, chocolates, etc.) may irritate the bladder, they should be ingested in moderation or an attempt should be made to eliminate them from the diet. Bacteriuria, whether symptomatic or asymptomatic, cervicitis, and vaginitis must be treated. Medications which the patient takes and which may contribute to her urinary incontinence (e.g., diuretics, phenothiazines, etc.) should be scrutinized. Special attention should be given to the treatment of chronic respiratory and metabolic diseases. These problems often necessitate consultation with other physicians. Bladder retraining may be necessary to adjust the patient's voiding schedule. She also may have to limit some activities associated with her daily lifestyle (i.e., jogging, tennis, etc.), and she should embark upon an honest attempt at Kegel's exercises (3, 4).

Kegel's perineal resistive exercises should be taught to postpartum patients as prophylaxis against the development of urinary stress incontinence. They will help many patients with urinary stress incontinence compensate to such a degree that surgery may be postponed. The first step in teaching a patient Kegel's exercises is to teach her awareness of the function of the pubococcygeus muscle. Once this is learned, with the examining finger on the medial margin of the pubococcygeus at the level of the urethra, the patient should be told to ''(1) squeeze the vaginal muscles upon the palpating finger, (2) draw up or draw in the perineum, (3) contract or draw up the rectum as though checking a bowel movement, and (4) contract [the perineal muscles] as though interrupting the flow of urine while voiding''. Once learned, the pubococcygeus should be contracted for 3 to 4 seconds, 15 times in a row, at least 6 times a day for at least 3 months. In addition, the patient should learn to contract the pubococcygeus *prior* to physical efforts which may cause sudden increases in intra-abdominal pressure (e.g., coughing, laughing, sneezing, lifting, awkward movements, etc.).

The alpha-adrenergic stimulating drugs, phenylpropanolamine, imipramine, and phenylephrine, and the general adrenergic stimulator, ephedrine, can increase the smooth muscle tone of the urethra and be useful in treating urinary stress incontinence. The beta-adrenergic blocker, propranolol, has theoretic usefulness but is rarely used for this problem.

Tampons, Smith-Hodge and ring pessaries, and other devices have been recommended for the relief of urinary stress incontinence (6). Their success in providing socially acceptable continence is variable and unpredictable. In order to buy time, they may be tried if care is taken to prevent excessive drying of the vagina, pressure necrosis, and the inflammation and ulceration which may be associated with their use.

In cases of socially disabling urinary stress incontinence, I prefer a modification of the Burch colpourethropexy (1) as the primary surgical procedure. I am even more convinced that this is the procedure of choice for the patient who insists upon preserving her childbearing potential. The operation was designed to correct mild and moderate cystocele; its durability can be improved by using permanent suture materials.

In this particular case, the surgeon would have to use his best judgment about entering the peritoneal cavity to obliterate the cul-de-sac and/or suspend the uterus prophylactically. Although these procedures may realign the uterus and prevent the development of an enterocele, which is a recognized complication of a Burch procedure, they may cause adhesions and infertility. Likewise, the surgeon would have to use his judgment about the need for correction of the ''moderate rectocele.'' If a rectocele repair were to be done, I would not do it until all other procedures had been complete.

I am not aware of any articles in medical literature which deal specifically with the route of delivery of an infant in a patient who becomes pregnant and must be delivered after successful surgical correction of urinary stress incontinence. Krantz (5) has stated that after the Marshall-Marchetti-Krantz procedure ''pregnancy may be anticipated without difficulty and vaginal delivery, while not preferred, is not contraindicated.'' Given what we know about the etiology and pathophysiology of urinary stress incontinence and the importance attached to cure by the first operation, I would not hesitate to recommend an elective cesarean section, preferably prior to the onset of labor, for all patients needing delivery who have had a successful operation and cure of their urinary stress incontinence.

References

1. Burch JC: Urethrovaginal fixation to Cooper's ligament for correction of stress incontinence, cystocele and prolapse. *Am J Obstet Gynecol* 81:281–290, 1961.
2. Crystle CD, Charme LS, Copeland WE: Q-tip test in stress urinary incontinence after repair operations. *Obstet Gynecol* 38:313–315, 1971.

3. Kegel AH: Progressive resistance exercises in the functional restoration of the perineal muscles. *Am J Obstet Gynecol* 56:238–248, 1948.

4. Kegel AH: Stress incontinence and genital relaxation. In Walton JH (ed): Ciba Clinical Symposia. Summit, NJ, Ciba Pharmaceutical Products, 4:35–51, 1952.

5. Krantz KE: The Marshall-Marchetti-Krantz procedure. In Stanton SL, Tenagho EA (eds): *Surgery of Female Incontinence.* New York, Springer Verlag, pp 47–54, 1980.

6. Norton C: Pads and mechanical methods. In Stanton SL (ed): *Clinical Gynecologic Urology.* St. Louis, CV Mosby, 1984, pp. 499–510.

CHAPTER 58
Inability to Void Following Vesicourethral Sling Procedure

DAVID H. NICHOLS, M.D.

CASE ABSTRACT

Severe and socially disabling recurrent urinary stress incontinence was found in an obese patient with chronic bronchitis and emphysema.

A vesicourethral sling procedure was advised and this was accomplished using a modified Goebell-Frangenheim-Stoeckel technique employing a strip of fascia lata.

The transurethral catheter was removed on the fourth postoperative day, and although otherwise comfortable, the patient was unable to void. She was catheterized repeatedly during the next 24 hours, at the conclusion of which time, the transurethral catheter was replaced. It was removed again on the morning of the eighth postoperative day, and despite a strong desire and conviction that the bladder would function, the patient was still unable to void. Although straining hard as by a Valsalva maneuver, only a few drops of urine could be expressed.

DISCUSSION

Inability to void following a retropubic suburethral sling procedure generally occurs when the tension under which the sling has been fixed is too great, and an actual mechanical obstruction of the urethra has been produced. In most instances the sling has been initially fixed too tightly either as an error in the operator's judgment as to the proper tension, or more likely that the sling itself is too short and the excess tension has been produced consequent to fixing the ends of the to the rectus aponeurosis.

This problem might be avoided by more thoughtful judgment as to the initial tension at which the sling should be placed—observing Moir's suggestion that it be placed only tightly enough to "take out the wrinkles and ruckles that are present" within the sling (Fig. 58.1).

If the sling has been fashioned from a strip of Mersilene mesh (never tape!) it may be precut to any desired length up to 32 cm. If, however, the operator has chosen fascia lata, and the strip is too short and can be fixed in place only by applying an excess degree of tension, it is possible to lengthen the sling before it has been fixed in place as shown in Figure 58.2.

Although there is considerable postoperative edema immediately following a surgical sling procedure, this generally subsides by the fourth or fifth postoperative day and is of itself not a common cause of postoperative inability to void. Replacing the catheter (preferably using one which is silicon coated to reduce mucosal edema) for a day or two will allow residual edema to subside further, but if the patient is still unable to void and the bladder is neurologically normal, one must presume a mechanical obstruction from the sling. Because there are a few persons who habitually void by contracting their rectus abdominis muscles instead of relaxing them, one should ascertain from the patient's history that this is not the case, for if it is, the voiding habits of such a person must be changed and the patient taught to relax when voiding.

The treatment of a significant mechanical obstruction requires that it should be relieved promptly and this is accomplished by freeing *one* end of the sling from its attachment to the

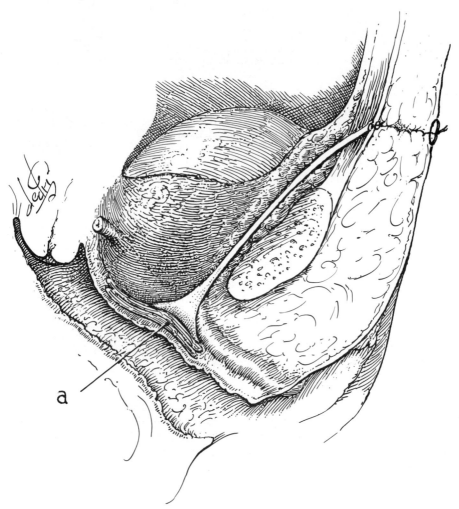

Figure 58.1. The gauze-hammock is shown fixed in place beneath the vesicourethral junction and the bladder. The ends have been attached to rectus aponeurosis, and the incision in each groin closed. The vaginal portion of the hammock has been insulated from the vagina by a two-layer vaginal lapping procedure, as noted in *a*.

rectus aponeurosis within a few days of the initial surgery; if this was the cause of the inability to void, the patient will invariably be relieved. Interestingly, the patient will generally remain continent, because by the fifth or sixth postoperative day there is enough healing around the sling to hold its central belly more or less in place. The opposite end of the sling still elevates the vesicourethral junction, but the pathologic obstruction has been relieved.

Beyond two months from the original surgery, it is likely that the fibrosis and healing around the sling will be so great that the ten-sion may not be relieved by cutting or freeing the sling at the site of its attachment to the rectus aponeurosis. If this is the case, the sling may be transected through a transvaginal incision lateral to the midline thus avoiding the site of the previous incision into the vagina. If necessary, this may be followed by stretching the urethra with an appropriate sized dilator, which will also permit "rocking" of it beneath the pubis. Transvaginal cutting of the sling does increase the potential risk of infection by exposing the wound to the considerably mixed bacterial flora of the vagina.

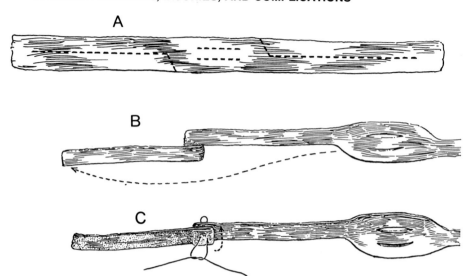

Figure 58.2. A means of increasing the length of the fascia strip is shown. Incisions are made along the path of the *dotted lines* shown *(A)*. This is folded back without loss of continuity as depicted *(B)*, and folded fascia in place *(C)*. A single stitch is placed as shown, to fix the folded fascia in place. The same procedure is accomplished on the opposite end of the fascial strip. If an increase in the thickness of the central belly of the strip is desired, it may be incised, as shown by the *two dotted lines* in the center of the strip *(A)*. This widened belly may be anchored in place by a few sutures beneath the vesicourethral junction at the time the vaginal portion of the sling is placed.

This complication should not exist if the sling had not been initially placed under too great tension. The degree of tension requires a nicety of judgment, because if too loose the incontinence will not be relieved, and if too tight the patient will be unable to void comfortably.

Replacement of the vesicourethral junction to a proper retropubic pelvic position may be achieved by insertion of a firm intravaginal packing at the conclusion of the vaginal portion of the operation and prior to fixation of the abdominal ends of the sling to the rectus aponeurosis. When the vaginal portion of the operation has been completed, the abdominal ends of the sling may be fixed to the rectus aponeurosis with minimal tension.

Mild or partial degree of obstruction appears to be generally transient, as over a period of time the patient tends to develop increased detrusor tone sufficient to permit intravesical pressure to exceed intraurethral pressure at the time of voiding. Patients so inclined may be taught self-catherization, using the flexible plastic ''Mentor'' catheter for the female urethra. The technique is ''clean,'' but not sterile, and the patient may boil and reuse the

catheters as necessary. This is particularly helpful for the patient in whom inability to void adequate amounts is thought to be the result of transient postoperative edema, which will subside with healing. Some operators prefer to use a suprapubic catheter regularly instead of a transurethral one. This is certainly an acceptable approach to postoperative bladder drainage but would of itself not relieve urethral obstruction. If the latter were present, and the patient persistently unable to void following clamping of the suprapubic catheter, the treatment of the problem would be outlined as above.

Selected Readings

Moir JC: The Gauze-Hammock Operation. *J Obstet Gynaecol Br Commonw* 75:1, 1978.
Nichols DH: The Mersilene mesh gauze-hammock in repair of severe or recurrent urinary stress incontinence. In Taymor ML, Green TH, (eds): *Progress in Gynecology,* Vol. V, New York, Grune & Stratton, 1970.
Nichols DH: The sling operations. In Cantor EB (ed): *Female Urinary Stress Incontinence.* Springfield IL, Charles C. Thomas, 1979.
Ridley JH: *Gynecologic Surgery—Errors, Safeguards, Salvage,* 2nd ed. Baltimore, Williams & Wilkins, 1981.

SECTION 6
Intestinal Problems and Injuries

CHAPTER **59**

Injury to the Bowel During Pelvic Surgery

GEORGE W. MITCHELL, JR., M.D.
FREDDY M. MASSEY, M.D.

CASE ABSTRACT 1: TRANSABDOMINAL INJURY

A total abdominal hysterectomy with bilateral salpingo-oophorectomy was being performed on a 36-year-old patient with severely symptomatic disability from advanced pelvic endometriosis.

Because of the long-standing severity of the condition, the hysterectomy was difficult, especially as surgical dissection proceeded in the tissues around the cervix. The cul-de-sac had been obliterated by the disease, and cleavage planes were difficult to establish. As soon as the uterus had been removed, it was evident that a 2-cm longitudinal rent had been made through the full thickness of the anterior rectal wall near the vaginal apex.

DISCUSSION

When a difficult pelvic operation is in prospect, it is essential for the surgeon to determine, to the extent possible, whether or not the bowel is likely to be involved. This is particularly true when endometriosis is palpable in the posterior pelvis adjacent to the rectal wall, when the secondary manifestations of pelvic inflammatory disease are known to be present and adherent masses palpable, when the presence of ovarian carcinoma is suspected, and in all instances when the patient has had multiple previous pelvic surgical procedures. Pelvic operations may also be necessary on patients who are known to have intrinsic bowel problems such as Crohn's disease, ulcerative colitis, and diverticulitis. In all of these circumstances, some type of preoperative bowel work-up is indicated, and this should include proctoscopy and barium enema as a minimum. Selected patients should also have an upper gastrointestinal series and colonoscopy.

If direct bowel involvement is diagnosed preoperatively or there is a strong possibility of bowel injury during surgery, preoperative preparation of the bowel is indicated. Even if no bowel problems are anticipated, decompression of both the large and small intestine greatly facilitates pelvic surgery and is routinely accomplished by a mild cathartic the evening before and an enema the morning immediately prior to surgery. Nurses should be instructed to be certain that all of the fluid injected into the rectum is recovered before discontinuing the enema. More rigorous bowel preparation consists of cleansing enemas until clear and the oral administration of a drug such as neomycin which will lower the intraluminal bacterial content of the intestine. Various different solutions have been proposed for the enemas, including some containing antibacterial drugs, but the probability is that plain water is just as effective. A good rule is to prepare the bowel when there is the slightest doubt about the need to do so.

At the operating table, the pelvic surgeon should have in mind at all times the necessity to protect the intestine from injury. Even relatively minor nicks and abrasions have been shown to increase the risk of postoperative intestinal obstruction. In packing the bowel out of the operating field, care should be taken not to exert undue pressure, not to handle the bowel directly with forceps, and not to release intestinal adhesions by blunt dissection. If the rectosigmoid is prolapsed and adherent to the lower pelvis, its attachments to the pelvic organs should be severed by careful sharp dissection and the lateral peritoneal reflection cut as high as is necessary to allow adequate upward mobilization. Attempts to free the intestine by avulsing it from its attachment often cause injury either to the bowel wall or to the mesentery. Packing should be accomplished when the patient has had enough relaxing drug to permit it to be done easily. The anesthesiologist is responsible for this and should be kept informed of problems. To attempt to pack the bowel against persistent downward pressure will increase the chances of postoperative ileus, if it does not cause immediate bowel injury. As in the case of the rectosigmoid, adherent ileum in the pelvis should be mobilized by sharp dissection and bleeding points carefully ligated following relocation upward.

Direct injury to the bowel may be quite accidental, making the need for constant inspection of the viscera adjacent to the operative site imperative, or it may be the result of a calculated risk when tissue planes are absolutely unreadable and progressive dissection is essential for the successful completion of the operation. An intrafascial enucleation of the cervix is helpful in preventing rectal injury. This is particularly true when there are dense endometrial adhesions between the anterior surface of the rectum and the posterior surfaces of the cervix and vagina, as in the case described. Early recognition of such injury is important to avoid spillage of bowel contents, and closure should be undertaken immediately unless the primary surgical procedure is at a critical stage or there is an additional emergency, such as excessive blood loss, which takes priority.

In the case under discussion, the 2-cm vertical rent in the anterior surface of the rectum should have been closed in the same plane with interrupted sutures about 3 mm apart, set in such a way that the mucosa and the immediately adjacent seromuscular layer will be inverted. A two-layer closure of an opening this small would be technically difficult and would add little to the competence of the closure. The caliber of the rectum is so large that a vertical closure seldom constricts the lumen significantly. Most surgeons would use nonabsorbable suture material for the closure, some preferring nylon or other synthetic material and some preferring silk. The preference here is for the latter. The other difficult question in this type of situation is whether the rectal tissues being closed are so disrupted or fibrous, as a result of endometriosis, that they will not heal. The odds are that a small opening will heal well but, if the opening were large, creating a tissue deficiency, or if serious disease such as carcinoma were present, making successful closure unlikely, an attempt might be made to approximate the edges and cover the closure with a portion of the greater omentum, but a temporary diverting colostomy at the level of the transverse colon should also be done. Diverting sigmoid colostomies have the advantage of better patient acceptance because of the passage of formed stools, but the disadvantage that their location might eventually complicate the process of secondary rectal repair requiring mobilization of the sigmoid colon.

Following closure of an unplanned opening through the full thickness of the rectal wall or elsewhere in the colon, most surgeons would institute some type of drainage, especially if there had been overt spillage of feces into the peritoneal cavity. When the opening is low, good dependent drainage can be obtained by bringing the drain out through the vagina. For most purposes, a 1-inch Penrose drain stuffed with gauze will provide an adequate opening in the vaginal cuff. For injuries higher in the colon or when the primary operation is not hysterectomy, it is advisable to make the incision for the drain in either lower quadrant or, in some circumstances, in the upper abdomen. Drains should never be brought out through the original incision and should be left in for no longer than 24 hours, since they serve only to provide an immediate portal for infected material which might otherwise collect to form an abscess. If left in longer, they act as foreign bodies and channels for the re-entry of bacteria.

Injuries to the small intestine in the course of pelvic surgery should also be closed as soon as possible. Horizontal tears are best closed in the same plane, but vertical or diagonal tears, if they are long and through the full thickness of the bowel wall, should be closed in the horizontal plane to avoid constriction of the lumen. In most instances, a single layer closure will suffice, using interrupted nonabsorbable suture material and carefully inverting the edges of the mucosa and the adjacent seromuscular layer. Necrotic tissue should be trimmed before the closure. The patency of the lumen should be tested by squeezing the thumb and forefinger together from either side of the suture line. Occasionally, injuries occur as a result of the necessity to separate small bowel loops damaged by irradiation. The blood supply to damaged loops should be evaluated to determine whether the bowel is viable and whether a closure will remain competent. If this is questionable, or if the injuries are multiple but confined to a specific segment, resection of that segment and end-to-end anatomosis constitute the procedure of choice.

Attempts have been made to determine the viability of injured bowel by sending biopsies to the pathology laboratory, but this is usually not helpful. Ten cubic centimeters of 10% fluoroscein may be given intravenously and a Wood's light used to evaluate the vascularity of the affected area. When the patient's condition is poor, resection of the small bowel difficult, and injuries multiple - a combination most often associated with irradiation damage - sidetracking the involved area by side-to-side anastomosis of the proximal and distal loops, leaving the damaged intestine in situ, may be expedient. Obviously, this is not possible if the affected area is necrotic. While the abdomen is still open for verification of placement, the anesthesiologist can insert a nasogastric tube.

Prior to closure, the peritoneal contents should be irrigated, especially if there has been gross spillage of fecal material. Although some surgeons prefer to use antibiotics in the irrigating solution, there are no data to suggest that this is superior to normal saline. It is appropriate, however, to start such patients intraoperatively on antibiotic therapy on the assumption that peritonitis is certain to occur otherwise. Although the predominant organism is *Escherichia coli*, good broad-spectrum coverage can be obtained with a combination of a cephalosporin and an aminoglycoside. Intravenous fluids should be continued for at least 3 days, and the patient is permitted nothing by mouth until normal bowel sounds have returned and she is passing flatus per rectum. Vital signs should be monitored for the early possibility of septic shock, should some virulent organism such as beta-hemolytic streptococcus be the invader. Peritoneal signs should also be carefully followed and the wound inspected daily. After a contaminated case, some surgeons prefer to leave the skin and subcutaneous tissues open, with sutures placed for secondary closure. Others drain the subcutaneous space superficially at either end of the closed incision. The preference here is for primary closure unless the contamination at the time of injury has been great and, in those circumstances, for secondary closure. The risk of postoperative wound infection is significantly increased and should be promptly treated when it occurs. Local redness, heat, pain and swelling, and an elevation of temperature suggest the need for drainage. The incidence of dehiscence of the wound is also increased.

When normal bowel sounds return and the patient begins to pass gas per rectum, a liquid diet may be started. If this is well tolerated, the diet may be graduated rapidly to soft and then to regular fare. If ileus persists or there is evidence of partial mechanical obstruction, the patient should continue to be permitted nothing by mouth, and a nasogastric tube should be inserted for continuous decompression. Failure to use a nasogastric tube for abdominal distention or persistent ileus can result in perforation of the intestinal closure. On some services, postoperative enemas are used routinely to expedite evacuation of gas and the return of normal peristalsis. These and cholinergic drugs are strictly contraindicated when there has been an injury to the large or small bowel or when the appendix has been removed. When symptoms of obstruction persist or when there is evidence of spreading peritonitis, long tube drainage and surgical re-exploration of the abdomen should be considered. Total parenteral nutrition should be instituted when it seems likely that oral feeding will have to be long deferred.

CASE ABSTRACT 2: ACCIDENTAL PROCTOTOMY AT VAGINAL TUBAL LIGATION

A vaginal tubal ligation had been scheduled for a 28-year-old multipara. The initial incision in the vault of the vagina was made directly into an unprepared rectum, covering the operative field with fecal material. As the operator attempted to close the defect with some side-to-side interrupted stitches in the rectum, it was evident that a small opening had been made into the peritoneum of the cul-de-sac.

DISCUSSION

Tubal ligation by the vaginal route has been almost completely superseded in the modern era by laparoscopic techniques and mini-laparotomy. If the approach has to be made through a more contaminated area, locating the tubes may be difficult, especially if the uterus is high and anterior and there have been previous operative procedures; mobilization of the tubes to do one of the standard interruptions may endanger the blood supply or result in a faulty ligation. As a consequence of the latter, bilateral fimbriectomies, which are effective in preventing future pregnancy but which preclude the success of future operations to restore patency, may be done. In the case described, the surgeon succumbed to his own inclinations instead of listening to the voice of reason, a not infrequent happening.

To enter the posterior cul-de-sac with precision, using needle, scalpel, or scissors, it is logical first to identify as nearly as possible the approximate inferior margin of the cul-de-sac of Douglas. This can be done in several ways, the most efficient being to circumcise the cervix at the junction of the posterior portio with the vaginal mucosa and, with strong upward traction on the incised cervical margin, to sweep the vagina and rectum away from the isthmus, using a forefinger covered by a layer of gauze. With this method it is difficult to miss the right plane, and the peritoneum will eventually protrude between the rectal muscle and the posterior surface of the uterus. In order to provide the necessary mobility when the cul-de-sac is shallow, it may be necessary to sever the lateral vaginal mucosa from its cervical attachment as well. This technique should be used for posterior colpotomy for tubal ligation, but, since it takes time and colpotomy can usually be accomplished without it, many experienced surgeons prefer to estimate the most likely spot for the incision.

While the posterior lip of the cervix is drawn toward the pubis with heavy traction, a midline vertical fold of vagina, about 2 inches from the portio, is pulled downward toward the introitus with forceps. The point of pick-up must be above any obvious high rectocele. A triangle of vaginal mucosa, outlined by the tenaculum, the forceps, and the posterior wall of the cervix, is thus exposed. The incision is made with curved scissors, points turned upward, into the vertical fold about midway between the tenaculum and the forceps and directed toward the posterior cervix. Some surgeons prefer to enter the peritoneum with one swoop of the scissors, but safety dictates a more cautious approach, first cutting through both layers of the vagina, noting whether rectal fibers are present and then proceeding upward, exploring with the scissors and using blunt dissection to mobilize rectal muscle downward until the peritoneum is opened. Bleeding points on the rectal muscle are fulgurated or ligated. A retractor can then be inserted into the peritoneum and any type of exploration feasible for that area carried out.

A third method, suitable for beginners or when disease or anatomic defect seems to obliterate the posterior cul-de-sac, is to proceed as above but to explore the rectum directly through the anus, with the left forefinger covered with a second glove. This will assure the surgeon that the planned culdotomy is well above the rectal mucosa or that he should modify his approach to suit the anatomic situation.

In the event the rectal wall is entered but not the rectal mucosa, a few interrupted absorbable sutures, placed to invert the torn edges, should serve to close the defect. Mattress or figure-of-eight sutures are desirable because they hold better in muscle, and, to avoid pulling through, they should not be tied at maximum tightness. A smooth approximation is all that is needed. When the injury penetrates the rectal mucosa, a similiar closure is done through all layers. One layer of sutures is sufficient unless the margins of the rent are badly mangled, in which case the rectum should be widely mobilized from the undersurface of the vagina and closed with as many sutures as necessary to assure competence. The vagina mucosa, when closed, acts as a backup layer. Catgut or polyglycolic acid sutures of 2-0 size are best for this type of repair, and the fewer the better.

Since inadvertent proctotomy in the course of posterior culdotomy is uncommon, major preoperative bowel preparation is not ordered routinely for such cases, but enemas should be given, not only to clear the bowel of feces, but to avoid rectal distention. In the case under discussion, the immediate contamination of the field by feces suggests that enemas were not given or that they were not properly evacuated. When gross contamination occurs, it should be sucked out of the field as rapidly as possible and an attempt made to seal the defect temporarily, either with a finger or a loosely placed figure-of-eight suture, while the extent of the damage is considered and a decision made regarding what should be done next. Most accidental rectal openings are below the peritoneal reflection; in fact, it is difficult to make a surgical opening in the intraperitoneal portion of the rectum. Opening the peritoneum at the same time that the rectum was opened strongly suggests a careless initial incision by the surgeon, and this action introduces the possibility of postoperative peritonitis.

An immediate decision should have been made not to do the tubal ligation, in order to avoid further contamination higher in the pelvis. The rectal opening should have been closed as outlined above, removing any temporary suture that might have been placed, unless it was presumed to be adequate. A difference of opinion exists as to whether the peritoneum should be drained or closed primarily. The authors' preference is for the insertion of a small Penrose drain for 24 hours. To prevent its slipping

out, the drain can be kept in place by a single, fine, plain catgut suture through the drain and the edge of the peritoneum, not more than 2 mm from the edge, from which it can be easily pulled out. After the rectal closure, the vagina should be closed around the drain with interrupted sutures and a loose vaginal pack left in the posterior vagina to obliterate dead space. Temporary diverting colostomy is seldom indicated when inadvertent proctotomy occurs below the peritoneal reflection, since the closure will heal without fistula formation in the overwhelming majority of cases. Only if a significant opening is made above the peritoneal reflection, the local damage around the proctotomy site is extensive, or the tissues have been irradiated should colostomy be considered.

Postoperatively, the patient who has suffered such a surgical accident will soon be wide awake and inquiring about her operation. An immediate full disclosure of exactly what happened is indicated. The patient should be told that, even though another hospitalization will be required and another anesthesia, the tubal interruption must be postponed until after any possible complications. The patient should not be fed solid food until wound healing is assured. For the first week, an elemental diet that is largely absorbed in the jejunum should be given, and for 2 weeks thereafter, a low-residue diet. The drain and vaginal pack should not be left in longer than 24 hours. In the authors' opinion, antibiotics should be given but should not be continued for more than 24 hours. The authors' preference is to administer therapeutic antibiotics should the temperature remain elevated for 2 successive days or should signs of pelvic peritonitis develop.

CHAPTER **60**

Unexpected Clamping of Small Bowel During Hysterectomy

JOHN H. ISAACS, M.D.

CASE ABSTRACT

A 70-year-old patient with procidentia was undergoing a vaginal hysterectomy. A partial colectomy because of diverticulitis of the sigmoid colon had been performed 5 years previously. There were adhesions of small bowel to the left cornual angle prior to the removal of the uterus. The operative procedure, being photographed, was momentarily halted while the photographer changed film and refocused the camera. When surgery was resumed, 10 minutes later, it was evident that the Heaney forceps on the right cornual angle of the uterus had included 2 inches of small bowel that previously had not been noticed at this site. The bowel had not been opened.

DISCUSSION

This mishap might have been avoided if the surgeon had had good visualization. Before the first Heaney clamp was placed across the cornual angle of the uterus, care should have been taken to dissect any adhesions that are attached to the uterine fundus or to the proximal portion of the round ligament, ovarian ligament, or fallopian tube. Since these adhesions can be either on the anterior or posterior surface of any of these structures, careful scrutiny of the area is mandatory before the Heaney clamp is applied. One safeguard is to ligate the first pedicle leaving the suture long and tagged with a hemostat. In this way, there is no clamp in the way that might add further difficulty in clamping the opposite cornual angle. In spite of these precautions, accidents do happen and must be rectified.

The situation in this case is an area of bowel that has been crushed and consequently devitalized (Fig. 60.1). This tissue if left as is will undoubtedly necrose and the bowel will perforate in 24 to 48 hours with a resulting entero-vaginal fistula at best or an operative death at worst. Major small bowel fistulae are associated with a mortality rate of approximately 20% to 30%.

Since we must assume that the surgeon is aware of the gravity of the situation, methods of correction must be considered. In checking various textbooks, there are no specific guidelines that state how this situation should be

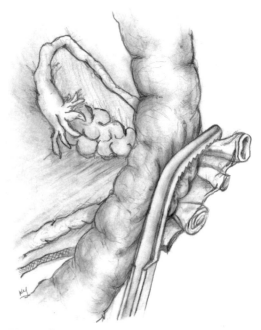

Figure 60.1. Heaney clamp across the round ligament, ovarian ligament, fallopian tube, and including a segment of small bowel.

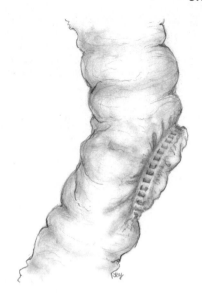

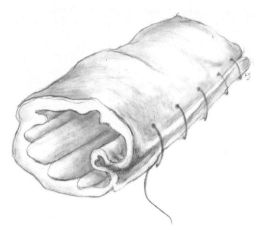

Figure 60.4. Cross-section of the small bowel after the devitalized area has been invaginated.

Figure 60.2. The damaged section of small bowel showing the crush mark produced by the Heaney clamp.

managed. Three possibilities exist: First, to open the abdomen and resect the damaged portion of bowel and do an end-to-end anastomosis. This, in my view, would represent far too much surgery for the problem at hand and should be done only if it is technically impossible to re-pair the damage via the vaginal route. Second, to resect the crushed section of bowel, as it is exposed through the vagina, and close the bowel in two layers. This would cause contamination of the operative field and would increase the chances of postoperative morbidity plus the added risk that the repaired enterostomy site might not heal with resulting leaking and subsequent complications therefrom. Third, the ideal choice would be to remove the Heaney clamp and dissect the remaining adhesions between the small bowel and the adnexa. The Heaney clamp could be reapplied to the adnexal pedicle and ligated. The portion of bowel which has been damaged could be steadied with two Babcock clamps and the damaged area inspected closely (Fig. 60.2). Since the bowel has been crushed but not opened, the damaged portion could be inverted using several interrupted 00 black silk sutures through the seromuscular layers of the normal bowel on each side of the devitalized portion (Fig. 60.3) of ileum. This should promote secure healing since the healing process depends on approximation of the serosal surfaces. This technique may reduce the lumen of the small bowel (Fig. 60.4) but should not really interfere with normal bowel function. Over time the bowel lumen will enlarge to be equal to that of the adjacent bowel.

Selected Readings

Barber HR, Graber EA: The intestinal tract in relation to obstetrics and gynecology. *Clin Obstet Gynecol* 15:650, 1972.

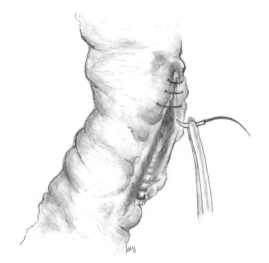

Figure 60.3. The devitalized bowel has been invaginated and healthy serosal surfaces are approximated with interrupted 00 black silk sutures.

Hardy JD: Surgical complications. In: Sabiston D (ed): *Textbook of Surgery.* Philadelphia, WB Saunders, 1981.

Howkins J, Stallworthy J: *Bonney's Gynaecological Surgery,* 8th ed., Baltimore, Williams & Wilkins, 1974.

Irvin TT: Techniques of anastomosis in gastro-intestinal surgery. In: Rod G, Smith R (eds): *Atlas of General Surgery,* 3rd ed. London-Boston, Butterworths, 1981.

Käser O, Iklé FA, Hirsch HA: *Atlas of Gynecological Surgery.* New York, Thieme Stratton Inc., 1985.

Simmons SC, Luck RJ: *General Surgery in Gynaecological Practice.* Oxford & Edinburgh, Blackwell Scientific Publications, 1971.

CHAPTER 61
Rectovaginal Fistula

JOHN J. MIKUTA, M.D.

CASE ABSTRACT

Spontaneous delivery and right mediolateral episiotomy and repair were followed by considerable rectal pain throughout the patient's hospitalization. A fecal impaction was broken up the day before discharge, and there was considerable edema and tenderness of the anterior rectal wall noted. At a dimple at the base of the anterior rectal wall, a small loop of suture was palpable. The patient was discharged.

She complained at her 6-week postpartum checkup that she had difficulty controlling rectal gas, and there was a copious purulent and almost constant vaginal discharge that required sanitary protection.

Although the episiotomy had healed, a 0.5-cm defect surrounded by granulation tissue was noted between the vagina and the top of an anal crypt.

DISCUSSION

The sequence of events in this particular case suggests very strongly that the causative factor in this patient's case was probably a combination of a rectal suture and the trauma that was associated with a fecal impaction as well as its removal. Rectal sutures following episiotomy repair are not at all uncommon. Discovered at the time of the completion of the repair it can be a relatively simple matter to cut the suture and leave it be. On the other hand, there are probably many times when there are unidentified sutures in the rectum at the time of episiotomy repair which are never discovered and appear to cause no significant problems.

A fistula that is discovered 6 weeks after delivery and episiotomy should not be repaired immediately, but the repair should be delayed anywhere from 4 to 6 months. This will allow reduction of the inflammatory reaction, an increase in the blood supply to the area, and time for maximal scar tissue delineation to occur prior to making the attempt at repair. In the meantime, again depending on the size of the fistula, the patient may be made more comfortable by being placed on a low-residue diet and by the reduction of foods that have a tendency to produce intestinal irritability and may in-

crease the amount of gas or create a more liquid type of stool. Another problem is that of resumption of sexual activity where the patient may be concerned about the esthetic effect of the fistula or by the escape of gas during intercourse. Such factors may be controlled by either the use of condoms by the male or by the use of enemas or douches prior to intercourse.

For a very small fistula as described here, it is very important to know whether the fistulous opening leads into the bowel at an angle or whether it is straight and also whether it involves the anal sphincter. In the former case, the repair is relatively straightforward. The latter would require incision through the muscle of the anal sphincter in order to remove all of the scar of the fistula prior to performing the repair.

Assuming that the anal sphincter is intact, one can prepare the patient for the standard layer by layer repair. After the appropriate waiting period and a careful examination with probing of the fistula to determine its direction and length, it is very helpful to proctoscope the patient to be sure that there is no instrinsic bowel disease. A fistula associated with Crohn's disease may be very difficult to repair successfully and may be associated later with other fistulas in the perianal area.

Preoperative preparation should include mechanical cleansing of the bowel with laxatives and enemas to remove as much fecal material as possible. Bowel preparation using neomycin orally may be given over a period of 3 days, although some individuals recommend instillation of neomycin just prior to surgery after a thorough mechanical cleansing of the bowel has been done for several days. A liquid diet 24 hours prior to surgery will help to reduce bowel contents.

The surgical principles involved in a repair of a rectovaginal fistula include having a wide enough ellipse of normal vaginal mucosa removed to guarantee that the underlying tissues that remain will be free of scar and freely mobile. The rectal mucosa then is closed by 3-0 chromic catgut, avoiding entry into the lumen of the bowel and inverting the rectal mucosa into the rectal lumen. A second layer approximates the rectal muscularis and fascia, and the final layer approximates the vaginal mucosa. The second layer is generally of a longer standing material such as Vicryl or Dexon.

Postoperatively the patient is kept on a low-residue diet for several days until spontaneous evacuation of the bowel occurs. Laxatives and enemas are avoided as is digital examination of the rectum.

There may be variations in the technique depending on the location of the fistula. At times a fistula that involves the anal sphincter is best handled by producing a fresh fourth degree tear, excising the fistula completely, and then doing a fresh repair approximating the rectal mucosa, the anal sphincter, and reconstituting the perineal body. In patients who have an old third or fourth degree laceration where the anal sphincter has retracted laterally on either side, the Warren flap operation has for years been a standby, with the creation of a flap which essentially constitutes the posterior vaginal wall with part of the base of the triangle being the areas at which the anal sphincter edges create a puckering of the perianal tissues. A flap is created from this mucosa over which the sphincter edges are approximated. The sphincter edges must be free of scar and fully mobilized. The rectal fascia and the levator ani muscles are approximated over this midline, and then the perineal body is reconstituted to complete the repair.

Today, many people, in carrying out this complete perineal repair, will use a simple layer method where, instead of creating the flap, the tissue is just removed, the sphincter ends are identified, and the denuded tissue is then approximated to reconstitute the anterior rectal wall down to the level where the sphincter has been placed.

There are times when the sphincter has been retracted for such a long period of time that approximation of the sphincter ends creates a significant narrowing of the anal canal. A suggestion made by Miller in the 1930s that a counter sphincterotomy be made away from the site of the repaired sphincter edges and removing the tension from the repair site is an excellent way of avoiding this problem.

The final aspect is when to do a colostomy. Fecal diversion may be necessary in patients who have a fistula of significant size in whom constant soilage is occurring and where a waiting period must be observed before making attempt at repair. This would be especially true of large fistulas or a fistula located high up in the vagina. This type is usually produced by entry into the rectum at the time of abdominal or vaginal hysterectomy. These colostomies are generally undertaken for patient comfort and can be replaced after the successful repair of the fistula.

There are also times when the repair fails and where, in order to have optimal bowel preparation and the healthiest possible environment for the repair, a colostomy should be carried out. While this may be disagreeable to the patient, the fact that it may improve the potential for successful repair may provide a sufficient incentive for the patient to agree to the procedure.

Selected Readings

Mengert WF, Fish SW: Anterior rectal wall advancement. *Obstet Gynecol* 5:262, 1955.

Miller NF, Brown W: The surgical treatment of complete perineal tears in the female. *Am J Obstet Gynecol* 34:196, 1937.

Nichols DH, Milley PS: Surgical significance of the rectovaginal septum. *Am J Obstet Gynecol* 108:215, 1970.

Nichols DH, Randall CL: *Vaginal Surgery*, ed. 2. Baltimore, Williams & Wilkins, 1983.

Warren JC: A new method of operation for the relief of rupture of the perineum through the sphincter and rectum. *Trans Am Gynecol Soc* 72:322, 1882.

CHAPTER 62
Postpartum Rectovaginal Fistula

BRUCE H. DRUKKER, M.D.

CASE ABSTRACT

A 22-year-old primigravida was delivered by spontaneous vaginal delivery of a 7 1/2 pound female infant following an uneventful labor of 6 hours' duration. At the time of delivery, the patient appeared to have sustained a second degree laceration of the perineum which was repaired at the time of delivery. By the second postpartum day, it was evident that the patient was passing fecal material through the vagina and pelvic examination showed a 3-cm laceration of the anterior rectal wall communicating with a defect in the lower posterior wall of the vagina. The perineum and perineal body appeared to be intact. The patient requested immediate repair.

DISCUSSION

Development of signs such as passing flatus or stool per vagina during the immediate or late postpartum period is a disturbing and unpleasant surprise for the patient and her physician. Postpartum rectovaginal fistula is not a common problem and most are preventable. Most commonly these fistulae occur following unsuspected perineal lacerations following vaginal or forceps delivery. The next most frequent cause can follow a median episiotomy with or without fourth degree extension. This type of extension has been reported to occur between 3% and 11% of the time during median episiotomy (4). Finally, but infrequently, fistulae can follow a mediolateral episiotomy, either right or left. The changing trends toward noninterventional obstetrics favors spontaneous vaginal delivery, infrequent episiotomy, alternative delivery locations and alternative delivery position. These changes may lead to an increase in rectovaginal fistula. This increase also may be related to attempted repair of perineal lacerations or episiotomies in positions permitting less than adequate exposure and visualization. Every effort must be made to avoid repair of an episiotomy or spontaneous perineal laceration in a compromised situation without proper lighting, instruments, position, and assistance when needed.

The clinical situation presented of an early

postpartum retovaginal fistula can be classified as a type III rectovaginal fistula (2). This occurence can be attributed to delivery through an introitus and perineum not sufficently "stretchable" to permit passage of the head and shoulders without damage. How could this be prevented? Judgment of perineal and introital capacity is the discerning factor. If following perineal distention there is not adequate "give" of the tissue, a precise midline episiotomy is preferable to the situation which developed in the patient described in this chapter, i.e., spontaneous perineal tear. When making the episiotomy, recall the position of the anterior rectal wall which can be tightly applied to the perineum. The instrument for episiotomy incision, either scissor or scalpel, must be carefully placed. Personally, I prefer a sharp scalpel blade with a wooden tongue depressor placed against the posterior vaginal wall, distending the perineal body and protecting the fetal scalp. An episiotomy, although common, should be regarded with caution.

Repair of spontaneous laceration or episiotomy must be done with the patient in a location and position with adequate exposure and light to permit careful inspection and surgical repair. Often a birthing bed or birthing chair does not permit appropriate exposure. Small, separate, or contiguous anterior rectal wall openings can often be visualized during repair by inserting a gloved index finger into the rectum, separating the perineal tissue, vulva, and posterior vaginal wall and exploring for an opening. If a separate opening is found, the rectum should be incised distal to the opening and a surgical fourth degree episiotomy be completed. Following complete delineation and opening of the rectum to the point of the aperture, closure should begin, inverting the edges with 3-0 polyglycolic acid interrupted suture using a fine taper needle. Sutures should be placed at 0.5 cm intervals inverting the rectal mucosal edge. A second inverting layer of similar suture is advisable, being placed through the perirectal fascia. Therafter, the episiotomy or laceration can be repaired in a routine fashion with 2-0 interrupted polyglycolic acid sutures through the fascial covering of the sphincter muscle. These basic steps should significantly reduce the potential for fistula.

When fistula appears within 24 hours after delivery, for example, assessment for closure is necessary. Although tradition mitigates against primary closure proximate to the diagnosis of the fistula, this narrow time frame coupled with precise surgical technique offers an opportunity for successful closure with sufficient success to permit attempting the procedure. It must be done quickly, however, to remain within the time frame. To attempt closure at this time, the patient requires a rapid bowel prep with an oral purgative and mechanical cleansing of the colon. At the time of transvaginal surgery, immaculate perineal and vaginal cleansing using a povidone iodine solution is mandatory. A minimally moistened, tightly rolled laparotomy pad can be placed in the the recently distended vagina against the cervix to prevent uterine contamination during vaginal prepping. The packing can remain in place during the surgical procedure if it does not compromise exposure. The pad should be removed, of course, immediately following surgery.

The basic principles of surgery to effect closure at this time include development of healthy vascular, non-necrotic tissue planes, absence of contamination, and absence of tissue tension. Since bacterial contamination is a major deterrent to success, prophylactic intravenous antibiotics should be started prior to any incision to assure satisfactory peak serum levels at the time of operation. An appropriate intravenous prophylactic, short-term antibiotic regimen should follow the initial operative dosing. At surgery, the recently repaired episiotomy or primary perineal and vaginal laceration incisions should be opened, all remaining sutures removed, necrotic tissue resected, and edges freshened to obtain healthy tissue. The rectal sphincter should be opened at the sight of previous repair and the rectum opened, too, and slightly above the area of the fistula. The fistula track then should be removed and the entire area copiously irrigated with saline to assure significant reduction in bacterial tissue contamination. These maneuvers essentially convert the perineum, vagina, and fistula into a new fourth degree laceration with good vascularity and healthy tissue. Repair should begin using 3-0 polyglycolic acid suture on the rectal wall, inverting the freshened mucosal edge. Sutures should be interrupted and placed at 0.5 cm intervals. The perirectal fascia should be closed in a similar fashion after mucosa has been completely closed from the apex of the fistula to the anal opening. The rectal sphincter should be approximated by placing interrupted polyglycolic acid 2-0 suture through the muscular fascia, thus bringing into apposition the fresh edges of the sphincter muscle located within the facial ring. Often five or six sutures are necessary with care taken to place these sutures in both cephalad and caudad positions of the fascial ring. Do not rely on one or two sutures to maintain the fascial integrity. No sutures are required in the muscle per se. The remaining portion of the perineal defect can be repaired similar to an episiotomy, using absorbable suture and closing the perineum with a subcuticular 3-0 polyglycolic acid suture. A very small, low pressure suction drain placed just below the vaginal wall can be used but is rarely necessary. If it is used, it should be left in place for only 24 hours. Postoperatively, a low residue, high fiber, nonconstipating diet with a stool softener (3) should be used for 14 days. Sphincterotomy by scalpel at the 5:00 to 6:00 position can be considered if the rectal mucosal defect is of significant length, i.e., greater than 4 cm, or if there is any suggestion that there will be increased pressure on the anterior rectal wall due to a tight sphincter. This type of sphincterotomy heals spontaneously without fecal incontinence. If a fistula redevelops following this closure, another repair should be delayed until all infection and induration have subsided and complete scarification has occurred. Delay of 12 to 16 weeks is usual. Prior to surgery, colon cleansing, as previously described, is necessary. Surgical repair can take a number of approaches. Isolation loop colostomy is not routinely necessary for closure at this time.

If the fistula is located proximate to the introitus and external to the hymenal tags, it can be repaired by recreating a fourth degree midline episiotomy, excising the fistula track, reapproximating the rectal mucosa and repairing the sphincter as previously described. The remaining closure is similar to an episiotomy. For a fistula located higher in the vagina, the so-called type III, a transvaginal approach without creation of an episiotomy is appropriate. In this situation, a circumferential incision through the vaginal mucosa around the fistula opening is dissected, and the fistula track identified, including its attachment to the rectum. With meticulous care, the entire fistula tract is removed, thus creating an opening to the anterior rectal wall somewhat larger than the fistula tract. Meticulous closure of the rectal wall is necessary using interrupted 3-0 polyglycolic acid sutures on a small taper needle. Suture placement should be 0.5 centimeter apart or closure can be affected by a purse string suture that does not crimp the anterior rectal wall too tightly. The perirectal fascia is closed in a linear fashion and vaginal mucosa can be closed with interrupted 2-0 polyglycolic acid sutures. If additional reinforcement of the repair is necessary, a bulbocavernosus fat pad flap can be created from either labia and sutured over the perirectal fascia closure. A transperineal repair has also been described which may give more mobilization of tissue proximate to the fistula, improved visualization of the rectal orifice of the fistula and decrease the occasional tendency for vaginal constriction. This approach should be considered seriously if a very large fistula is present (5). Repair of fistulae close to the introitus will, in some situations, result in a thin perineal body. In these situations, initial development of cruciate incisions across the perineal body with advancement of skin flaps following levator plication and sphincter apposition will recreate normal distance between the anus and intoitus (1). It is important to restore as much muscular integrity of the perineum as possible, if the area is shortened or defective.

Unfortunately, rectovaginal fistula repair will fail, on rare occasion, despite meticulous preparation and careful technique. Should a fistula repair fail following a second attempt, isolation loop colostomy should be considered before embarking on a third repair. The colostomy should be fashioned to prevent seepage of colonic contents from one stoma to another which can occur with proximate stoma locations often created by loop colostomies. If colonic contamination is prevented, spontaneous fistula closure will, in some situations, occur following diversion. If spontaneous closure does not occur, surgical correction in a clean field will yield excellent results following basic surgical principles for fistula repair. After the fistula has healed completely and there has been documented evidence of integrity of the anterior rectal wall and posterior vaginal wall, colon reanastomosis can be accomplished at a convenient time, ususally 3 to 4 months later.

References

1. Corman ML: Anal incontinence following obstetrical injury. *Dis Colon Rectum* 28:86, 1985.
2. Rosenshein NB, Genadry RR, Woodruff JD: An anatomic classification of rectovaginal septal defects. *Am J Obstet Gynecol* 137:439, 1980.
3. Rothenberger DA, Goldberg SM: The management of rectovaginal fistulae. *Surg Clin North Am* 63:61, 1983.
4. Shieh CJ, Gennaro AR: Rectovaginal fistula: A review of 11 years experience. *Int Surg* 69:69, 1984.
5. Thompson JD, Masterson BJ: Transperineal repair of rectovaginal fistula. *Ob/Gyn Illustrated*, The Upjohn Company, 1985.

CHAPTER **63**

Napkin-ring Constriction of Descending Colon

CLAYTON T. BEECHAM, M.D.

CASE ABSTRACT

A 50-year-old nulligravida, with a lifelong history of incapacitating dysmenorrhea, recently developed rectal tenesmus, constipation, and lower abdominal cramps. These are accentuated at the time of her menstrual period and coincide with pain in her back and pelvis—both radiate down the medial surface of her left thigh. Pelvic examination discloses the internal genitalia to be "frozen," and barium enema study demonstrates a "napkin-ring" constriction of the descending colon below its midportion.

DISCUSSION

The Problem

1. Long-standing pelvic pain.
2. Pelvic examination is consistent with advanced endometriosis.
3. Bowel symptoms with x-ray demonstration of descending colon constriction are not unexpected with this protracted clinical entity.
4. Provide relief.

Approach to the Problem

The crescendo of pain is consistent with untreated endometriosis. Coalesced and solidified endometriotic lesions have obliterated the posterior cul-de-sac and made identification of the pelvic viscera next to impossible. To the examiner, only one other entity could simulate this picture, i.e., ovarian carcinoma. While both lesions can "feel" alike, ovarian carcinoma is not tender to touch nor does it give the ligneous impression which characterizes endometriosis. And the medical histories of the two diseases are not comparable. Demonstration of an encircling constriction of the pelvic colon adds confirmation to the clinical diagnosis of stage 4 endometriosis.

Solution to the Problem

No further diagnostic studies are indicated. Sonography and laparoscopy would add expense, delay, and little, if any, information to what has been learned by history, pelvic examination, and x-ray studies.

Accordingly, after routine preoperative studies plus bowel preparation, a pelvic laparotomy should be carried out. All manner of elaborate colonic routines have been described for anticipated bowel surgery; however, we find mechanical cleansing adequate: one dose of magnesium citrate with cleansing enemas twice a day for 1 day, while the patient maintains a clear liquid diet.

At surgery, upon assessment of the endometriotic involvement, one must first be assured that he is dealing with endometriosis. If the colonic lesion is a direct extension of the pelvic disease, there can be little doubt; however, should the constricting lesion be separate from the internal genitalia and appear to exist as an isolated enitity, a biopsy with immediate frozen section study must be carried out.

After verification of the diagnosis, a total hysterectomy and bilateral salpingo-oophorectomy with resection of the colonic lesion is optimum treatment. At age 50 years, there is no place for conservative surgery.

Hysterectomy in the presence of broad ligament and cul-de-sac endometriosis should follow the principles described in the chapter on crushed ureter. Liberal use of dessicating electrocoagulation will be useful in the depths of the broad ligament. Careful avoidance of the ureter is essential.

After the hysterectomy and after the adnexa have been removed, a bowel resection with end-to-end anastomosis should be carried out. It has been suggested that removal of the adnexa alone will result in endometrial necrosis; therefore, the bowel resection would not be necessary. However, the amount of fibrosis and collagen formation in and around the bowel, the adnexa, cul-de-sac, and uterus in a lesion this massive contraindicated anything less than total removal. Bowel obstruction, due to residual disease, sometime postoperatively is too much of a hazard to risk less than complete removal.

As the surgery is being completed and hemostasis assured, the vaginal apex is best left open but peritonealized. This simple step provides adequate drainage.

The natural, water soluble, conjugated estrogen Premarin 1.25 mg with methyl testosterone 10 mg (available in a combined tablet) should be administered starting the second postoperative day and continued indefinitely. This medication has many advantages: (a) It prevents menopausal symptoms without stimulating endometiotic implants, moreover, it allows them to atrophy. (b) Prevents osteoporosis. (c) Reinforces anabolism in the patient's aging metabolism.

Selected Reading

Beecham CT: Endometriosis: When is surgical treatment indicated? *Postgrad Med* 63:221, 1978.

CHAPTER **64**

Carcinoma of the Vulva with Coexistent Genital Prolapse

GEORGE W. MORLEY, M.S., M.D.

CASE ABSTRACT

A 39-year-old, married homemaker with multiparous relaxation of the vagina, mild urinary stress incontinence, and a retroverted, slightly enlarged uterus, has a 1.5-cm invasive squamous cell carcinoma of the right labium majus. A single, hard, not movable lymph node is palpable in the right groin.

DISCUSSION

It is interesting to note that this patient is only 39 years of age since invasive carcinoma of the vulva is seen more commonly as a clinical entity in the older age population. This lesion is, however, seen occasionally in younger patients; therefore, one should be prepared to carry out appropriate diagnostic tests when a lesion of this type is seen in this age group. This patient's lesion is classified as stage 2 since the groin lymph node appears to be suspicious. The treatment of choice for this patient is radical vulvectomy and bilateral groin lymph node dissection and pelvic lymph node exploration. Certainly a frozen section should be carried out on the suspicious groin lymph node; should this be positive, then most gynecologic oncologists would carry out a retroperitoneal pelvic lymph node dissection immediately. The issue of whether this patient should be treated with postoperative pelvic irradiation is not within the scope of this discussion.

The question raised in this abstract is an interesting one in that it becomes a question of clinical judgment as to whether surgery for two different and unrelated problems should be performed at "one sitting." In this day and age, with more sophisticated anesthetic methods and with improved surgical techniques,

certainly this question enters the realm of possibilities, and it deserves our focus of attention. Much experience has been reported in the surgical literature throughout the past decade, and many authors feel that "double" surgery for unrelated pathologic conditions carries with it very little risk. This seems to be especially true when one considers intra-abdominal procedures, e.g., hysterectomy and cholecystectomy, etc.

In regard to this specific patient, the answer seems quite simple since the patient has only "mild" urinary stress incontinence and the uterus is only "slightly" enlarged. In this patient, I would be much more concerned with possibly altering our surgical techniques as they relate to the primary problem in an attempt to preserve the clitoral tissue without jeopardizing her chance for survival. This, of course, would increase the operating time. It is possible that too much tissue is removed in performing the radical vulvectomy part of the procedure since the disease extends primarily through lymph channels once the primary lesion has been surgically controlled. This question can only be resolved by gynecologic oncologists who see a significant number of these patients each year and in clinics where close follow-up is a major part of their effort. It must be remembered, however, that the conventional therapy as indicated above is the treatment of choice until such time that the results from these principal investigators are in!

If one is considering more surgery for this patient, then certainly "cosmetic" vulvoplasty should be given our attention. Certain rotational or transpositional flap techniques could be included in the primary procedure in an attempt to gain an improved cosmetic result. To date, most gynecologic oncologists have deferred this part of the procedure because of: (a) lack of experience, (b) limited technical possibilities, and (c) poor results. Furthermore, a number of these patients develop functional abnormalities—such as misdirected micturition, introital stenosis, or marked pelvic relaxation—which requires surgical correction in the future. It is at this time that some type of vulvoplasty can be considered.

As I pondered this abstract, I altered it in the following way: moderate stress urinary incontinence and grade 2 uterine prolapse with a symptomatic rectocele, and the patient wants something done. This makes the discussion more controversial. If the patient were 75 years of age, the answer would be easier and I would probably deny her request.

Even in the 39-year-old patient, given the risk of additional surgery and another anesthetic and in realizing that abdominal and pelvic surgeons are less hesitant today to do unrelated surgeries at one time, there is one overwhelming point that supports the decision not to perform combined surgery in this patient. It has often been reported that wound infection and wound disruption are the most common complications following radical pelvic surgery for an existing invasive carcinoma of the vulva. This mitigates against doing any additional elective surgery on these patients. The rectal area is difficult to sterilize, and, in its close proximity to the operative site, this may, in itself, be a reason for the high incidence of groin wound breakdown. One could, however, do a perineorrhaphy at the time of closure of the posterior vulvar wound to correct this patient's symptomatic rectocele. In addition, one might consider an anterior colporrhaphy in an attempt to correct the stress urinary incontinence symptoms. I confess I would have to draw the line at this point. Objectively speaking, I would be strongly opposed to entering the peritoneal cavity via the vaginal hysterectomy and to entering the space of Retzius with all its vascularity in performing a retropubic urethropexy.

In the future, should the incidence of wound disruption in radical vulvectomy and groin lymph node dissection decrease significantly, then the treatment of the symptomatic pelvic relaxation could be seriously considered—especially in a 39-year-old patient. This patient may want something done, but her desires could suddenly change should she experience a significant postoperative complication. This combined surgical approach would be difficult to defend in other arenas.

I am certain there are a number of less conservative gynecologic surgeons who would not hesitate to do a radical vulvectomy and groin lymph node dissection followed by a vaginal hysterectomy, and anterior colporrhaphy or possibly a retropubic urethropexy, a posterior colpoperineorrhaphy, and even a sacrospinous ligament suspension of the vaginal apex if indicated—especially in a a 39-year-old patient. More than likely, the patient would do well; however, if she becomes morbid, it could be very significant. Age itself would probably influence me only a very little in my decision, and I have heard physicians say that they took a chance in a young patient and did thus and so. We must remember it is the patient who takes the chance!

Finally, and on a somewhat philosophic note, it seems wiser to avoid the "blue-plate special" or the "package deal" as a convenience to the patient when one might place the patient in significant jeopardy.

CHAPTER 65

Radical Vulvectomy — One Node Positive

PHILIP J. DiSAIA, M.D.

CASE ABSTRACT

A 70-year-old patient, in otherwise good health, has had a radical vulvectomy with bilateral superficial node excision because of a grade 2 invasive squamous cell carcinoma of about 1.5 cm in diameter involving the inner surface of the right labia majora. Although no nodes were palpable, a bilateral inguino-femoral lymph node dissection was accomplished and one node of 20, from the patient's right, but not the node of Cloquet, was positive for metastatic disease.

DISCUSSION

The patient described has a small invasive squamous cell cancer of the vulva and is discovered to have only one positive lymph node in the ipsilateral groin dissection. Several questions arise: (a) Should the contralateral groin have been dissected? (b) Should the deep pelvic nodes be excised, and if so, should the dissection be done on one or both sides? (c) Are further diagnostic studies appropriate? (d) What additional therapy should be advised?

Over the last decade, clinicians have been tailoring therapy in vulvar cancer to the diseased state, often avoiding extended surgical procedures. This statement is especially true for small lesions such as this case presents. Our preference for this case would have restricted the groin dissection to the right side (ipsilateral) because her lesion was less than 2 cm and lateralized. Our experience has shown that with lateralized lesions less than 2 cm in diameter, the contralateral groin nodes are rarely involved, unless extensive lymph node involvement is found with a small central lesion, it is invariably an anaplastic primary tumor which is the source. If the contralateral side had not been dissected, a program of close observation for at least 2 years would be practiced at our institution because our experience has shown that good salvage can be attained with delayed

inguino-femoral node dissections in patients who subsequently develop palpable groin nodes.

In our experience, the prognosis for patients with clinically negative groins who are found to have one positive inguinal node, is very similar to that of patients with negative nodes. A similar outcome was reported by Boyce et al, in a review of all patients with one positive groin node where a 78% 2-year survival was compared to an 82% recurrence-free interval in all patients with negative nodes. Based on these observations, our recommendation would be to omit the pelvic lymphadenectomy on the uninvolved side, since several studies have shown that pelvic node involvement does not occur in the absence of ipsilateral inguinal nodal metastasis.

Further diagnostic studies should be considered. Since this patient is asymptomatic and undoubtedly had a preoperative chest x-ray, the only recommendation we suggest would be a CT scan of the abdomen and pelvis with intravenous contrast to outline rare distant metastases. The cost effectiveness of even this recommendation could be questioned. Lymphangiography should not be considered since an inguino-femoral lymphadenectomy results in ligation of the main lymphatic channels from the leg to the pelvis and periaortic nodes, resulting in a very poor study.

Adjuvant therapy in the form of chemotherapy or radiation therapy is not necessary in this case. Chemotherapy for vulvar squamous cancer is not very effective and hardly appropriate in a patient with such a good prognosis. The issue of adjuvant radiation therapy to the groins and pelvis is not nearly as well defined. Preliminary analysis of a Gynecologic Oncology Group study suggested that survival with postoperative radiation therapy for patients with positive groin nodes in whom the deep pelvic nodes were not dissected survived as well as patients who underwent pelvic lymphadenectomy. The real issue is the probability that the patient has a positive pelvic node balanced against the morbidity and expense of radiation therapy. The probability of a positive pelvic node in all patients with positive inguinal nodes is 20%. With only one positive inguinal node and a small central lesion, this probably falls to less than 5%. In addition, experience has shown that only 20% of patients with positive pelvic nodes survive 5 years following therapy. Therefore, our preference in this case would be to omit all adjuvant therapy unless the CT scan was positive.

Selected Readings

Boyce J, et al: Prognostic factors in carcinoma of the vulva. *Gynecol Oncol* 20:364-377, 1985

Figge D, Tamimi H, Greer B: Lymphatic spread in carcinoma of the vulva. *Am J Obstet Gynecol* 152:387-392, 1985.

Franklin EW, Rutledge FN: Prognostic factors in epidermoid carcinoma of the vulva. *Obstet Gynecol* 37:892-901, 1971.

GOG Statistical Report, July, 1985

Morris JM: A formula for selective lymphadenectomy: Its application to cancer of the vulva. *Obstet Gynecol* 50:152-158, 1977.

CHAPTER 66
Carcinoma of the Vulva with Postoperative Inguinal Wound Breakdown

GEORGE W. MORLEY, M.S., M.D.

CASE ABSTRACT

A radical vulvectomy with en bloc bilateral superficial inguinal lymphadenectomy had been performed on a 62-year-old, 276-lb, diabetic through a large "butterfly"-type incision, with primary closure of all exposed surfaces. Preoperative biopsy had shown an invasive, well-differentiated squamous cell carcinoma, 1 × 2.5 cm, on the medial aspect of the left labia majus.

On the third postoperative day, the inguinal skin flaps were swollen and inflamed and the incisional edges were dusky colored. The patient was, and remained, afebrile.

When the skin sutures were removed on the fifth postoperative day, the wounds were grossly purulent, and the skin flaps in the inguinal areas pale white, becoming necrotic, and well demarcated from the adjacent viable skin. After debridement, the underlying soft tissues, covered with thick, creamy, purulent exudate, were widely exposed. A foul-smelling odor was present.

DISCUSSION

First of all, it must be remembered that wound breakdown in a patient who has undergone a radical vulvectomy and bilateral groin lymph node dissections is the most common complication encountered in the treatment of invasive carcinoma of the vulva (3). This complication is frightening to the patient and worrisome to the more junior physicians caring for the patient, but it must be realized that it is not that bad a complication and the patients respond satisfactorily to appropriate conservative measures once the wound is adequately exposed and treated accordingly. It must be remembered that this patient had a significant lesion of the vulva classified as Stage II since the lesion was greater than 2 cm (Fig. 66.1) in diameter and it was necessary to do an extensive procedure to control the malignant process.

From a review of the literature and from personal communications, the inguinal wounds following this procedure break down to some degree in approximately 50% to 75% of the cases. It has been stated that if the wound does not break down to some degree then an adequate enough procedure probably has not been performed!

In our own series at the University of Michigan, approximately 50% of the wounds break down to some extent. Oftentimes, these wounds become infected locally without any associated febrile episodes. It is important, however, that one open the wound more adequately once this complication is recognized so that appropriate treatment can be carried out. All of our patients undergoing this procedure are treated with prophylactic broad-spectrum antibiotics. Infrequently, a significant cellulitis will occur, and these patients must be treated more aggressively utilizing appropriate therapeutic doses of chemotherapeutic agents.

In discussing this complication of radical vulvectomy and groin lymph node dissection,

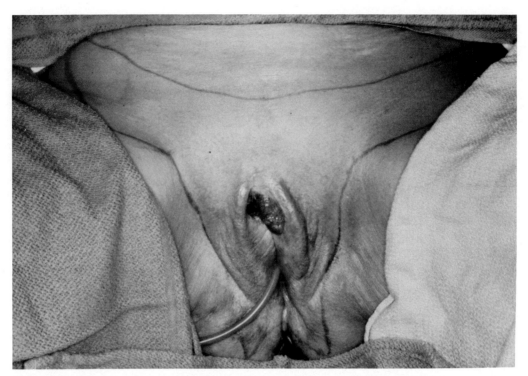

Figure 66.1.   Invasive carcinoma of the vulva. Stage II (lesion greater than 2 cm in diameter, involving the clitoris and paraclitoral tissue). "Butterfly" incision is also outlined in this figure.

one must first consider the question, "Could it be prevented?" In a review of the literature, there are many techiques described for the type of incision to be used in performing the groin lymph node dissection on these patients. Whether one selects a "butterfly"-type of incision or uses separate inguinal incisions for the lymph node dissection does not seem to play any significant role. Personally, I have used the "butterfly" incision (Fig. 66.1) for the past 25 years, and this continues to be the incision of choice in our institution (2).

In the future, with patients seeking medical attention earlier, we will see early Stage I disease more frequently. In these cases, it is perfectly appropriate to use the "3-in-1" incision with the vulvar tissue and the right and left groin lymph node tissue being removed through three separate incisions.

During my residency training and shortly thereafter, I used separate groin incisions with undermining of the skin flaps. It is my belief that if one uses the full-thickness type of dissection as described in the "butterfly" technique, this complication can be significantly

reduced. In doing an adequate full-thickness dissection, one must be certain that the width of the skin incisions is 7 to 8 cm at its greatest point to ensure an adequate dissection of the lymph node-bearing area. On the other hand, if the undermining technique is utilized, then one must be certain to remove all of the tissue lying deep to Camper's fascia, again to ensure removal of all of the superficial groin lymph nodes. As stated above, this technique does give rise to an increased incidence of skin flap loss through infection and necrosis.

We carry out several steps in an attempt to reduce significantly the incidence of wound breakdown. First of all, while in the operating room, we "freshen up" the skin flaps and the underlying subcutaneous tissue after completion of this rather lengthy dissection. The incisions are then closed in layers using one of a variety of absorbable sutures. The skin edges are approximated at wide intervals between the sutures to encourage adequate drainage of the wound. A pressure dressing is then applied in an attempt to reduce fluid accumulation and to immobilize the wound flaps as effectively as

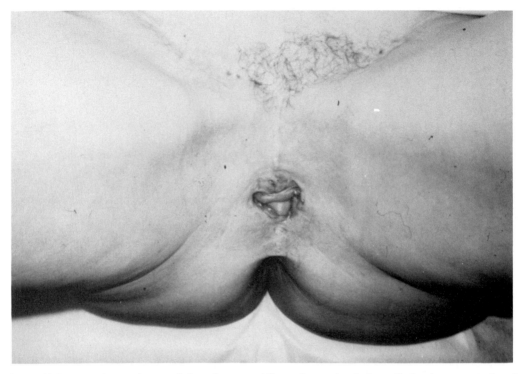

Figure 66.2.   Invasive carcinoma of the vulva treated 3 months previously by radical vulvectomy and groin and pelvic lymphadenectomy. Note linear scarring which represents complete healing.

possible to encourage wound healing. A number of surgeons dress the wounds open to allow closure by secondary intention.

The patients are placed in a semi-Fowler's position for 48 hours to reduce the tension on the suture line. They are strictly confined to bed for approximately 72 hours. All of these patients had been placed on prophylactic anticoagulant therapy, and they are urged to move around in bed at frequent intervals.

One of the most controversial issues encountered in this type of discussion is whether to drain the wounds once the procedure is completed. I do not use drains in these wounds and have no reason to regret this decision. This approach to the "drains" issue is supported by a number of gynecologic oncologists. On the other hand, there are a number of surgeons who believe to the contrary.

A word of caution must be registered in regard to the dissection of the mons veneris tissue overlying the symphysis pubis. It seems advisable to leave a small amount of fatty tissue on the periosteum in this area so that the periosteum is not traumatized. There have been

a few isolated reports of osteitis pubis secondary to an overly aggressive dissection of this area, and this complication is extremely difficult to treat satisfactorily. Frequently, the area overlying the symphysis cannot be closed primarily. This should cause no concern, and this part of the wound is dressed with appropriate packing.

The use of skin grafts in this area is not recommended since all of these wounds ultimately heal primarily with linear scarring overlying the symphysis similarly as seen in the groin wounds (Fig. 66.2). The use of skin graft not only further prolongs the operative procedure in these elderly patients but the end result is somewhat disfiguring since there is no underlying fatty tissue in the region of the skin grafts.

If the wound has not healed satisfactorily and the common complication of wound breakdown is encountered, then an aggressive approach to its treatment is to be outlined. As stated before, these wounds should be opened up completely to the extent of the infection so that adequate therapy can be applied. Debridement is carried out periodically to "freshen up" the wound edges to rid the exposed area of the necrotic membrane. These wounds are packed three times daily, and the patients are placed in a whirlpool bath for 30 minutes twice daily to stimulate wound healing. Silver nitrate, potassium permanganate, Elase, and various antibiotic ointments have been utilized in the past, but their efficacy has been challenged. Applications of honey to these open wounds is recommended periodically by the more junior staff caring for these patients, and it does have some merit. In the undiluted form, honey is considered to be bactericidal, and it is thought not to support pathogenic organisms (1). Skin grafts should not be used in these areas, at least until the infection is cleared and the wound is granulating in well. The indications for the use of skin graft at this time seem to be very limited.

One must exercise great caution, however, in the debridement of the diabetic patient since the potential for wound healing is compromised in these people. Although debridement is good 90% of the time, there is a 10% untoward response, since debridement itself also causes some tissue destruction. In the diabetic patient, one must be sure that the necrotic area is well demarcated before carrying out aggressive debridement.

Once the wounds have started to heal and the infection is cleared, then the patients become increasingly active in the self-care of their wounds. The nurse in charge instructs the patient on the dressing changes and packing of the wounds. Once the patient is comfortable with this self-care program, she is ready for discharge from the hospital. The median hospital stay for these patients is about 21 days; however, if the wounds do not break down, the patient can usually be discharged approximately 2 weeks after surgery.

There are other complications that should be mentioned in the postoperative care of these patients. Rarely do any of these patients encounter a thromboembolic complication to the surgery. This is somewhat surprising since these patients are not only elderly and are strictly confined to bed postoperatively for a short period of time, but the surgery directly involves the femoral and oftentimes the pelvic venous system. One should always be alerted to the possibility of pulmonary embolization and act accordingly. As stated above, all of these patients are treated with prophylactic anticoagu-

lant therapy, which is continued until they are actively ambulated in the postoperative period.

The risk of hemorrhage, particularly from the groin region, is ever present in these patients, but this again is an unusual complication. The major blood supply to the leg is exposed when performing the deep groin lymph node dissection and certainly must be protected following the initial dissection. This is accomplished with closure of the cribriform fascia over the vessels, or, if the dissection is extensive, the sartorius muscle can be transplanted from its lateral insertion into the anterior iliac spine and lateral third of the inguinal ligament medially with an attachment to the inner portion of Poupart's ligament, thus overlying these vessels.

On infrequent occasions, a groin lymphocyst will be encountered in the postoperative period. These "cysts" usually can be prevented by being certain that all of the vessels are clamped and tied throughout the dissection. If this complication does occur, it can be treated rather conservatively with intermittent aspiration of the lymph fluid followed by pressure dressings. The surgical approach to the control of this complication is rarely, if ever, necessary.

In regard to delayed complications, chronic lymphedema of the lower extremities seems to be the only one that appears with any significant frequency. Although most of these patients do not complain of any particular discomfort from this complication, they are terribly self-conscious about the resultant deformity and appearance of the "fat" leg. In an attempt to avoid this, elastic stockings (at least up to the knee) should be worn postoperatively every day for at least 6 months, and other conservative precautions should be outlined for the patient. Recently, we have been preserving the saphenous vein during the groin lymph node dissection; whether this will aid in the reduction of the incidence of chronic lymphedema remains to be seen.

In closing, it must be remembered that the breakdown of the wounds in patients undergoing radical vulvectomy and groin lymph node dissection is the most common complication encountered in patients going through this procedure; yet, it must be realized that the 5-year survival rate of women treated in this way is most satisfactory. From a collaborative review, one estimates that the 5-year survival rate for patients having no positive inguinal lymph nodes is approximately 90%. If one groin lymph node is involved with metastatic disease, the 5-year survival rate is reduced to approximately 85%. If more than one node is involved, the overall survival rate is reduced to around 50%. In the future, not only do we still have to improve the survival rates, but we must focus our attention on various surgical techniques and care of wounds so that we can reduce the incidence of this fairly common complication.

If one does review the various modifications being reported concerning surgical techniques, probably the most significant contribution has been in the area of incisions. In the past 10 to 15 years, fortunately, the lesions seen are much more often either classified as Stage I or early Stage II. In this group of patients, the separate "3-in-1" incision is preferred to the "butterfly" incision. With this preservation of normal tissue, one notes that the postoperative morbidity and complications are lessened significantly.

References

1. Cavanagh D, Beazley J, Ostapowicz F: Radical operation for carcinoma of the vulva: A new approach to wound healing. *J Obstet Gynaecol Br Commonw* 77:1037, 1970.
2. Morley GW: Infiltrative carcinoma of the vulva: Results of surgical management. *Am J Obstet Gynecol* 124:874, 1976.
3. Way S: Carcinoma of the vulva. *Am J Obstet Gynecol* 79:692, 1960.

CHAPTER 67
Vulvar Paget's Disease

JOHN McLEAN MORRIS, M.D.

CASE ABSTRACT

A 48-year-old multipara has a vulvar biopsy which shows Paget's disease. Examination shows a healing scar surrounded by a reddened area in the right labial area. There are several shotty nodes in each groin.

DISCUSSION

Diagnosis

This case has been appropriately approached by vulvar biopsy. Extramammary Paget's disease occurs in areas in which apocrine glands are present, including the axilla, perianal region, vulva, auditory canal, nasal vestibule, and eyelids. Histochemical staining may be necessary to differentiate Paget's disease from disorders such as amelanotic melanoma.

Because of the frequent occurrence of other cancers in such patients, particularly breast cancer, any necessary steps should be taken to rule out concomitant carcinoma elsewhere (4, 11).

Treatment of the Vulvar Lesion

Clinically, Paget's disease may show areas of erythema or hyperkeratosis, but Paget cells may be also found just above the basal layer of the epidermis when the overlying skin appears perfectly normal. Even wide vulvectomy may show the process extending to the margins of the resection. Local recurrence, sometimes extending as far us as the umbilicus, may require repeated re-excisions. Extension to the perianal area is not uncommon and may ultimately require posterior resections with or without colostomy. Therefore, in this patient, in spite of her relatively young age, a wide vulvectomy is indicated.

Careful sectioning will frequently show the disorder extending down apocrine gland ducts and into underlying apocrine glands. Underlying apocrine gland invasive carcinoma will be found in approximately 25% of cases of vulvar

Paget's disease (1, 5, 8, 11). Over a 20-year period at Yale, eight patients with vulvar Paget's disease were encountered. Two of these had underlying apocrine gland cancer. For this reason, skinning vulvectomy is not adequate, and the dissection must be carried down to the underlying fascia. Local excision as well as laser or cryosurgical techniques are not acceptable.

Vulvectomy in such patients does not preclude the resumption of sexual activity. While ordinarily vulvar cancers are encountered in elderly patients, younger patients undergoing vulvectomy have reported satisfactory sexual relationships associated with orgasm. On occasion, patients have said that intercourse was more satisfactory because of elimination of pain or irritation from the disease process.

Treatment of the Nodes

The presence of shotty nodes in both groins raises the question as to whether further evaluation of the groin areas should be carried out, including lymphangiograms, node biopsies, radical node dissections, or radiation therapy to inguinal and pelvic node areas. As vulvar Paget's disease is usually an intraepithelial form of malignancy, it would seem inappropriate to carry out any such studies unless the final sections of the vulva show underlying apocrine gland cancer. This may require multiple sectioning of the specimen and, except in unusual circumstances, should not be attempted by frozen sections at the time of surgery.

Should invasive carcinoma be found in the specimen, the question of the enlarged nodes would have to be re-evaluated. Lymphangiography has generally been abandoned as being inaccurate, with dye uptake in only approximately half of the nodes in a given area, as well as misleading in a high proportion of cases. With large nodes needle biopsies may be helpful, but with a small superficial inguinal node, excision of the node may be more satisfactory in helping establish a diagnosis.

The more important question that arises if invasive apocrine gland carcinoma is found in the vulvectomy specimen is whether lymphadenectomy should be carried out. If so, should it be unilateral or bilateral? Should dissection be confined to the inguinal nodes, or should it include the pelvic nodes, the common iliac, and lower para-aortic nodes? For the gynecologic surgeon who believes-as some do-that "excision must be as ruthless as the disease itself," the wider and more extensive the dissection, the greater the theoretical cure rate. In a young patient of 48 years of age, the mortality of the procedure should not be excessive. Unfortunately, however, the fact that there was only one 5-year survivor among 17 patients reported in the literature who were found to have node metastases in Paget's disease with underlying apocrine gland carcinoma leaves the value of routine lymphadenectomy open to question (1, 5, 8).

A formula has been suggested (6) which can be applied to node dissection in which the benefit factor equals the percent of patients with positive node lymphadenectomy. This is balanced against the operative mortality, complications, and the cure rate by other modalities (radiation therapy).

The reported incidence of positive nodes in apocrine gland carcinoma of the vulva is approximately 40%. If one assumes a cure rate of 10% in cases with positive nodes, the benefit factor would be four patients saved per 100 operations. The operative mortality in 445 cases of vulvectomy with inguinal and pelvic node dissection reported in the literature in the years 1970 through 1980 was 4.5% (7). While in this relatively young patient, the figure would undoubtedly be very much lower, subtracting the mortality from the possible cure rate would, perhaps, be in the vicinity of 2%. She could probably withstand the complications. These include wound breakdown, lymphocysts, postoperative edema of the lower extremities, and erysipelas. The question can be raised as to whether radiating the node areas with a dose of 4000 to 4500 rads might not achieve an equal or better result. If, of course, the patient presented any significant surgical risk, such as recent myocardial infarction or other problems, the formula would show a far better result if radiotherapy was substituted for radical lymphadenectomy.

If the ipsilateral superficial nodes are negative, the chance of deep or contralateral node involvement is so small (less than 4%) and the cure rate so low that the benefit factor (less than 0.5%) would be definitely outweighed by the risks of bilateral inguinal and pelvic lymphadenectomy.

Removal of the superficial nodes on the ipsilateral side in cases of early vulvar cancer and doing nothing further if these nodes prove negative offers the best benefit-risk ratios to the patient (3). This would seem to be a sensible course of action in this case, carrying out either further bilateral inguinal and iliac node dissections should frozen sections show node involvement or, as an alternative, postoperative radiation therapy to the nodal areas. Removal of para-aortic nodes has been advocated by some in vulvar cancer, but the advocates fail to recognize that they have not cured any of the patients in whom the nodes are involved.

Follow-Up

Multiple local recurrences, as well as the development of other primary tumors, are extremely common events in cases of vulvar Paget's disease. Careful follow-up over a period of many years is essential. Vulvar cytology or toluidine blue tests are unsatisfactory in indicating sites or extent of recurrence. Biopsies of hyperkeratotic or erythematous areas may show tumor, which may be a recurrence or may be a separate second primary tumor. There are many reports of cases with subsequent involvement of the vulva, perianal area, rectum, vagina, cervix, urethra, bladder, bowel and other sites with Pagetoid or other histologic tumor types including squamous cancer, transitional cell cancer, and adenocarcinoma.

Because of the inaccuracy of methods for clinical estimation of the extent of the disease, laser or cautery are generally not suitable methods for treatment. Occasional remissions or cures have been achieved with radiation therapy or local 5-fluorouracil applications, but re-excision is preferable (2, 9, 10).

References

1. Boehm F, Morris JM: Paget's disease and apocrine gland carcinoma of the vulva. *Obstet Gynecol* 38:185, 1971.
2. Creasman WT, Gallager HS, Rutledge R: Paget's disease of the vulva. *Gynecol Oncol* 3:133, 1975.
3. DiSaia PJ, Creasman WT, Rich WM: An alternate approach to early cancer of the vulva. *Am J Obstet Gynecol* 133:825, 1979.
4. Friedrich EG, Wilkinson EJ, Steingraeber PH, et al: Paget's disease of the vulva and carcinoma of the breast. *Obstet Gynecol* 46:130, 1975.
5. Lee SC, Roth LM, Ehrlich C, et al: Extramammary Paget's disease of the vulva: A clinicopathologic study of 13 cases. *Cancer* 39:2540, 1977.
6. Morris JM: A formula for selective lymphadenectomy and its application to cancer of the vulva. *Obstet Gynecol* 50:152, 1977.
7. Morris JM: Risk/benefit ratios in the management of gynecologic cancer. *Cancer* 48:642, 1981.
8. Parmley TH, Woodruff JD, Julian CG: Invasive vulvar Paget's disease. *Obstet Gynecol* 46:341, 1975.
9. Pitman GH, McCarthy JG, Perzin KH, et al: Extramammary Paget's disease. *Plast Reconstr Surg* 69:238, 1982.
10. Sillman FH, Sedlis A, Boyce JG: A review of lower genital intraepithelial neoplasia and the use of topical 5-fluorouracil. *Obstet Gynecol* 40:190, 1985.
11. Tsukada Y, Lopez RG, Pickren JW, et al: Paget's disease of the vulva, a clinicopathologic study of eight cases. *Obstet Gynecol* 45:73, 1975.

CHAPTER 68

Vulvar Paget's Disease Involving Anal Skin

JOHN H. ISAACS, M.D.

CASE ABSTRACT

The vulvar biospy of a 42-year-old married woman with a long history of vulvar pruritis was diagnosed as typical extramammary Paget's disease. A skinning vulvectomy was planned. The area to be excised extended over the perineum and perianal skin.

DISCUSSION

The treatment of Paget's disease of the vulva is to remove all of the involved area plus a margin of at least 2 cm of normal skin surrounding the entire lesion. Since the Paget cells may well extend along the hair follicles, the apocrine and eccrine sweat glands, the sebaceous glands, the depth of the skinning vulvectomy should extend deep enough into the superficial layer of the subcutaneous fat in order to remove all of the adnexal structures.

For the sake of discussion, it must be assumed that in this patient there is no underlying separate adenocarcinoma of the vulva, since this would require a more radical procedure. We must further assume that this is a typical Paget's disease, which is usually a slowly progressive indolent localized process.

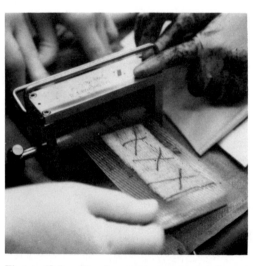

Figure 68.1. The donor skin has passed through the Meshgraft Skin Expander. Note the meshing pattern on the donor skin.

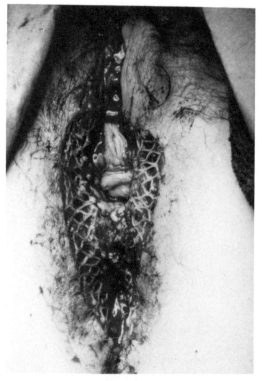

Figure 68.2. Meshed skin graft fixed in place over the raw surface of the vulvar and perianal area.

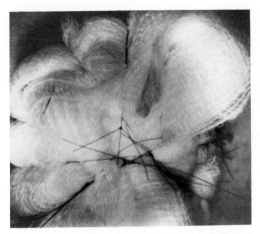

Figure 68.3. Gauze stent covering the skin graft and held in place with black silk sutures.

After the involved area has been completely excised, a large raw surface, which includes the area around the perineum and anal skin, must be covered. Such an area can be covered with a split thickness skin graft taken from the buttock, lower abdomen, or upper thigh. The skin from the donor site should be placed on a Derma carriers II with a 1.5 to 1 expansion ratio and then meshed by running the skin through the Meshgraft Skin Expander (Fig. 68.1).

After the skin has been meshed, it is placed over the raw surface, including the raw area of the perineum and surrounding the anal canal. Since the blood supply is plentiful in this area, the chances of success are almost 80% to 90%.

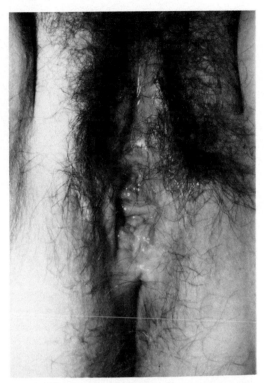

Figure 68.4. Vulvar and anal area approximately 3 months after the skin graft has been applied.

The graft is fixed laterally to the external skin margins, medially to the introitus, and posteriorly to the skin at the anal verge. It has been our custom to use 00 Dexon for this purpose. The graft is further stabilized by interrrupting stiches, fixing the graft to the underlying raw

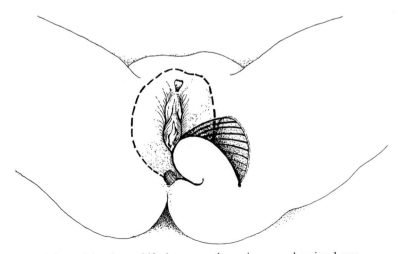

Figure 68.5. A pedicle graft has been shifted to cover the perineum and perianal area.

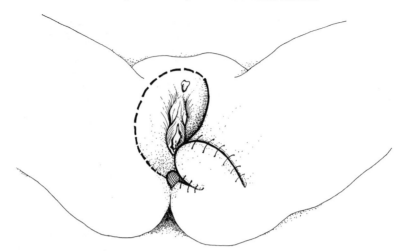

Figure 68.6. Pedicle graft sutured in place. A similiar pedicle graft can be raised for the contralateral side.

surface (Fig. 68.2). The skin graft is covered with multiple saline soaked gauze balls; gauze dressings are then placed over the gauze balls. This stent is held in place by heavy black sutures anchored to the skin (Fig. 68.3). The patient must remain at bed rest for at least 5 to 7 days with a Foley or suprapubic catheter in place. The bowel should have been thoroughly cleansed prior to surgery. An elemental diet and an antispasmodic should prevent a bowel movement for the first few days, thus reducing the chance of infection (Fig. 68.4).

We have used this technique on numerous occasions and have not had any severe complications or any vaginal or anal strictures. If there is a lack of "take" around the perineal area, a full thickness pedicle graft can be utilized (Figs. 68.5 and 68.6).

Since recurrences are not unusual, close follow-up is manadatory. Any recurrent sites may be treated with further excision and skin grafting with primary closure of pedicle grafts depending on the site of the recurrence. Small area of recurrence may also be treated by CO_2 laser, but whether this will cause complications later is as yet unknown.

Selected Readings

Blaustein A: *Pathology of the Female Genital Tract.* New York, Springer-Verlag, 1977.

DiSaia PG, Creasman WT: *Clinical Gynecologic Oncology,* 2nd ed. St. Louis, CV Mosby Co., 1984.

Friedrich EG: *Vulvar Disease.* Philadelphia, WB Saunders Co., 1976.

CHAPTER 69

Vaginal Hysterectomy for a Patient with Microinvasive Carcinoma of the Cervix and Symptomatic Pelvic Relaxation

GEORGE W. MORLEY, M.S., M.D.

CASE ABSTRACT

A 35-year-old asymptomatic, para 1, was found on recent colposcopy and conization to have a microinvasive carcinoma (3.0 mm in depth) of the uterine cervix. Margins were free of tumor. On pelvic examination, the uterus was freely movable, not enlarged, and there was some multiparous cystocele and rectocele. The patient had some symptomatic but not disabling urinary stress incontinence and was not required to wear sanitary protection. The incontinence was worse when the patient was exercising or when she had an upper respiratory infection. The surgeon thought a vaginal hysterectomy could easily be accomplished on this patient and wondered whether or not to perform coincident anterior and posterior colporrhaphy.

DISCUSSION

There are a number of different issues related to the presentation of this very interesting case. This combination of problems is not an uncommon situation. First of all, the definition must be accurate in making the diagnosis of microinvasive carcinoma (3) since serious recurrences have been reported simply because the treatment was based on an incorrect definition of this condition. The diagnosis of microinvasive or Stage IA carcinoma of the cervix is defined by most gynecologic oncologists as up to 3 mm depth of invasion from the basement membrane into the underlying stroma and that there is no evidence of angiolymphatic invasion. Given that these criteria are satisfied in making this diagnosis, one can then proceed with the discussion of several points to be considered.

In regard to the therapy directed toward the microinvasive disease, most gynecologic oncologists are in agreement with total hysterectomy as the treatment of choice. There is no need to have a preference between the transabdominal or transvaginal route for performing the hysterectomy since survival rates are the same and assessment of the regional lymph nodes is not required.

Now that the definition and the treatment of the malignant process has been established, one can then direct comments toward the second part of the question which is the coexistence of the cystocele and rectocele with or without symptoms of stress urinary incontinence. If the patient is totally asymptomatic; i.e., she does not complain of apparent pelvic relaxation and does not experience urinary loss with stress, then certainly there should be no surgical "correction" of the slight variations from normalcy. All too often, an anterior colporrhaphy and posterior colpoperineorrhaphy are performed in these situations and the patient ends up with symptoms of stress urinary incontinence or dyspareunia, etc. There also is no evidence that a repair of either the anterior or posterior vaginal wall gives better support to the vaginal apex following a vaginal hysterectomy. Furthermore, if the vaginal repair is performed in an *asymptomatic* patient in addition to the required surgery, the cost of the entire procedure would be significantly higher—a situation that must be avoided whenever possible. In summary, there is an old saying pertaining to these situations in general which is that, "If it works, don't fix it!" Also, simply stated, "Seldom does surgery help the asymptomatic patient!"

If, however, the patient complains significantly about symptoms of stress urinary incontinence or an annoying bulge of the anterior vaginal wall, then there is no contraindication to surgery directed toward correction of the posterior urethro-vesicle angle and the anterior wall relaxation through an anterior colporrhaphy. If, in addition, the patient has a symptomatic rectocele, then this too could be corrected transvaginally with a posterior colpoperineorrhaphy (2). In general, there is no contraindication to combining surgical procedures irrespective of the presence of a malignancy since there is essentially no increased risk and no decrease in survival rates. Any risk would be related to the procedure itself; not to the fact of combination therapy. Furthermore, there are increased risks in performing these procedures separately since two anesthetics would be required. In the past it has been said that "double-headers" should be reserved for baseball and not be applied to surgery. Certainly, this may have been appropriate in days past for a variety of reasons; however, this approach to surgery today does not seem necessarily appropriate.

If the patient had undergone an abdominal hysterectomy, then the urinary stress incontinence could be treated using a retropubic approach. If the physician's preference, however, were to treat the malignancy transabdominally and the pelvic relaxation transvaginally, this too would be appropriate and would be essentially at the discretion of the surgeon. This decision-making process is not to be looked upon with disfavor even though

there seems to be a less cumbersome way of handling these combined problems. Most commonly, I could think that the surgeon would choose either the transabdominal or the transvaginal route for the entire surgical procedure. To restate the obvious, all of these decisions related to the pelvic relaxation would have to be with the understanding and concurrence of the patient. If the symptoms of relaxation were not too bothersome, then it might be in the best interests of the patient to try medical management first and only operate for the malignancy at this time.

Finally, the question about when should hysterectomy be performed following the diagnostic conization is raised. A good guideline in response to this query is to perform the hysterectomy within 48 hours of the conization or to wait 6 weeks before proceeding with the more definitive therapy (1). When confronted with the treatment of a malignancy, however, most people would wait only about 4 weeks. There are others (4), however, who feel that it makes little or no difference when the postconization hysterectomy is performed and just depend on the liberal use of prophylactic antibiotic therapy. The author's bias is reflected in the first suggested approach to this question.

In summary, an appropriate decision as to route of surgery, the extent and timing of the surgery can be met after taking a detailed history, performing appropriate diagnostic tests, and discussing thoroughly all the facets of care with the patient. There is no one answer!

References

1. Malinak LR, Jeffrey RA Jr, Dunn WJ: The conization-hysterectomy time interval: A clinical and pathologic study. *Obstet Gynecol* 23:317, 1964.
2. Mattingly RF, Thompson JD: *TeLinde's Operative Gynecology*, 6th ed. Philadelphia, JB Lippincott, 1985.
3. Van Nagell JR Jr, Greenwell N, Powell DF, et al: Microinvasive carcinoma of the cervix. *Am J Obstet Gynecol* 145:981, 1983.
4. Webb MJ, Symmonds RE: Radical Hysterectomy: Influence of recent conization on morbidity and complications. *Obstet Gynecol* 53:290, 1979.

CHAPTER **70**

Microinvasive Cancer of the Cervix in Pregnancy

PHILIP J. DiSAIA, M.D.

CASE ABSTRACT

An 18-year-old, para 1, gravida 2, received a Papanicolaou smear as part of her initial physical examination. This was reported as abnormal with findings consistent with carcimoma in situ with possible microinvasion. A cervical conization was performed at 11 weeks' gestation. Although the entire lesion appeared to be within the conization specimen and edges were free of tumor, there were several nonconfluent foci of microinvasion noted between 1 and 3 mm in depth with no vascular involvement. The gestation is now of 15 weeks' duration.

DISCUSSION

Microinvasive carcinoma of the cervix is a subject that has been associated with several decades of confusion. The diagnostic issues have been confused and some investigators have reported conflicting results on what appears to be the same subset of patients. The terminology used by various authors has varied widely. Adding a first trimester pregnancy to this clinical dilemma seemingly "adds salt to the wound." The issues which must be addressed include abortion versus continuation of the pregnancy, treatment under either circumstance, and appropriate follow-up of the pregnancy if it is not terminated.

It is our belief that microinvasion should be strictly defined as invasion to a depth of no greater than 3 mm with no confluent tongues and no areas of lymphatic or vascular invasion. The volume of the invasive process is the key to predicting the aggressiveness of the disease and the treating physician must evaluate the histologic sections himself to make a judgment on a case basis. At our institution, the only indication for conization in pregnancy, is a colposcopically directed biopsy which suggests "possible microinvasion." We prefer the term "coin biopsy" (Fig. 70.1) to underscore the fact that the squamocolumnar junction everts during pregnancy and thus avoids the need for what may be a dangerous excision of canal tissue.

Some authors have shown that lesions in nonpregnant patients meeting the criteria outlined in our definition, can be adequately treated with conization alone. Based on these reports and our own observations with eight patients with microinvasion in pregnancy treated with conization only, we would recommend no further therapy for this patient at this time. We see no need for termination of this pregnancy, nor for immediate definitive therapy in the form of a hysterectomy.

The patient should be followed with inspection of the cervix in the second trimester accompanied by repeated cytology in the third trimester when regeneration of the cervical tissue is complete. No specific route of delivery is recommended. Six weeks postpartum, the cervix should be re-evaluated with cytology and colposcopy. If no further neoplastic disease is uncovered and the patient is desirous of further childbearing, it is our practice to withhold any further surgical therapy until such time as childbearing is complete or disease of a significant degree reappears. Whether or not simple hysterectomy should be recommended at the completion of childbearing in the absence of any recurrent disease is controversial. The pa-

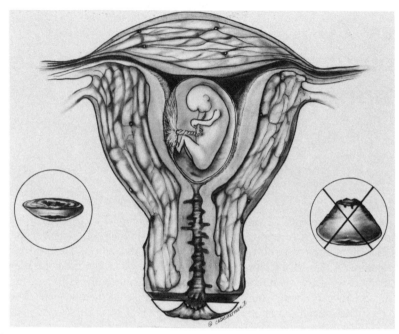

Figure 70.1. Demonstration of shallow "coin biopsy" appropriate in pregnancy. Reproduced with permission from DiSaia PJ, Creasman WT: *Clinical Gynecologic Oncology*, St. Louis, CV Mosby, 1984, p. 434.

tient undoubtedly is at some increased risk for a recurrence of cervical neoplasia and the decision for hyterectomy at this time should be made by the physician and patient taking into consideration the probabilty of good patient compliance for serial cytologic evaluation, the level of cancer phobia in the patient, and other benign pathology which may coexist.

Selected Readings

DiSaia PJ, Creasman WT: *Clinical Gynecologic Oncology*, St. Louis, CV Mosby, 1984.
Marcuse PM: Incipient microinvasive carcinoma of the cervix. *Obstet Gynecol* 37:360-371, 1971.
Taylor H: Early invasive cancer of the cervix. *Am J Obstet Gynecol* 85:926-939, 1963.
Wheeler CB Jr: Carcinoma of the cervix with early stromal invasion. *Am J Obstet Gynecol* 72:119, 1956.

CHAPTER 71

Unexpected Uterine Malignant Tumor (Adenocarcinoma or Endometrial Sarcoma) Found When the Uterus Was Opened in the Operating Room

JOHN J. MIKUTA, M.D.

CASE ABSTRACT

A vaginal hysterectomy had been performed because of perimenopausal menorrhagia in a 53-year-old patient. The uterus was of average size and there were no technical difficulties during the hysterectomy. The ovaries were grossly normal, and one appeared to contain a small follicle cyst. As a matter of departmental policy, the uterus was opened, and following its removal in the operating room was found to contain a wide-based, hemorrhagic, somewhat necrotic tumor about 1 inch in diameter, located at the fundus of the uterus and grossly invading the inner third of the myometrium.

DISCUSSION

To begin with, this patient should not have had a hysterectomy without a preliminary dilatation and curettage to determine the cause of the perimenopausal menorrhagia. This could have been done as an office procedure, such as an endometrial biopsy or Vabra aspiration, or prior to the removal of the uterus by a diagnostic dilatation and curettage with a frozen section to determine whether there was any abnormality of the endometrium. There is frequently a tendency to avoid a dilatation and curettage in the absence of abnormal bleeding if there is an obvious indication for hysterectomy, particularly the presence of uterine myomata or adnexal masses. This is an erroneous concept, and the few minutes necessary to rule out the presence of endometrial disease may obviate the kind of problem that occurred in this patient. In addition, in this patient it is possible that the dilatation and curettage may have resolved the cause of the bleeding or, even without the discovery of an obvious cause, been helpful in correcting the menorrhagia.

In the situation described here the first step should be to identify the nature of the tumor. In this case, if it turned out to be the most likely lesion, an endometrial carcinoma or a sarcoma, one should proceed appropriately with the next step, the removal of the adnexa. This might be able to be done through the vagina. However, if this were not possible, it should be done after the completion of the vaginal operation by entering the abdomen through an appropriate incision which will allow one to complete the removal of the adnexa, having first obtained washings from the peritoneal cavity using heparinized saline solution. While peritoneal washings are routinely accepted in the management of adnexal masses and ovarian carcinomas, they must also be considered for patients who have carcinoma of the endometrium. Recent reports by Creasman et al. have shown an incidence of involvement of peritoneal washings with positive cytology as high as 17% with stage 1 carcinoma of the endometrium. Such patients apparently also have a poor prognosis in that they tend to have recurrences in the peritoneal cavity. In addition, careful palpation of the retroperitoneal nodes and node sampling should be done as indicated by the presence of enlarged nodes.

It should be emphasized that the gynecologist must also be mindful of the way in which the prospective surgery was presented to the patient. A blanket preoperative type of permission is generally not adequate in today's medical-legal climate. It is much better if the gynecologist explains to the patient that at times a particular approach, e.g., vaginal hysterectomy, laparoscopic tubal ligation, cannot be carried out due to technical difficulties or as in this case unexpected findings that would alter the nature of the procedure to be carried out. Prior to any surgery it is worth discussing with the patient what her wishes might be. She should have the choice of having the procedure stopped, recovering from anesthesia, and then having the possible procedure discussed with her. The advantages of using only a single anesthetic, reducing the possible spread of any malignancy

that may have been discovered, and getting earlier treatment are certainly advantages to be stressed to the patient.

Selected Readings

Brown JM, Dockerty MD, Symmonds RE, et al: Vaginal recurrence of endometrial carcinoma. *Am J Obstet Gynecol* 100:544, 1968.

Butler CF, Pratt JH: Vaginal hysterectomy for carcinoma of the endometrium: Forty years experience at the Mayo Clinic. In Gray LA Sr (ed): *Endometrial Carcinoma and Its Treatment*. Springfield, IL, Charles C Thomas, 1976.

Creasman WT, Boronow RC, Morrow CP, et al: Adenocarcinoma of the endometrium: Its metastatic lymph node potential. A preliminary report. *Gynecol Oncol* 4:239, 1976.

Creasman WT, DiSaia PJ, Blessing J, et al: Prognostic significance of peritoneal cytology in patients with endometrial cancer and preliminary data concerning therapy with intraperitoneal radiopharmaceuticals. *Am J Obstet Gynecol* 141:921, 1981.

Jones HW III: Treatment of adenocarcinoma of the endometrium. *Obstet Gynecol Surv* 30:147, 1975.

CHAPTER 72
Undiagnosed Microinvasive Carcinoma of the Cervix with Vascular Involvement

WILLIAM E. CRISP, M.D.

CASE ABSTRACT

A positive Papanicolaou smear on routine annual pelvic examination was found in a 36-year-old gravida 2 para 2, and five colposcopically directed biopsies were obtained. One biopsy was reported as benign, but the other four were diagnosed as carcinoma-in-situ of the cervix. A vaginal hysterectomy was performed. On the morning of the fourth postoperative day as the patient was preparing to go home, her physician reviewed the pathology report of the hysterectomy specimen which identified "microinvasive carcinoma of the cervix to a depth of between 3 and 4 mm." In one section tumor cells were found within the lumen of a nearby blood vessel.

DISCUSSION

This 36-year-old woman had a positive Pap smear and a diagnosis of carcinoma-in-situ made in four of five cervical biopsies, which implies a relatively large lesion, followed by a vaginal hysterectomy. The problem is that the cervical lesion was not completely evaluated before treatment. It is imperative that before treatment is instituted in a woman who has had a positive Pap smear that certain criteria must be followed.

1. The entire distribution of the abnormal epithelium must be visualized by colposcopy.
2. The endocervical curettage must be negative for any abnormal epithelium.
3. There must be agreement between the cytologic findings, the colposcopic findings, and the histologic report of the directed biopsies and endocervical curettage.

When these diagnostic criteria cannot be met or there is a discrepancy in the findings, then a cold knife conization must be performed before any type of definitive therapy is done. This patient should have had an endocervical curettage and, depending on the findings, a cervical conization. It is also imperative that the entire lesion be seen by the colposcopist.

The hysterectomy specimen was reported as a microinvasive carcinoma of the cervix to a depth of 3 to 4 mm with vascular space invasion of one section.

In order to individualize treatment, which is paramount with a microinvasive carcinoma, the physician must ask the pathologist for more sections to ascertain the width and volume of the lesion and whether it is multifocal or confluent. These help to give the physician an idea of the aggressiveness of the tumor.

Although there has been much confusion over the definition of early stromal invasion or microinvasive carcinoma of the cervix, it has been more precisely defined by the Society of Gynecologic Oncologists as "one in which neoplastic epithelium invades the stroma in one or more places to a depth of 3 mm or less over the base of the epithelium and in which lymphatic or vascular involvement is not demonstrated." Even though many studies have been tabulated on microinvasive carcinoma of the cervix, most of these are not comparable because a standard definition was not applied.

There are, however, some generalized conclusions that must be applied in individual cases.

The recurrence rate, after simple hysterectomy, of microinvasive carcinoma using the above definition is less that 1.5%.

Sedlis's cooperative study showed vascular invasion in 23% of the cases, but there was no nodal involvement and no nodal metastasis in any of these cases studied by pelvic lymphadenectomy.

Other studies have indicated that there is approximately 1% nodal metastasis with lymphatic space involvement. This patient showed only one section where endothelial space involvement was noted; therefore, it is imperative that other adjacent sections be cut to give the physician some idea of the degree of vascular invasion.

Because microinvasive carcinoma may range from a minute single cluster of cells just penetrating the stroma to a significant volume of invasion with evidence of lymphatic invasion, treatment must be individualized.

Patients with less than 2 mm of penetration without lymphatic permeation can be treated with simple hysterectomy. All others should be treated by modified radial hysterectomy.

Serious morbidity and mortality associated with modified radical hysterectomy is less than 2% and the possibility of recurrence is remote.

In this patient who had already undergone a simple hysterectomy, her chances of cure are almost 99% even though a more radical surgical approach would have been preferred had the lesion been diagnosed accurately preoperatively.

If additional study of this lesion by pathology shows it to be superficial with only one small area of invasion then no further treatment is necessary except close follow-up. If, however, there is an unanticipated volume of invasion, or additional endothelial space invasion, additional treatment will be indicated.

The problem should be fully explained to the patient so that she will understand the necessity for adequate follow-up.

Selected Readings

Morrow CP, Townsend DE: *Synopis of Gynecologic Oncology*, ed. 2. New York, John Wiley & Sons, 1981.

Precis III: American College of Obstetrics and Gynecology. *Gynecol Oncol* 1986.

Sedlis A: Strategies for treating microinvasive cancers. *Contemp Ob/Gyn* 18:31, 1981.

CHAPTER 73

Undiagnosed Invasive Squamous Cell Carcinoma in Hysterectomy Specimen

HENRY C. McDUFF, JR., M.D.

CASE ABSTRACT

A 47-year-old patient with uterine fibroids and menorrhagia had been examined by endometrial biopsy and the curettings reported as "cystic hyperplasia." It was the examiner's opinion that the patient had a submucous fibroid. Because of some coexistent multiparous relaxation, a vaginal hysterectomy and anterior and posterior colporrhaphy were performed. The convalescence was unremarkable, but the day before discharge, the pathology report reached the surgeon: "early invasive squamous cell carcinoma of the cervix," with invasion greater than 5 mm.

DISCUSSION

Identification of the Problem

This 47-year-old woman with known uterine fibroids and heavy menstrual bleeding was evaluated in an office setting. An endometrial biopsy was performed and the pathology report indicated cystic hyperplasia. This is not a malignant condition, but it is a remote precursor of endometrial carcinoma, according to studies of Dr. Hertig (1). The patient was known to have fibroid tumors, and the physician presumed her bleeding was due perhaps to a submucous fibroid component. It would seem appropriate that a dilatation and curettage should have been done since a total evaluation of the endometrium might have identified some adenomatous or dysplastic components to her cystic hyperplasia. If that had been done and if dilatation and curettage performed had been fractional, the malignancy within the endocervix would have been recognized and appropriate treatment could have been instituted. As the patient now presents, she is at significant risk. An inappropriate operation has been performed in regards to the ultimate diagnosis (invasive carcinoma of the cervix). Beyond this, the patient also underwent a vaginal repair because of multiparous vaginal wall relaxations,

and thereby tissue planes immediately adjacent to the cervix were opened and traumatized. If the invasive characteristics of the cervical lesion also identified vascular and lymphatic invasion, a high potential for seeding malignant cells in the region of the repair must be given great consideration. If no further treatment is pursued, this patient undoubtedly will soon demonstrate a florid extension of her cervical cancer in the parametrium and the upper vagina. Further trauma to the parametrium and the adjacent vascular and lymphatic channels would hasten embolic involvement of the pelvic and periaortic lymph node areas.

How Might It Have Been Avoided?

This "surprise diagnosis" of invasive cervical cancer with extension greater than 5 mm posed a very significant problem in regards to further study and treatment (4). The appropriate diagnosis would have been made if preoperative surveillance had been more searching. One would have to imagine that a Papanicolaou smear had been performed and that it was reported as normal, otherwise further preoperative studies would have been carried out. If a Pap smear had not been done, the physician must be held truly accountable. This must have been an occult stage I-A lesion (2) that was not visible to the naked eye. The cervix was obviously easily visualized since there was a sufficient amount of relaxation to require repair during the performance of vaginal hysterectomy. Since the cervix was so available for study, the performance of the Pap smear should have included a swabbing of the endocervix, and this would hardly fail to identify at least the suspicion of a cervical malignancy. If the Pap smear had been reported abnormal, an office colposcopy, endocervical curettage, and biopsies would have been carried out. The invasive cervical cancer would then have been identified and appropriate treatment would have been carried out, either by radiation or radical surgery.

Historical Trend

Total abdominal hysterectomy had been the preferred management for surgical uterine disease for the past 40 years. Previously, the simpler procedure of supracervical hysterectomy was done. Before 1940, most clinics interested in the management of cervical cancer reported their experience in the intact uterus as well as cancer of the cervical stump which was seen in about 5% to 8% of any total series (2). In 1940, total hysterectomy replaced the supracervical operation, and, interestingly, the Pap smear was first popularized at about the same time. The advent of these two changes should almost write an epitaph to cervical cancer, because of early disease recognition by the Pap smear and definitive removal of cervix by total hysterectomy for benign disease. The incidence of cancer of the cervical stump is seen with decreasing frequency, and in its place we are seeing patients similar to the one under discussion, who are found to have invasive cervical cancer in the uterus which has been removed for another, nonmalignant condition. It is rare that this should occur, because the Pap smear should identify the presence of a problem in almost all instances. In this particular patient, I again believe we are dealing with an occult lesion and either a Pap smear was not done or it was reported as normal, so there was no clinical suspicion of cervical malignancy.

Further Study Recommended

Once a diagnosis of invasive cervical cancer had been made, certain further studies very obviously should be performed. These would include an intravenous pyelogram, cystoscopy,

sigmoidoscopy, a bipedal lymphangiogram, and remotely an intraperitoneal, periaortic, and pelvic node sampling (1). The sigmoidoscopy, cystoscopy, and intravenous pyelogram would be necessary regardless of the further recommended treatment. It is extremely important to evaluate the condition of these organs and the location of the patient's kidneys if deep x-ray therapy is to be recommended. There is a great deal of enthusiasm at the present time for "staging laparotomy" for cervical cancer. This involves an abdominal incision to sample pelvic and periaortic lymph nodes, to define whether the patient would be best treated surgically or by radiation. The patient under discussion, obviously represents a I-A occult lesion, and the potential for recovering any positive nodes is extremely remote. Bipedal lymphangiography gives some information concerning the status of the pelvic and periaortic lymph nodes, but it is associated with a high percentage of false-positives and false-negatives. Certain clinics continue to use this, however, emphasizing that they have improved their yield in evaluating the nodal phase of study and have acquired increasing expertise in the evaluation of the ductal phase, so that possibly lymphangiography would be a worthwhile procedure.

The areas of great concern in this patient, however, are the adjacent parametria and upper vagina, and the use of fine needle biopsy (1) to study these areas more clearly would be very helpful. Vigorous scrapings of the upper vagina for Pap smear evaluations would also be important.

Treatment Considerations

I believe that this patient could be managed either by radical vaginectomy (3) and pelvic node dissection or by external total pelvic irradiation plus a Delcos vaginal applicator. The surgical approach for a condition of this type is not easy, and great care is necessary because of the previous surgery. Total pelvic irradiation plus the vaginal Delcos applicator would, in time, lead to vaginal stenosis, the appearance of the cone-shaped vagina, and some difficulty with intercourse plus the problems of radiation cystitis and proctitis. These conditions should be thoroughly discussed with the patient before further treatment.

My solution to the study of this problem would include cystoscopy, sigmoidoscopy, intravenous pyelogram, bipedal lymphangiogram, and fine needle biopsy. The preferred treatment would be full pelvic irradiation, 4500 to 5000 rads (4), followed by the insertion of a Delcos vaginal applicator, 4000 rads on the surface of the applicator. Careful follow-up is important, and a repeat intravenous pyelogram should be obtained in 1 year and repeated again in 3 years.

Prognosis

The prognosis depends on the staging of the disease, the depth of invasion, and the presence or absence of lymphatic or vascular involvement. Proper treatment should result in a cure rate of between 85% and 90% if the disease is totally confined to the cervix, stage I.

Summary

Approximately 0.5% to 1.0% (4) of all hysterectomies done for benign disease have been reported to demonstrate the surprise finding of cervical cancer. Generally, this is a low-stage disease, stage 0 or stage I, and usually occult. Biopsy of the squamocolumnar junction or endocervical curettage should identify all of these lesions preoperatively. No further treatment is recommended for in situ lesions, but full pelvic radiation with or without the addition of vaginal source is recommended for all patients with invasive disease. The outlook for cure is good, 100% for in situ lesions and 85% to 90% for stage I disease (4).

References

1. DiSaia PJ, Creasman WT: *Clinical Gynecologic Oncology*, 2nd ed.. St. Louis, CV Mosby, 1984, pp. 122–145.
2. Finn WF: The postoperative recognition and further management of unsuspected cervical cancer. *Am J Obstet Gynecol* 63:717, 1952.
3. Masterson JG: Discussion of paper by W. F. Finn. The postoperative recognition and further management of unsuspected cervical carcinoma. Discussant John Masterson. *Am J Obstet Gynecol* 63:717, 1952.
4. McDuff HC, et al: Accidentally encountered cervical cancer. *Am J Obstet Gynecol* 71:407, 1956.

CHAPTER 74

Undifferentiated Adenocarcinoma of Endometrium Incomplete Staging and Surgery

STEPHEN L. CURRY, M.D.

CASE ABSTRACT

Total abdominal hysterectomy with bilateral salpingo-oophorectomy was being performed on an obese, 59-year-old, nulligravida in whom the uterus was slightly enlarged. A low transverse incision was used. A previous endometrial biopsy had been reported as "undifferentiated adenocarcinoma." The hysterectomy specimen was opened in the operating room disclosing a friable 2 X 3 cm endometrial tumor near the center of the posterior wall of the fundus invading the myometrium to its outer third. The surgeon had never seen nor performed a para-aortic or pelvic node dissection, but did not palpate any adenopathy. Gynecologic oncology consultation was obtained postoperatively.

DISCUSSION

Advances in the management of endometrial cancer over the last 15 years should have prevented the surgeon from being in the situation described above. Although endometrial cancer has a very high cure rate, it is now well know that the patients at greatest risk for recurrence are those with poorly differentiated lesions, extension to the lower uterine segment and cervix, and/or deep myometrial invasion.

This patient presented with the classic epidemiologic findings of endometrial cancer in that she was obese, postmenopausal, and of low parity. One would presume that the endometrial biopsy was carried out because of postmenopausal bleeding. Here is the first error in judgment. It is perfectly acceptable to carry out an endometrial biopsy for diagnostic reasons in a patient who presents to the office with abnormal perimenopausal or any postmenopausal bleeding. If the endometrial biopsy is positive for cancer and can be adequately graded, then this is sufficient in lieu of a formal dilation and curettage under anesthesia. However, it is now well accepted that all patients with the diagnosis of endometrial cancer should have a frac-tional curettage. This means that the endocervix is aggressively scraped prior to any passage of instruments through the internal os into the uterine cavity since this may result in contamination of the endocervical specimen and, thus, upstaging of the disease. Therefore, in the office prior to endometrial biopsy for any patient suspected of being at risk for endometrial cancer, the surgeon should do an endocervical curettage and then the endometrial biopsy; thus, if the diagnosis of cancer is made an appropriate and complete diagnostic procedure has been carried out.

If the patient is unable to tolerate office biopsy or if the pathology report returns not showing cancer, then the patient should always undergo formal fractional dilation and curettage. During this anesthesia it is critical that the surgeon carry out a careful examination under anesthesia to assess the remainder of the pelvic organs. Again, scraping the endocervix first and carefully sounding the uterus for size are important and should be a part of the dictated operative note.

Preoperative work-up should always include a stool guaiac, chest x-ray, and a mammogram. Alternate studies such as intravenous pyelogram, barium enema, ultrasound, and abdominopelvic CT scan are reserved for those patients with signs or symptoms indicating a need for further evaluation. Only if the serum alkaline phosphatase is elevated should a bone scan be done and likewise only if liver function studies are elevated should radiologic or nuclear scan tests be ordered.

Since up to 80% of patients have stage I disease and since most physicians agree that stages II and higher should be managed in comprehensive cancer centers, the remainder of this chapter will concentrate on the management of stage I disease; that is, disease thought to be localized to the fundus of the uterus.

Controversy continues as to whether or not some patients should receive preoperative radiation therapy prior to definitive surgery. However, it is now well accepted that patients with well differentiated endometrial cancer have a very low risk of deep myometrial invasion and, thus, extrauterine spread. Therefore, these patients can be treated with total abdominal hysterectomy and bilateral salpingo-oophorectomy with peritoneal washings. In the vast majority of cases a vertical or transverse muscle cutting incision must be made to ensure complete exploration and ability to perform extended surgery if necessary. Peritoneal washings are obtained by placing 100 cc of normal saline in the pelvis immediately after opening the abdominal peritoneum and sending this fluid to the cytology laboratory. Careful upper abdominal and retroperitoneal node palpation is always the next step. Only if there is deep myometrial invasion, unsuspected extension to the lower uterine segment or cervix, or extension to the adnexa, should these patients be considered for postoperative radiation therapy.

Patients with moderately differentiated endometrial cancer can be managed as above with the surgeon opening the specimen in the operating room and in conjunction with the pathologist assessing the depth of myometrial invasion to decide on the need for selective lymph node evaluation. Most gynecologic-oncologists carry out selective lymph node sampling in the para-aortic and bilateral pelvic areas on all patients. Again postoperative radiation therapy is tailored to those patients at high risk for recurrence.

Para-aortic sampling is carried out by opening the posterior peritoneum at the aortic bifurcation and, after identifying the ureter laterally and the vena cava and aorta deeply, a generous sampling of precaval and periaortic fat-containing lymph nodes is removed. The pelvic peritoneum is opened bilaterally over the external iliac artery and a large sample of node-bearing fat is removed from over and around this vessel. Finally, the obturator space is entered and after identifying the obturator nerve, the fat below the external iliac vein and above the nerve is generously removed. Adequate hemostasis should always be obtained. These procedures should never be attempted unless one is well trained in retroperitoneal surgery.

Although most investigators have shown that deep myometrial invasion is the most significant prognostic indicator in endometrial cancer, a pathologic report of poorly differentiated endometrial cancer prior to removing the uterus, should indicate to the surgeon a high risk of microscopic or macroscopic spread beyond the fundus of the uterus. Some authors continue to recommend preoperative radiation therapy followed by total abdominal hysterectomy, bilateral salpingo-oophorectomy, pelvic washings, and selective periaortic sampling. Others would argue that definitive surgical staging should be carried out and then postoperative radiation therapy tailored to the sites at risk. In this situation most investigators recommend total abdominal hysterectomy with bilateral salpingo-oophorectomy, pelvic washings, and selective para-aortic and pelvic lymph node sampling.

The treatment of positive peritoneal cytology and/or widespread disease continues to undergo investigation. However, the present standard of care is to utilize chemotherapy, with progesterone being the first line agent. Adriamycin has been shown to be effective in the management of patients with recurrent endometrial cancer.

Follow-up should include complete history and physical examination at least every 3 months for the first 2 years and then every 6 months thereafter. Particular attention should be paid to the lymph nodes, lungs, breast, abdominal, and pelvic examination. A yearly chest x-ray and mammogram should be obtained. Constant reassurance of negative findings is very important to the patient.

In summary, it is critical that all physicians understand the need for fractional curettage in all patients suspected of endometrial cancer, as extension to the lower uterine segment or cervix portends to a greater incidence of extrauterine spread and poor prognosis. Secondly, careful exploration including peritoneal washings through an adequate incision is critical. Patients with well-differentiated endometrial cancer localized to the fundus of the uterus can be managed with primary surgery. This should be followed by radiation therapy for that small group of patients who have indicators of poor prognosis. These include deep myometrial invasion (greater than one-half of the way through), extension to the lower uterine segment or cervix, or extrauterine spread.

Between 15% and 20% of patients with endometrial cancer will have a poorly differentiated lesion and consideration should be given for referral to a comprehensive cancer center in order to be sure that they receive the most up to date and aggressive evaluation and therapy as they are the patients with the highest risk of recurrence and thus make up the majority of deaths from this disease.

Selected Readings

Boronow RC, Morrow CP, Creasman WT, et al: Surgical staging in endometrial cancer. 1. Clinical pathologic findings of a prospective study. *Obstet Gynecol* 638:25-32, 1984.

Creasman WT: Surgical treatment of endometrial cancer. In Sciarra JJ (ed): *Gynecology and Obstetrics.* New York, Harper and Row, Vol. 4, Chap 19, 1980.

DiSaia PJ, Creasman WT: *Clinical Gynecologic Oncology.* St. Louis, C.V. Mosby, 1981, pp. 128-152.

DiSaia PJ, Creasman WT, Boronow RC, et al: Risk factors and recurrent patterns in stage I endometrial cancer. *Am J Obstet Gynecol* 151:1009-1015, 1985.

CHAPTER 75

Trauma to the Vena Cava During Para-Aortic Node Dissection

JEROME L. BELINSON, M.D.

CASE ABSTRACT

A 60-year-old woman with a grade 2 adenocarcinoma of the endometrium was undergoing a para-aortic dissection. Using Metzenbaum scissors, the peritoneum was dissected off of the nodal tissue and vena cava on the right side. A large amount of bleeding suddenly occurred. The nodal tissue was quickly lifted up, the bleeding markedly increased, and it was clear that the vena cava had been injured.

DISCUSSION

The inferior vena cava can be easily injured in the process of doing a para-aortic dissection. Even if one is careful, the variability of the venous system or the adherence of a node to the vena cava may not always be predicted. However, if one is observant and precise in his/her surgery, the caval injuries that occur can usually be solved without having to resort to inferior vena caval ligation.

There is a small vein that enters the inferior vena cava on its ventral surface just above the aortic bifurcation. This vein runs from the overlying nodes to the cava. Occasionally, it originates from the peritoneal surface running through the nodes to the cava. In my experience, this small vein is highly predictable in its location as well as being the most common cause for more serious injury to the vena cava. Generally, as one elevates the nodal tissue, the vein is either avulsed, or worse, tears a small strip in the wall of the cava. A similar injury can occur if the cava is tented slightly during dissection and cut with the scissors. It is important that one takes a calm stepwise approach to solving the bleeding since efforts poorly done will invariably convert simple problems to complex and dangerous ones. On a more general note, if the attachment of a variety of structures is not appreciated, the surgeon who elevates these tissues and then cuts or probes too quickly will discover that the vena cava has been tented up and a large hole has been created. This type of injury will, of course, result in massive bleeding, and in my opinion, is totally avoidable. First, one elevates the peritoneum or the nodes off from the cava very gently. Attachments that are identified are isolated and controlled. I prefer the use of hemostatic clips for this purpose, although clamping and tying or the use of electrocautery will certainly work (Fig. 75.1). If cautery is used, it must not be set too high or the damage will run quickly down the vein and create a hole in the cava.

In the case presented, it appears that the nature of the injury is similar to the small venous injury previously described. This, as mentioned, must be taken very seriously since it can bleed significantly and can lead to more damage. Unless the bleeding is initially quite severe, I prefer to try and isolate the bleeding site first. This generally means elevating the nodal tissue off the cava. Once the bleeding site is identified, direct pressure is then applied for 5 to 10 minutes depending upon the size of the injury. If pressure alone will stop the bleeding, then use pressure alone. The more one has to do to stop caval bleeding, the greater the risk of further injury. If one is forced to use pressure before dissecting away surrounding tissue, keep in mind that as the nodes are removed the bleeding is likely to restart, although often at a much slower rate.

If the bleeding continues, my next choice is

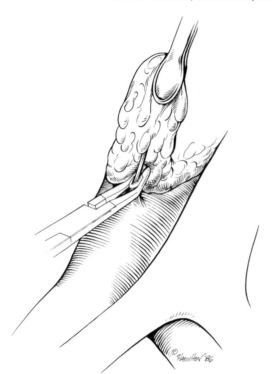

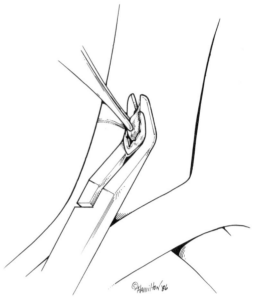

Figure 75.2. The defect is held closed with vascular pick-ups and then a hemostatic clip is applied.

Figure 75.1. The small vein is identified and clipped as one elevates the nodal tissue off the vena cava.

to try using hemostatic clips. The clips will be most effective if one can control the bleeding with a pair of vascular pick-ups. Then, while holding closed the defect with the pick-ups, a clip is placed parallel to the surface of the cava just below the pick-ups (Fig. 75.2). Be careful not to allow the tip of the hemostatic clip to cause a rent in the cava as it is being closed.

On occasion, it is fully evident that an injury to the vena cava will have to be sutured. I prefer to control the hemorrhage first with a vascular spoon clamp. Then, using a 4-0 monofilament vascular suture, the defect is closed. If there is a small amount of oozing when the clamp is removed, I again use pressure. The secret of using the spoon clamps is to include a small margin of normal caval wall around the vascular defect. The defect is then repaired within the arc of the clamp (Fig. 75.3). The repair of the slit-type injury is also quite effectively managed using an Allis clamp, especially when the exposure is good. The Allis is used to pinch the defect closed and then a 4-0 or 5-0 monofilament suture is placed running

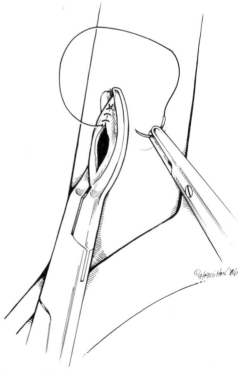

Figure 75.3. Larger defects can be clamped and sutured using a vascular spoon clamp.

just beneath the clamp. In situations where one is having difficulty controlling the bleeding and exposing the injury for repair, a Fogerty catheter can also be quite handy. A number 4 or 5 Fogerty catheter is pushed through the defect and the balloon inflated. Gentle traction on the catheter then controls the bleeding and allows one to improve the exposure.

Rarely, the inferior vena cava will be torn so severely that the anatomy is lost, alignment is impossible, and hemorrhage is overwhelming. Under these circumstances the only choice may be to ligate the vena cava above and below the injury. Fortunately, we have this last resort option available, since we are rarely working above the renal veins. Keep in mind that after ligating the cava, there may still be a lumbar vein entering the injured segment that will need to be ligated. Caval ligation may be accomplished by a number of techniques. Under emergency circumstances, passing a 0 silk suture under the cava and tying it may be the quickest. The use of staples or caval clips can also be quite expeditious and is certainly acceptable.

Selected Readings

Belinson JL, Goldberg MI, Averette HE: Paraaortic lymphadenectomy in gynecologic cancer. *Gynecol Oncol* 7: 188-198, 1979.

Schwartz SI (ed): *Principles of Surgery*, 4th ed. New York, McGraw-Hill, 1984, pp. 257-259.

CHAPTER 76
Myomectomy with Unexpected Leiomyosarcoma

ARLAN B. FULLER, JR., M.D.

CASE ABSTRACT

The uterus of a 26-year-old infertility patient, with troublesome menorrhagia, had multiple uterine leiomyomata, one of which was encroaching significantly on the endometrial cavity. Transabdominal multiple myomectomies were accomplished and all visible leiomyomata were removed. The patient's recovery was remarkably smooth and the pathology report was received on the morning of her planned discharge from the hospital. It reported that the largest tumor contained a leiomyosarcoma.

DISCUSSION

A 26-year-old infertility patient undergoes a procedure intended to improve her chances of childbearing and emerges with a diagnosis that threatens her fertility, her femininity, and even her life.

The diagnosis and classification of smooth muscle tumors of the female genital tract represent a challenge to the pathologist and clinician alike. Controversy surrounds the diagnostic criteria for classification of benign tumors of the uterus, borderline tumors, and leiomyosarcomas. Review of the criteria that may predict the clinical behavior of this tumor will permit a decision regarding preservation of reproductive function and prognosis for this patient. As specific information about the histologic characteristics of the tumor are not available, discussion must be inclusive.

Leiomyomas are the most common tumors in the female pelvis and are frequent cause for hysterectomy in the United States. However, only 5% to 10% of infertility patients may have fibroids as a causative factor in their infertility, presumably a consequence of tubal obstruction (necessarily bilateral) or severe hypermenorrhea as a consequence of its submucous location.

Alternatively, myomectomy may be performed in a young woman in order to preserve fertility. If one or more fibroids are documented on successive examinations to be rapidly enlarging in a young woman not yet desirous of pregnancy, timely intervention may allow resection of that myoma prior to its further distortion of uterine architecture and before the procedure might become technically difficult or unnessarily morbid. Hopefully, this is an area where medical therapy with compounds such as GnRH may have an increasing role in the future, particularly in the patient with multiple benign leiomyomas.

Meigs observed an incidence of "malignant degeneration" of 0.6%, or nine of 1330 patients with leiomyomas. Unfortunately, this figure remains frequently quoted today; in a recent symposium on management of uterine myomas, the risk of malignant transformation was stated to be between 0.1% and 0.5%. If as many as 30% of women may have benign leiomyomata, and the incidence of leiomyosarcoma is in the range of 0.67%/100,000 women over the age of 20 years, then the true risk of malignant change may be between 1 in 10,000 and 1 in 100,000.

The diagnosis of leiomyosarcoma on gross examination is difficult because of both the gradation of malignancy (Table 76.1) and the overlap of degenerative changes in both benign and malignant lesions. Although sarcomas typically have a necrotic or hemorrhagic center,

Table 76.1
Smooth Muscle Neoplasms Diagnostic
Criteria (adapted from Kempson and Bari:
***Hum Pathol* 1:331-349, 1970).**

Mitoses per 10 HPF	Cytologic Atypia	Diagnosis
0–4	No	Cellular myoma
0–4	Yes	Atypical myoma
5–9	No	Borderline
5–9	Yes	Leiomyosarcoma
10 or more	Either	Leiomyosarcoma

so too may the necrotic myoma with carneous degeneration. Alternatively, the sarcoma may have merely lost the typical, whorled appearance of a benign myoma and acquired the pale grey, gelatinous appearance of a benign tumor that has outgrown its blood supply. Significantly, Silverberg has examined the clinical impressions of the gynecologist and pathologist as a prognostic factor for patients with leiomyosarcomas. When the gross impression of the tumor was that of a leiomyosarcoma, only 20% of the 10 patients studied were alive at 5 years. Conversely, when the diagnosis was not suspected clinically, 80% of the 20 patients available for follow-up were still alive.

The histologic diagnosis of leiomyosarcoma is based on the observations of hypercellularity, nuclear atypia, pleomorphism, and number of mitoses according to Woodruff. The clinical behavior documented in any series of patients with a diagnosis of uterine sarcoma greatly depends on the criteria for inclusion of patients in the study. If one has loose criteria, including all patients with even very few mitoses, then the natural history of the disease, time to recurrence, sites of recurrence, and response to conservative therapy will differ significantly from another series in which criteria for numbers of mitoses and cellular atypia might be more strict. In his series of 43 patients, Woodruff required at least two mitoses in any high power field to designate a tumor as a leiomyosarcoma; in some other series, the minimal criteria for inclusion are not even identified.

The intraoperative diagnosis of leiomyosarcoma would necessitate the frozen section examination of all myomas at the time of laparotomy. Many malignant tumors can be identified by their gross appearance on cut section. Frozen section examination can then be performed only on those tumors with necrotic centers, hemorrhage, or evidence of hyaline degeneration.

However, given the rarity of leiomyosarcomas, the uncertain reliability of frozen section diagnosis, and the desire to employ myomectomy in young women wishing to preserve childbearing, even if malignancy was suspected, few gynecologists would perform an abdominal hysterectomy and bilateral salpingo-oophorectomy based on frozen section diagnosis alone! These are indeed the women who would have the most to lose with hysterectomy and would be the group who would most easily tolerate a second operation, if necessary. Moreover the most critical case would be that of a patient with a low grade sarcoma, where the differential diagnosis would be difficult; the high grade sarcomas will be rapidly fatal to a large population of patients, regardless of what procedure was employed.

If the diagnosis of leiomyosarcomas were to be made preoperatively (by curettage showing necrotic, atypical smooth muscle cells, or frank cancer), the appropriate procedure would involve both surgical resection of the entire tumor and precise surgical staging in order to determine the anatomic and pathologic extent of disease. This extent of disease evaluation would have involved examination of both pelvic and para-aortic nodes as well as evaluation of the extent of transcelomic spread and parenchymal organ metastases to liver and lung. Patients with disease extending beyond the uterus at the time of diagnosis have a uniformly poor prognosis in multiple series, with no survivors.

Meigs stated that "if myomectomy has been done...immediate reoperation and total hysterectomy are necessary." The vast majority of patients cited in the literature have had at least total abdominal hysterectomy and bilateral salpingo-oophorectomy as primary treatment. Little information is available concerning the management of patients with incidental cancer found after myomectomy.

Woodruff, however, does report the outcome of nine patients treated by myomectomy alone. Three had immediate re-exploration with hysterectomy and did well. Of six others treated "conservatively," five remained free of disease, while one recurred locally at 2 years in the uterus and abdomen and was still alive with disease at 6 years following initial therapy.

There is little evidence that postoperative pelvic radiation therapy changes the prognosis, or even the site of recurrence. The majority of recurrences are identified at extrapelvic sites in patients with anaplastic tumors.

Chemotherapy for advanced disease has produced few, if any, real successes. Reports ascribing benefit to adjuvant chemotherapy in this disease have employed historical controls and are open to the criticism. Better survival in patients with stage I disease could be attributed to variations in staging of the tumor, particularly in light of the uniformly high risk of recurrence in patients with extrauterine spread of disease. Nevertheless, van Nagell and others have described fewer recurrences in stage I patients with uterine sarcomas treated with combined chemotherapy employing vincristine, actinomycin D, and cyclophosphamide (VAC).

More than 10 mitoses per 10 High Power Field (HPF) carries a poor prognosis for patients with frank leiomyosarcoma; tumors with less than 5 mitoses per 10 HPF rarely metastasize and are almost never associated with recurrence and death. These latter are the lesions that commonly occur in young women and may explain the better prognosis in premenopausal women. Woodruff reported 100% 5-year survival for patients with 1-4 mitoses per 10 HPF, 75% survival if the mitotic count was 5-9 per 10 HPF, and only 20% if there were more than 10 mitoses per 10 HPF.

Silverberg and Woodruff have both reported, as have others, that the prognosis of tumors arising de novo in the myometrium have a much poorer prognosis than tumors arising within a leiomyoma. Survivals in the 75% range have been noted for malignant tumors in pre-existing fibroids vs. a 25% survival for tumors arising in myometrium.

Silverberg noted the markedly favorable prognosis in premenopausal women; 16 of 18 premenopausal women available for follow-up were alive and well, while only two of 12 postmenopausal women enjoyed the same outcome.

It is known that leiomyomas contain high levels of estrogen and progesterone receptors relative to normal myometrium, in some cases reaching levels near that of normal endometrium. Although extensive receptor data are not available, it seems that anecdotal evidence for receptors in some uterine sarcomas does exist. One potential explanation, then, for the better prognosis in premenopausal patient may be related to the removal of both ovaries occurring at the time of hysterectomy for an estrogen-dependent tumor.

Clearly, almost all of the favorable prognostic factors are interrelated. The premenopausal patient is more likely to have a tumor with a low mitotic index, less pleomorphism and atypia, and to have a tumor arising in a leiomyoma. Although survival after myomectomy alone is not uniform, individualized selection of "conservative" therapy may be warranted in the properly informed patient with favorable prognostic indices.

Selected Readings

Fuller AF, Patterson DC, Shimm DS: Sarcomas of the female genital tract. In Raaf J (ed): *Management of Sarcomas*; in press.

Kempson RL, Bari W: Uterine sarcomas: Classification, diagnosis, and prognosis. *Hum Pathol* 1:331-349, 1970.

Meigs JV: *Tumors of the Female Pelvis*, New York, Macmillan, 1934.

Silverberg SG: Leiomyosarcoma of the uterus. *Obstet Gynecol* 38:613-627, 1971.

Van Dinh T, Woodruff JD: Leiomysarcomas of the uterus. *Am J Obstet Gynecol* 144:817-823, 1932.

Van Nagell JR, Hanson MB, Donaldson ES, et al: Adjuvant vincristine, actinomycin D and cyclophosphamide therapy in stage I uterine sarcomas. *Cancer* 57:1451-1454, 1986.

Wallach EE, Hammond CP, Goldfarb AF, et al: Symposium: Problems linked to uterine myomas. *Contemp Ob Gyn* 265-279, 1983.

Wilson EA, Yang F, Rees LD: Estradiol and progesterone binding in uterine leiomyomata and in normal uterine tissue. *Obstet Gynecol* 55:20-24, 1980.

CHAPTER 77

Unexpected Carcinoma of the Fallopian Tube at Vaginal Hysterectomy

CHARLES E. FLOWERS, JR., M.D.

CASE ABSTRACT

Vaginal hysterectomy with repair was recommended to a 43-year-old patient complaining of chronic menometrorrhagia. Immediately after removal of the uterus, a 3-cm nonadherent hemorrhagic mass was noted within the right fallopian tube. The left tube appeared "normal," as did both ovaries.

DISCUSSION

The findings of a 3-cm nonadherent mass on a fallopian tube dictate that immediate diagnosis be made in order that the patient can be appropriately treated. The differential diagnosis is: (1) an ectopic pregnancy; this usually appears as a slightly cyanotic mass with small areas of hemorrhage beneath the mucosa, (2) a hemorrhagic salpinx secondary to trauma or previous inflammatory disease, and finally (3) the most unfortunate diagnosis— carcinoma of the fallopian tube. The diagnosis is made from a frozen section of the fallopian tube. The fallopian tube should be appropriately clamped, removed, and sent to pathology for a frozen section. If there is any question concerning the diagnosis, treatment should await permanent sections.

It is not necessary to delay the operation while the frozen section is being evaluated. If one of the first two diagnoses is correct, the patient has been appropriately treated. If the third diagnosis is made, a laparotomy must be performed, but the completion of the vaginal hysterectomy does not interfere with the management of the patient. Thus, the vaginal hysterctomy is completed and the diagnosis from the pathologist awaited. It is always preferable to obtain consent for a laparotomy in patients who are to have a vaginal operation. If their permission has been obtained then the laparotomy is immediately performed using a Maylard or midline incision. A staging procedure similar to that done for ovarian carcinoma is done. If permission for a laparotomy has not been obtained, the patient can be reoperated after consent is obtained. If there is any question concerning the diagnosis, the laparotomy must be delayed until the question is resolved.

Carcinoma of the fallopian tube unfortunately may frequently metastasize through the bloodstream, the lungs, and the central nervous system. Therefore, the use of postoperative radiation in this patient is not indicated: chemotherapy is the treatment of choice.

CHAPTER **78**

Unexpected Carcinoma of the Ovary Reported by Pathology 5 Days Following Unilateral Salpingo-oophorectomy for Presumed Endometrial Cyst

DENIS CAVANAGH, M.D., Ch.B. (Glas.), F.A.C.O.G., F.A.C.S., F.R.C.O.G.
DONALD E. MARSDEN, M.D., M.R.C.O.G., F.R.A.C.O.G.

CASE ABSTRACT

A unilateral oophorectomy for presumed endometriosis had been performed in a 23-year-old patient. At surgery, the ovary measured 12 cm in diameter, and there was no evidence of endometriosis on the opposite side nor, for that matter, elsewhere in the pelvis. Some light, filmy adhesions between the tumor and the surrounding intestine had been severed easily at the time of surgery. The tumor had been removed in its entirety, along with the tube, which was uninvolved. There was no spillage of tumor.

On the fifth postoperative day, the pathology report indicated an adenocarcinoma of the ovary, existing in a specimen with an intact capsule, and no gross evidence of serosal penetration was described.

DISCUSSION

Identification of the Problem

The extreme seriousness of the problem must be clearly understood by all those involved in the management of this patient.

A superficial assessment might lead to the conclusion that this young woman, presumably wishing to retain reproductive potential, has had a stage IA carcinoma of the ovary completely excised and has, therefore, been adequately treated. On the basis of the information supplied, such an assumption is completely unfounded and carries grave risks for the patient.

The prognosis and treatment of ovarian carcinoma are directly related to the clinical stage, the amount of residual tumor, and the histopathology. In this patient there is inadequate information available on all of these subjects.

With respect to the clinical staging and amount of tumor possibly remaining in this patient, a number of observations relating to ovarian carcinomas actually or apparently belonging to Federation of International Gynecologists and Obstetricians (FIGO) stage I must be clearly understood.

1. Peritoneal washings will contain malignant cells in up to 36% of patients with stage I tumors with intact capsules (8), and their presence significantly affects the prognosis (3, 14) and hence the treatment.

2. The contralateral ovary, although normal to gross inspection, will harbor microscopic carcinoma in 12% to 18% of cases (9).

3. Diaphragmatic metastases have been found in over 10% of patients who, having been previously diagnosed as having stage I lesions, were subjected to surgery for restaging within a few weeks of initial diagnosis (10).

4. Para-aortic lymph node metastases have

been shown to be present in approximately 10% of women with stage I ovarian carcinoma, and pelvic nodes were involved in 8% of cases (10).

5. Omental metastases were present in 3% to 5% of patients with disease that had been thought to be stage I (2, 10). Routine omentectomy in such cases may well show this estimate to be conservative.

Considering all these facts, it is not surprising that the staging of early ovarian cancer is reportedly inaccurate in 30% of cases (5). In the patient we are considering, there is no mention of any extrapelvic structures being palpated or examined for even macroscopic evidence of tumor spread. Clearly the staging is totally inadequate.

Nor is the pathology report of "adenocarcinoma . . . with an intact capsule and no gross evidence of serosal penetration" sufficiently precise in this situation. Of particular importance here is the accurate identification of tumor type, its degree of differentiation, and microscopic evidence of serosal penetration. In a tumor of this size these judgments must be based on the examination of multiple sections from all areas of the tumor by an experienced gynecologic pathologist. Decker et al (4) reported an 87% 5-year survival in stage I, grade I papillary cystadenocarcinomas, compared to a 54% 5-year survival in stage I, grade III papillary cystadenocarcinomas.

The seriousness of the situation for this young woman is, therefore, due to major inadequacies in the assessment of possible residual tumor, the staging of the disease, and the pathologic assessment of the tumor. Given these obvious deficiencies, no rational plan of therapy can be formulated.

Avoidance of this Problem

In the clinical evaluation of any female with a pelvic or adnexal mass, the possibility of ovarian malignancy must be considered. In the 20- to 30-year age group approximately 10% of ovarian tumors are malignant (13). Although only about 8% of epithelial cancers of the ovary occur in women under age 35, the proportion may be increasing (1).

With this in mind, preoperative evaluation should include, in all cases:

1. A complete history and physical examination, including cervical cytology and rectovaginal examinations.

2. Complete blood count, serology, serum electrolytes, renal and liver profiles.
3. Urinalysis and pregnancy tests.
4. Human serum beta chorionic gonadotropin and alpha-fetoprotein.
5. Chest x-ray.
6. If pregnancy has been excluded, an intravenous pyelogram should be done.

Other tests such as barium enema, upper gastrointestinal series, liver scan, sigmoidoscopy, or colonoscopy may be indicated by features such as dyspepsia or bowel disturbances revealed on history or by findings on physical examination. Biopsy specimens should be obtained from enlarged groin or supraclavicular nodes. If a pleural effusion is found, thoracentesis should be performed to allow cytologic examination of the effusion. On the other hand, even if ascites is present, abdominal paracentesis should be avoided because fluid will be obtained more safely at the time of laparotomy.

Sonograms, computerized axial tomography scans, and lymphangiograms are rarely helpful and are occasionally misleading (12).

The definitive investigative procedure for ovarian masses over 5 cm in diameter, or persistent masses of smaller size, or in any case where malignancy is suspected is laparotomy. Laparoscopy may be misleading or even dangerous in the presence of ovarian carcinoma and provides inadequate information for staging.

With a mass the size that this patient had, or when there is the slightest suspicion of malignancy, a vertical incision should be used.

Immediately after the peritoneal cavity is opened the nature and volume of any ascites are noted, and samples are aspirated and sent for cytology. If ascites is not present, irrigation of the peritoneal cavity with 300 cc of saline should be performed and the fluid aspirated and sent for cytology. A soft rubber catheter and bulb syringe are used to irrigate the space between the right hemidiaphragm and the liver, which is a common site of miliary metastases.

The upper abdomen is explored first, with palpation of the retroperitoneal structures and palpation and examination of all peritoneal surfaces and intraperitoneal organs. Special attention is paid to the liver and undersurface of the diaphragm. Use of a sigmoidoscope or laparoscope may aid in obtaining sufficient illumination and better visualization of this important area. The stomach, bowel, mesentery, and omentum are all palpated and inspected. Biopsy specimens are obtained from any suspicious lesions. The para-aortic region is palpated and biopsy specimens are obtained from any palpable nodes. Even in the absence of palpable tumor deposits within it, the greater omentum should be removed if ovarian malignancy is present or strongly suspected.

When the upper abdomen has been thoroughly explored, attention is directed to the pelvis. The gross appearance of the uterus, tubes, and ovaries is noted. Adhesions, excrescences, bilaterality, and tumor rupture are suggestive of malignancy and indicate a poorer prognosis.

If at this stage there is no indication that the disease has spread beyond one ovary and the patient is young and desiring further children, consideration can be given to conservative therapy.

The criteria for conservative therapy in such a case as this are:

1. Stage IA lesion (FIGO)
2. Histopathology of tumor
   (a) Grade I epithelial carcinoma
   (b) "Borderline tumors" ("low malignant potential")
   (c) Dysgerminoma
   (d) Granulosa cell tumor
   (e) Arrhenoblastoma
3. Tumor encapsulated and free of adhesions
4. No invasion of the capsule, lymphatics, blood vessels, or mesovarium
5. Peritoneal washings showing no malignant cells
6. Omentectomy specimen normal
7. Sections from remaining ovary histologically negative for tumor
8. Pelvis otherwise normal

Now it is clear that not all of these criteria can be fulfilled at the initial laparotomy. If reliable frozen section services are available, upper abdominal biopsies and omental and para-aortic nodal biopsies containing tumor on frozen section would indicate the need for the maximum surgical effort. If these are negative or reliable frozen sections are not available, decisions must be made on clinical grounds, pending permanent section results.

If conservative management still appears feasible, salpingo-oophorectomy is carefully performed to avoid rupture or leakage of the tumor. Should there still be uncertainty as to its nature, it should be cut in the operating room (away from the operating table) and checked for signs of malignancy. Again, frozen sections, if available and reliable, may be immensely useful. If malignancy appears to be or is shown on frozen section to be present, the other ovary is bivalved and wedge biopsy performed. Once more, a positive frozen section would indicate the need to abandon conservatism. The ovary should be carefully repaired using 5-0 polypropylene sutures as the aim of conservatism is primarily to preserve fertility, and adhesion formation would defeat that aim.

Biopsy specimens should be obtained from any suspicious pelvic lesions or pelvic nodes.

Assuming there is still no contraindication to conservative management, the abdomen is closed, and careful and detailed operative notes are made.

The patient must be given a detailed evaluation of the situation. Should subsequent pathology or cytologic reports indicate that any of the criteria for conservative management have not been fulfilled then reoperation with maximal surgical effort must be advised, with suitable adjunctive therapy.

If all the criteria are shown to have been fulfilled, the patient is followed carefully. When the desired family size has been achieved, total hysterectomy and removal of the remaining ovary are then carried out (1). The same careful total abdominal assessment advised for the first operation is mandatory.

Only by such a fastidious approach to this type of patient can we hope to avoid misdiagnosis, optimize treatment, and improve survival and cure rates. Nothing short of the ideal should be an acceptable goal.

This Patient's Problem and Its Management

By now it will be clear that the patient has received far from optimal management.

Several things must be done immediately:

1. The operative specimen and slides should be seen and assessed by a competent gynecologic pathologist and, if necessary, further sections made as described above.
2. Any relevant investigations that were not done preoperatively should be performed.
3. The patient should be strongly advised to have a staging laparotomy performed, in the

manner described above. Laparoscopy would not be appropriate in this situation.

Should the patient refuse repeat surgery, the dangers inherent in such a decision must be made clear to her, and monthly follow-up for 1 year, with subsequent visits every 3 months advised.

If the patient agrees to re-exploration, it would seem to be wisest to have it performed in a center where a skilled gynecologic pathologist can perform reliable frozen sections to minimize the chance of a repeat laparotomy, if sections show more advanced disease than had been suspected.

Patients with stage IA "borderline" or grade I carcinoma of the ovary appear to do equally well whether treated by unilateral salpingo-oophorectomy or total hysterectomy and bilateral salpingo-oophorectomy (7, 9). However, it has been pointed out that these reports are from older series, and survival rates were not optimal in either the conservatively or radically treated groups (11).

In the event that the criteria for conservative management are not fulfilled, the patient should have total hysterectomy, bilateral salpingo-oophorectomy, omentectomy, and appendectomy. The aim is to reduce tumor bulk as much as possible and leave no residual tumor nodule over 1 cm in diameter ("maximal surgical effort").

Subsequently, any patient with stage I disease with poorly differentiated tumor, bilateral ovarian involvement, ascites, or positive peritoneal washings, and any patient with stage II, III, or IV disease, should receive combination chemotherapy from an experienced oncologist, using cyclophosphamide, doxorubicin, and cis platinum. This therapy is given once every 4 weeks for approximately 12 courses, with careful surveillance for hematologic, cardiologic, hepatic, and renal complications. Regular gynecologic examinations, including vaginal vault cytology, and rectovaginal examinations are essential.

After approximately 12 courses of chemotherapy, if there is no clinical evidence of recurrence, a "second look" laparotomy, performed as for the staging procedure previously described, should be done. If there is no residual tumor and peritoneal washings are negative, the patient should continue on oral cyclophosphamide, 150 mg/m^3, for 8 days per month for an additional 3 months. Thereafter the chemotherapy is discontinued, but regular gynecologic follow-up is still essential.

The place of radiotherapy in the management of ovarian carcinoma is controversial at the present time, and opinions differ widely (6, 15).

References

1. Barber HRK: *Ovarian Carcinoma: Etiology, Diagnosis and Treatment.* New York, Masson, 1978.
2. Buchsbaum HJ, Keetel WC: Radioisotopes in treatment of stage IA ovarian cancer. *Natl Cancer Inst Monogr* 42:127, 1975.
3. Creasman WT, Rutledge F: The prognostic value of peritoneal cytology in gynecologic malignant disease. *Am J Obstet Gynecol* 110:773, 1971.
4. Decker DG, Malkasian GD, Jr, Taylor WF: The prognostic importance of histologic grading in ovarian carcinoma. *Natl Cancer Inst Monogr* 42:9, 1975.
5. Decker DG, Webb MJ: Prophylactic therapy for stage I ovarian cancer. *Gynecol Oncol* 1:203, 1973.
6. Dembo AJ, Bush RS, Beale FA, et al: The Princess Margaret Hospital study of ovarian cancer: stages I, II and asymptomatic III presentations. *Cancer Treat Rep* 63:249, 1979.
7. Julian CG, Woodruff JD: The biologic behavior of low grade papillary serous carcinoma of the ovary. *Obstet Gynecol* 40:860, 1972.
8. Keetel WC, Pixley EE, Buchsbaum HJJ: Experience with peritoneal cytology in the management of gynecologic malignancies. *Am J Obstet Gynecol* 108:878, 1970.
9. Munnell EW: Is conservative therapy ever justified in stage I(IA) cancer of the ovary? *Am J Obstet Gynecol* 103:641, 1969.
10. Piver MS, Barlow JJ, Lele SB: Incidence of sub-clinical metastasis in stage I and II ovarian carcinoma. *Obstet Gynecol* 52:100, 1978.
11. Smith WG: Surgical treatment of epithelial ovarian carcinoma. *Clin Obstet Gynecol* 22:939, 1979.
12. Watring WG, Edinger DD, Anderson B: Screening and diagnosis in ovarian cancer. *Clin Obstet Gynecol* 22:745, 1979.
13. Way S: *Malignant Disease of the Female Genital Tract.* Philadelphia, Blakiston, 1951.
14. Webb MJ, Decker DG, Mussey E, et al: Factors influencing survival in stage I ovarian cancer. *Am J Obstet Gynecol* 116:222, 1973.
15. Young RC: Ovarian carcinoma: An optimistic epilogue. *Cancer Treat Rep* 63:333, 1979.

CHAPTER 79

Nonresectable Adenocarcinoma of Ovary Which Shrinks During Chemotherapy

WILLIAM T. CREASMAN, M.D.

CASE ABSTRACT

A 15-cm fixed pelvic mass, separate from the uterus, was found in an asymptomatic 57-year-old multipara with a tentative diagnosis of ovarian carcinoma. The abdomen was opened through a midline incision. There was free peritoneal fluid from which washings were obtained, and the initial diagnosis was substantiated. There was extensive carcinomatosis. The disease was bilateral, fixed to the sidewalls of the pelvis, the broad ligament, the posterior surface of the uterus, the mesosalpinx, the descending colon, and various loops of small intestine. There were countless subserosal 1- to 2-mm nodules of metastatic tumor on the small bowel and diaphragm. Representative biopsies from the tumor were obtained. It was the opinion of the operator that the tumor was nonresectable. The abdomen was closed and the patient placed on chemotherapy involving courses of adriamycin and cis-platinum. During the course of the chemotherapy there was a good clincial response as measured by a dramatic reduction in the size of the tumor. Upon pelvic examination it now appeared to be movable and the surgeon wondered about the propriety of re-exploration and possible resection.

DISCUSSION

The situation presented by this patient was unusual when single agent chemotherapy was standard therapy. Today, with combination chemotherapy particularly if cis-platinum is included there appears to be an increased number of patients exhibiting the clinical picture of the patient described. Yet uninhibited enthusiasm should be tempered. There is no question that patients who are optimally debulked (tumor residual equal to or less than 2 cm) have a greater chance of achieving a complete response, come to a second look, have a surgical pathologically complete response, and are longer survivors than the patient not optimally debulked. With the use of multiple agent chemotherapy there appears to be an increasing number of patients (both optimally and suboptimally debulked) who are experiencing a clinical response. Some preliminary data suggest that as many as 80% to 85% of patients are responding to chemotherapy. One must be extremely careful in interpreting this data, as two-thirds to three-quarters of the responders are only partial responders and their survivals have minimal or no increase compared to those that have no change in clinical disease.

Approximately one-third of patients with stage III or IV disease who are treated with chemotherapy will come to second look because of a response to the treatment. If only complete responders (CR) are included, the number is less. Of the patients undergoing second look operation, only one-quarter to one-third will have surgical pathologic CRs. The rate of surgically confirmed response in two large series was 7.3% and 12.3%, respectively. Those patients with surgical CRs can expect a 20% to 40% recurrence. The overall prognosis of these patients with current modalities is, therefore, very dismal.

Since there is such a poor overall survival in this group of patients, approaches are now being evaluated which were considered at one time radical. The first question this patient poses is whether or not she could have been optimally debulked by a more experienced surgeon. Apparently only a biopsy was obtained. It is recognized that there are some situations in which no surgeon can adequately debulk a patient. Preliminary data do suggest that a significant number of patients said to be unresectable were re-explored and optimally debulked. Some required removal of part of the gastrointestinal tract with reanastomosis. The amount of tumor remaining behind after the surgical procedure continues to be an extremely important (if not the most important) prognostic criteria for prolonged survival. Even in "unresectable" cases the adnexal masses and partial omentectomy can be performed in essentially every situation. Approaching the pelvic mass(es) retroperitoneally always facilitates removal as well as decreasing blood loss considerably. The decision to re-explore the patient immediately after the initial exploration many times is difficult. Clinical judgment, reports from the primary surgeon and political consideration are all taken into the decision-making process. In some instances it has been decided not to re-explore the patient immediately even though it was felt that optimal debulking may be achieved. The patient is given three courses of chemotherapy and if there has been a clinical response, re-exploration at that time has been performed. In several instances, optimal debulking, even down to "no gross remaining disease," has been accomplished. The number of cases are few and definitive statements concerning what if any role this protocol will accomplish cannot be made.

There is an increasing body of information suggesting that converting a partial responder to CR by surgery (at the time of second look surgery) does not improve survival. These patients do not have an increased survival compared with those with tumor incompletely removed at second look. The role of cytoreductive surgery done early in the planned chemotherapy course may be different than reductive surgery at the time of second look, particularly since those patients who respond early may self-select and have a better chance for long-term survival.

Most protocols evaluating patients such as presented will usually suggest at least six to eight courses of chemotherapy and if there has been a CR, suggest a second look laparotomy. If there is a surgical pathological CR, the chemotherapy is usually stopped. There have, however, been some studies which because of the high recurrence rate have continued chemotherapy for up to a year after a negative second look. Disease has recurred even with this regimen. Whether or not there will be fewer recurrences with adjunctive chemotherapy is unknown.

In patients with minimal residual disease after second look operation, radiation to the whole abdomen and pelvis has been suggested as a possibly effective rescue modality. In several small studies where this has been tried, the results have been very disappointing and the complications (mainly gastro-intestinal) have been disastrous. Some patients who have had no disease or microscopic disease only at the time of second look operation have had the instillation of P32 postoperatively in an attempt to decrease recurrences and improve survival. The data are limited but results are comparable to those following external radiation with considerably less toxicity.

In patients with good response, this information should be conveyed to them and guarded optimism expressed. Given the above dismal situation in patients with suboptimal stage III disease, nevertheless, individuals who have a CR, particularly if confirmed at second look surgery, are the privileged few. Unfortunately, at the present time if a patient does not show a response to her first chemotherapy regimen, the chance of responding to the next single or combination regimen is minimal. Only time will tell whether or not the role of intraperitoneal chemotherapy will be of benefit in the future. The use of markers such as OC-125 which may help us to monitor our patients better and suggest other treatments earlier, await future study.

Whether this patient would benefit from exploratory laparotomy because of a clinical response "during" chemotherapy is unknown. Data concerning second look laparotomy at the completion of chemotherapy would suggest that only those patients with complete response possibly will benefit from such a procedure. If a complete response is obtained and since this patient had extensive disease we would approach this patient first with open laparoscopy, looking at areas of known residual disease with special attention to the diaphragms. If disease remains, then the exploratory laparotomy is not done. In patients not on a protocol the role of second look laparotomy is not done. In patients not on a protocol the role of second look laparotomy has not been defined. Second look laparotomy is not standard therapy at the present time. Preoperative evaluation has not included any special exams. CT scans have not been of benefit in these patients. The role of OC-125 is being evaluated but definitive statements cannot be made at this time.

Selected Readings

Cohen CJ, Goldberg JD, Holland JF, et al: Improved therapy with cis platinum regimen for patients with ovarian carcinoma (FIGO Stage III and IV) as measured by surgical end staging (second look operation). *Am J Obstet Gynecol* 145:955-967, 1983.

Richardson GS, Scully RE, Nikrui N, et al: Common epithelial cancer of the ovaries (Part I and Part II). *N Engl J Med* 312:415-424, 474-483, 1985.

Wiltshaw E, Kankipatis R, Dowson I: The role of cytoreductive surgery in advanced carcinoma of the ovary: An analysis of primary and second surgery. *Br J Obstet Gynecol* 92:522-527, 1985.

CHAPTER 80

Unexpected Adenocarcinoma of Ovary and Uterus

JOHN L. LEWIS, JR., M.D.

CASE ABSTRACT

A 38-year-old nulligravida with acute abdominal pain and a shock-like state was diagnosed as having pelvic inflammatory disease, peritonitis, and sepsis and responded to intravenous and intramuscular antibiotics. One week later a 15-cm midline pelvic mass was noted, of irregular shape, firm to palpation anteriorly, and soft and cystic posteriorly. Sonography and barium enema confirmed its presence, and the report suggested that it was adnexal in origin, having a multiloculated cystic appearance.

Previous gynecologic history included a diagnosis of endometriosis made by pelvic examination 18 years previously, and a 20-year history of uninvestigated primary infertility.

At surgery both fallopian tubes were markedly inflamed, both grossly and microscopically. The right ovary measured 8 × 10 cm and was firmly adherent to the tube, uterus, and cul-de-sac. A total abdominal hysterectomy and bilateral salpingo-oophorectomy were performed. The uterus weighed 170 gm and contained multiple leiomyomata measuring up to 5 cm. The right ovary contained benign endometrial cysts and contained a focus of endometrioid cystadenocarcinoma which extended to but not through the capsule of the ovary. The left ovary was unremarkable. Microscopic examination of the uterus disclosed an unexpected and separate well-differentiated adenocarcinoma of the endometrium with no myometrial invasion.

DISCUSSION

This 38-year-old nulliparous female presented with acute abdominal pain and a shock-like state which apparently subsided with conservative management including intramuscular and intravenous antibiotics. Her past medical history included the clinical diagnosis of endometriosis made 18 years earlier on the basis of a pelvic examination only and a 20-year history of infertility which had never been evaluated. We have no information concerning menstrual pattern or whether she had ever taken any type of hormones. Apparently she was well enough a week later to be considered a candidate for exploration to evaluate an irregularly shaped, 15-cm pelvic mass which on palpation was felt to be firm and cystic and on sonogra-

phy to be a multiloculated adnexal cyst. The barium enema apparently showed only the presence of a mass.

The findings at the time of surgery were (a) inflamed fallopian tubes (apparently accounting for the acute symptoms of the week before); (b) an 8 × 10 cm right ovary adherent to the tube, uterus, and cul-de-sac (pathology showing apparent endometriosis with a focus of endometrioid cystadenocarcinoma which extended to but not through the capsule); (c) fibroid uterus; (d) grade I adenocarcinoma of the endometrium with no myometrial penetration; and (e) normal left ovary. The obvious problem here is to try to determine whether this represents a stage III carcinoma of the endometrium or synchronous stage I cancers of the endometrium and ovary. Since we will have no more information made available to us that is in the protocol, it seems appropriate to make a choice of therapy based on the likelihood of these diagnoses.

For purposes of organization, comments on this case will be divided into those relating to preoperative evaluation, surgery, working diagnosis, subsequent therapy, and prognosis.

Preoperative Evaluation

Although it cannot be assumed that the people caring for this patient had seen her prior to the time of her admission with acute abdominal pain and a shock-like state, it is obvious that 20 years of infertility should have been evaluated. Because we are going to be faced later with the surprise diagnosis of an endometrial adenocarcinoma in a woman below the age of 40, it would be very surprising if she had not had problems consistent with anovulatory cycles or hormonal therapy either with sequential oral contraceptives or estrogens alone. For purposes of this discussion, this is purely theoretical, but it is almost unheard of for a female to have endometrical cancer below the age of 40 without some condition producing anovulatory cycles, use of exogenous hormones, or an estrogen-producing tumor. The preoperative sonogram and barium enema were important to help determine the nature of the mass and also to rule out diverticulitis as a source of the acute symptoms of a week before. The barium enema was also indicated even if there had not been acute symptoms because of the finding of colon cancer metastatic to the ovary in those patients who either have a history of familial polyposis of the colon or a family history of colon cancer. I also think she should have had an intravenous pyelogram to determine the number and position of ureters and whether they were involved in the mass. This is particularly true in a patient with a clinical diagnosis of endometriosis. Finally, proctosigmoidoscopy and cystoscopy are important parts of our evaluation of all pelvic masses.

Surgery

The obvious need for a dilatation and curettage in this patient comes not from her symptoms but from the fact that it is another way to evaluate the nature of a pelvic mass prior to laparotomy. In her case, a fractional dilatation and curettage and sounding, with frozen section evaluation of the endometrium, would have taken away the surprise of at least one of the two diagnoses. Hopefully, this diagnosis of cancer would have led to a more thorough evaluation of the abdomen at the time of surgery.

It goes without saying that any laparotomy on a patient with an adnexal mass should be done through a vertical incision that can be extended as far toward the xyphoid as is necessary to evaluate the upper abdomen. Because of the finding of an adnexal mass of unknown nature, it is important to take washings from the pelvis and abdominal gutters prior to proceeding with any surgical procedure. The reactive changes in mesothelial cells that begin soon after the laparotomy are difficult to evaluate the longer one waits to take washings after entering the abdomen. If the right ovarian cyst had been sent for frozen section and the true nature of the malignant change within it had been detected, proper evaluation would have consisted of palpation, inspection, and biopsy of any abnormal areas on the diaphragm, a partial omentectomy, and surgical evaluation of the para-aortic nodes, particularly at the level of the renal vessels. Since this was not done, we have to assume that no gross lesions were found and ascites was not identified.

Working Diagnosis

The problem of establishing the correct diagnosis is important because it affects the choice of subsequent therapy. Ideally, the differentiation between adenocarcinoma of the endometrium metastatic to the ovary, ovarian cancer metastatic to the endometrium, or synchronous well-differentiated cancers in both organs would be helped by careful pathologic evaluation. However, even when very careful analysis is made, including search for in situ changes in both organs, it is not always possible to make this differentiation. Such seems to be the problem we are presented with in this case. I favor the choice of there being two synchronous tumors. In a series of more than 500 patients with clinically apparent stage I adenocarcinoma of the endometrium treated at this institution, only 3% had spread to the adnexa (2). It is highly unlikely that a well-differentiated adenocarcinoma of the endometrium with no myometrial penetration would have metastases. It is also unlikely that if there was spread to the ovary that there would not also be concomitant spread to the fallopian tube or broad ligament on that side. As mentioned before, the endometrial adenocarcinoma would be consistent with a history of prolonged infertility, although that is purely conjectural. On the other hand, the finding of adenocarcinoma of an endometrioid type arising in an ovary involved with what seem to be endometrial cysts (endometriosis if stromal reaction was found) is plausible. Because there is no extension of the ovarian lesion through the capsule and no projections on the outside of the capsule, we are apparently dealing with a stage IA (i) endometrioid cystadenocarcinoma of the ovary and a stage I, grade I adenocarcinoma of the endometrium. Whether the endometrial cavity sounded to a depth greater than 8 cm is not known, but I would not think it was very important since the increased size would seem to be accounted for by the fibroids rather than by endometrial cancer.

If we make the assumption that the patient has two synchronous cancers, one of which is an ovarian epithelial cancer, the next question which comes up is whether another surgical procedure should be carried out now to properly stage the cancers. This would include the procedures listed above. Because the ovarian tumor is well differentiated, has no apparent extension through the capsule, and there is no mention of ascites, I would not recommend further surgery at this time. On the other hand, I would recommend subsequent chemotherapy.

Subsequent Therapy

Although one could be tempted to advise no further therapy in this patient because both her endometrial cancer and her ovarian cancer are in categories with a good prognosis, there still is evidence that treating all established epithelial cancers of the ovary with therapy after surgery is appropriate. The cooperative study reported by Hreshchyshyn et al (3) showed that, in stage I epithelial carcinoma of the ovary, 6% of patients treated with Melphelan developed recurrence compared to 17% of those receiving no therapy and 30% of those receiving pelvic radiation. Piver has reported an even more dramatic difference in patients with stage IA ovarian cancer treated with radioactive colloids or no therapy after surgery (4). Of those receiving postoperative intraperitoneal radioactive colloids, 94% survived free of disease, whereas only 22% of a similar group treated with surgery alone were alive free of disease.

With these data in mind, it seems obvious that an alkylating agent is the treatment of choice because of its effectiveness and low rate of toxicity. The selection of a progestational agent to go along with this is purely empirical and is based on the histologic type of the tumor, the likelihood that both well-differentiated tumors will have estrogen and progesterone receptors, and the virtual absence of toxicity from these agents. We would continue therapy with an alkylating agent (either Melphelan in monthly cycles or Leukeran daily) and a progestational agent (daily oral doses of Provera or Megace) for 18 months. If there is no clinical evidence of disease at that time, we would recommend a "second look" laparotomy in order to determine if it is appropriate to stop therapy. In an unreported series of patients undergoing "second look" laparotomies, we found that more than 10% of those who had been categorized as having Stage I disease by proper surgical techniques had microscopic disease at the time of "second look" laparotomy. Since the patient we are discussing was not properly staged at the time of surgery, it seems even more appropriate to do this.

Prognosis

As best as one can predict from the information given, the patient should have more than a 90% chance of being free of disease at 5 years. This is based on the survival rate of 95% of stage I, grade I adenocarcinoma of the endometrium with no myometrial invasion and the success rate of stage IA ovarian cancer treated with subsequent chemotherapy. It is obvious that the good prognosis is based on the fortuitous fact that she developed acute pelvic inflammatory disease and came to the hospital for evaluation.

References

1. *Annual Report Gynecological Cancer*. Federation of International Gynecologists and Obstetricians, vol. 17, 1979.
2. Homesley HD, Boronow RC, Lewis JL Jr: Treatment of adenocarcinoma of the endometrium at Memorial-James Ewing Hospitals, 1949–1965. *Obstet Gynecol* 47:100, 1976.
3. Hreshchyshyn MM, Park RC, Blessing JA, et al: The role of adjuvant therapy in stage I ovarian cancer. *Am J Obstet Gynecol* 138:139, 1980.
4. Piver MS: Radioactive colloids in the treatment of stage IA ovarian cancer. *Obstet Gynecol* 40:42, 1972.

SECTION 8
Problems of Minor Gynecologic Surgery

CHAPTER **81**
Perforation of Uterus at Dilation and Curettage

JOHN C. LATHROP, M.D.

CASE ABSTRACT

Fractional D & C was recommended for a 65-year-old patient with a 1-year history of watery vaginal discharge which had recently become bloody. Menopause had been at age 50 years, and supplemental estrogen administration of 2 years' duration had been given immediately after the menopause.

The patient was a moderately obese multipara, but was neither diabetic nor hypertensive.

The endocervical portion of the fractional curettage proceeded easily enough producing scant, grossly benign curettings. However, when the uterine sound was introduced to measure uterine depth, its passage appeared to encounter little resistance. A curette was introduced, and the tip proceeded with ease well beyond the estimated depth of the cavum, suggesting perforation of the wall of the uterus.

DISCUSSION

Given the history of a watery, bloody discharge and her age, this patient must be considered as a likely candidate to have endometrial carcinoma. In order to establish the diagnosis and institute appropriate therapy, sampling of the endometrium is essential. Since it is probable that the sound and the curette have both perforated the uterus, the surgeon is understandably reluctant to persist in further attempts to complete the procedure in the usual fashion. Regardless, efforts to obtain endometrial tissue must be pursued in spite of the recognized perforation.

Uterine perforation at the time of curettage may occur for a variety of reasons. In a 65-year-old lady, the endometrium has become atrophied and the myometrium is thinner. If malignancy is present in the uterine wall, the likelihood of perforation is even greater (5). Marked degrees of unrecognized anteversion or retroversion of the fundus allow perforation to occur more readily by permitting misdirection of the sound of curette (Fig. 81.1) In keeping with the principles of performing a D & C, as outlined by Word et al (7) it is imperative that the position of the uterus be determined by bimanual examination before any instruments are inserted. Adherence to this guideline will reduce the incidence of perforation to a minimum. When instruments are inserted, care must be taken to avoid the overzealous use of force in their manipulation.

Upon recognition of the perforation of the uterus, subsequent management is considered in two phases: (a) treatment of the perforation; (b) establishment of the histologic diagnosis.

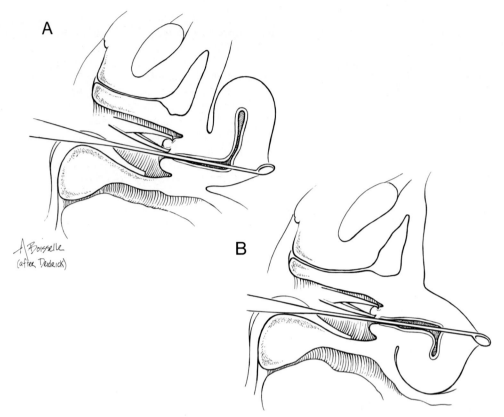

Figure 81.1. Perforation of the posterior wall of an anteflexed uterus is shown in *A*, while perforation of the anterior wall of a retroflexed uterus is shown in *B*.

Most uterine perforations occurring during diagnostic D & C in postmenopausal patients cause no significant clinical problems. A simple, noninvasive test, real-time ultrasonography, may be employed to scan the cul-de-sac for accumulation of blood. A negative scan in the presence of a clinically stable patient would permit management by simple observation over a period of 1 or 2 days for signs of bleeding, infection, or adjacent organ injury (6). If intraperitoneal bleeding to a significant degree is suspected, clinically or by real-time ultrasonography, a culdocentesis may be readily carried out for confirmation. Should gross blood be aspirated of if there is a serious concern regarding adjacent organ injury, laparoscopy would be advisable to evaluate the necessity of a formal celiotomy. In the event that severe bleeding or trauma to adjacent organs was demonstrated, laparotomy would be indicated in order to control the bleeding promptly or repair the injury. If infection occurred, antibiot-

ics could be utilized and colpotomy performed later if an abscess presented in the cul-de-sac.

The management of a perforation produced by a uterine sound does not differ significantly from the injury produced by a curette in the atrophic postmenopausal uterus. One might anticipate a somewhat lower incidence of complications following perforation with a sound because of its size, shape, and lack of sharp edges. In patients suffering perforation by a Heyman capsule, management is somewhat different. Roentgenograms confirming the mishap must first be obtained. The capsules are then removed in the routine manner. Should it not be possible to remove the capsule manually in the extrauterine position, laparotomy must then be promptly carried out to retrieve the radiation source.

Hysteroscopy, utilizing either gas or liquid as a distention system, is contraindicated in the presence of a uterine perforation since it would not be possible to distend the uterus (4). Contact hysteroscopy might be of some value in identifying the perforation site, although there has not been wide experience with this method at this time. It would be of greater usefulness in assessing the nature and anatomic location of intrauterine pathology. It has no value in determining the extent of extrauterine injury.

Perforations occurring in the presence of cervical carcinoma are managed according to the principles applying to any other type of uterine perforation at curettage. In this instance, however, it would be prudent to make no further attempts at endometrial sampling since the primary diagnosis is already established and the histologic evaluation of the endometrium will have little or no influence on the determination of treatment of the primary disease.

The question of dissemination of endometrial carcinoma to an intraperitoneal location is often considered in discussions of uterine wall perforation at the tumor site. Assuming that the primary diagnosis of malignancy is established, the initiation of therapy in the form of external radiation or surgery is usually undertaken promptly according to the appropriate clinical findings. Studies have shown that there is no significant survival difference for these patients as a result of the perforation. For this reason, the principles of management of the incident would be similiar to those described for the nonmalignant state.

In younger patients having curettage performed for a pregnancy situation, such as an incomplete or therapeutic abortion or a hydatidiform mole, the anatomic location of the perforation would have greater significance. Midline perforations in the anterior or posterior wall could be treated conservatively with observation for complications. Lateral perforations with their greater likelihood of injury to the uterine vessels, dilated in the gravid state, would indicate laparoscopic examination if there was any indication of broad ligament hematoma formation or laparotomy if significant intraperitoneal hemorrhage appeared to have occurred (3).

In the patient in question, diagnosis of her primary disease process must be promptly established by obtaining for study tissue samples of the endometrium. This could be done by first carefully reassessing the position of the fundus with a repeat bimanual examination.

If the operator is an experienced hystero-scopist, the contact hysteroscope may be gently inserted into the endometrial cavity to identify accurately the geographic location of the tumor (1). This would facilitate and minimize the amount of curetting necessary to obtain an adequate specimen and reduce the risk of reperforation of the uterus. It would also identify any bowel or omentum previously drawn into the uterine cavity by the curette at the time of perforation. Very cautious passage of the sound could then be executed in the appropriate axis of the uterus trying consciously to avoid the site of prior perforation. If this was successful, the cervix could then be dilated and the curette carefully passed into the endometrial cavity, again avoiding the site of perforation. Gentle and thorough curetting of the fundus should then be accomplished. An alternative possibility would be to perform a laparoscopic examination and then, with the laparoscope in place, execute the D & C under direct intra-abdominal vision (2). Evaluation of possible dissemination of a malignant process represents an added benefit of prelaparotomy laparoscopy but, by itself, is insufficient justification to warrant this procedure following simple perforation of the uterus.

In the absence of indications for emergency intervention, the standard order of diagnostic procedure should be carried out with the aim of establishing an accurate histologic diagnosis. Gross evaluation of the endocervical curettings is of no significance in this patient since their benign appearance does not eliminate the possibility of uterine malignancy. Should cancer prove to be present in the uterus, other forms of therapy, such as radiation or chemotherapy, might be more appropriate to consider as the first step in the optimal treatment plan for this patient. The interests of the patient are best served when laparotomy, if indicated, can be deferred to fit into a thoughtful and well-conceived plan of treatment.

References

1. Barbot J, Parent B, Dubuisson J: Contact hysteroscopy: Another method of endoscopic examination of the uterine cavity. *Am J Obstet Gynecol* 136:721, 1980.
2. Ben-Baruch G, Menczer J, Shalev J, et al: Uterine perforation during curettage: Perforation rates and postperforation management. *Isr J Med Sci* 16:821, 1980.
3. Berek JS, Stubblefield PG: Anatomic and clinical correlates of uterine perforation. *Am J Obstet Gynecol* 135:181, 1979.

4. Neuwirth RS: *Hysteroscopy*. Philadelphia, WB Saunders, 1975, p. 40.

5. Rutledge F, Ehrlich C: Adenocarcinoma of the endometrium. In Gray LA (ed): *Endometrial Carcinoma and Its Treatment*. Springfield, IL, Charles C Thomas, Chap. 12, 1977, p. 128.

6. Shalev E, Ben-Ami M, Zuckerman H: Real-time ultrasound diagnosis of bleeding uterine perforation during therapeutic abortion. *J Clin Ultrasound* 14:66, 1986.

7. Word B, Gravlee LC, Wideman GL: The fallacy of simple uterine curettage. *Obstet Gynecol* 12:642, 1958.

CHAPTER 82

Pelvic Mass Following Conization

BARRIE ANDERSON, M.D.

CASE ABSTRACT
Cold-knife conization of the cervix using a number 11 pointed scalpel blade had been
performed on a 52-year-old multipara to better evaluate and treat a severe cervical dysplasia which had extended into the endocervical canal. Deep hemostatic stitches of
chromic catgut had been placed at the 3 and 9 o'clock positions lateral to the cervix.
After conization, the vaginal edge was caught in a running locked hemostatic suture of
chromic catgut.

Postoperatively the patient felt weak and developed a persistent low grade fever and
troublesome backache, the latter thought to have been due to her position in the stirrups on the operating table at the time of the conization.

The symptoms persisted and the patient was examined in her doctor's office 2 weeks
postoperatively disclosing a marked tenderness around the cervix at the vault of the
vagina, and a raw purulent site of the recent conization. There was a hemoglobin of
10 gm. A local cellulitis was diagnosed and the patient placed on a broad spectrum
antibiotic. The symptoms of weakness, backache, and fever worsened progressively
and the patient was readmitted 5 weeks after surgery. The hemoglobin was now 8.5
gm. An IVP demonstrated compression and lateral displacement of the right ureter and
a CAT scan revealed a 6 × 8 cm cystic mass posterior to the cervix on the patient's
right. This was confirmed by pelvic examination under anesthesia.

Because of the distance of the mass from the vault of the vagina, a tentative diagnosis
of infected hematoma in this area was made, and through a flank incision a retroperitoneal exposure of this hematoma was accomplished with ease. The ureter was traced
for its length, found to be uninvolved. The hematoma was evacuated as well as possible, and a Jackson-Pratt drain placed in the cavity of the hematoma. The patient's
postoperative course was uneventful and she was discharged on her fifth postoperative
day.

DISCUSSION

The origin of the hematoma in the right broad
ligament and retroperitoneal area in this patient
resulted from lack of hemostasis in either the
descending cervical branch of the uterine artery or the uterosacral ligament branch of the
vaginal artery. This can occur during conization when the direction of the cervical canal is
identified incorrectly so that the incision per-
forates the cervix high in the endocervical canal,
in this case on the right and posteriorly. Bleeding in this area may not be expressed vaginally
and can be difficult to identify and to control.
Constant checking of the direction of the canal
and its relationship to the incision during the
procedure can prevent such perforations. This
can be facilitated by placing a sound in the endocervical canal and aiming the point of the
blade toward it at all times. In such a maneuver the handle of the knife will describe a very
large circle with the point remaining essentially stationary.

Another cause for bleeding in this area may

be inadequate ligation of the descending cervical branch of the uterine artery. In the postmenopausal woman, cervical atrophy and obliteration of the vaginal fornices may make it difficult to place a lateral suture high enough along the cervix to ligate this artery satisfactorily. Reflecting the vaginal mucosa away from the cervix, as at the beginning of a vaginal hysterectomy, can allow for better access to the descending cervical branch which should be ligated at the level of the internal os. Also, care must be taken to place the suture perpendicular to the endocervical canal. If the needle is angled too much, the cervical artery may be perforated or missed entirely with subsequent bleeding upon removal of the cone specimen.

In addition, better hemostasis may be obtained from the lateral sutures if they are not tied until after removal of the cone specimen. After decrease in cervix bulk following removal of the specimen, it is not uncommon for sutures to become less snug and therefore less hemostatic. This is particularly true in a small or atrophic cervix. To prevent this, lateral sutures can be placed and held with hemostats until completion of the surgical excision when they can be tied.

Finally, suturing of only the portio vaginalis may not be sufficient to control hemorrhage from deeper branches of the cervical artery but may place sufficient pressure to prevent vaginal exit of the blood, thus forcing it into a retroperitoneal location and delaying diagnosis. An alternate closure that allows better hemostasis and control of deeper vessels is the Sturmdorf closure, which has both a deep and a superficial component and approximates portio epithelium with endocervical epithelium (3, 4).Other methods of hemostasis include injection of the cervix with Pitressin or electrocautery. Any postoperative bleeding from the latter two methods would be immediately evident vaginally.

Differential diagnosis in this patient would have to include ureteral obstruction, retroperitoneal hematoma, and pelvic inflammatory disease. The presence of backache should direct attention to the retroperitoneal area and to the kidneys especially in the presence of fever. Ureteral obstruction could have resulted from a poorly placed lateral hemostatic suture at either 3 or 9 o'clock as the ureters pass from a lateral position near the cervix medially down the anterior vaginal wall to the trigone at a point about 3 to 4 cm below the anterior vaginal fornix. Atrophy in the postmenopausal cervix blurs landmarks and increases the risk of accidental ureteral compromise. Unilateral ureteral obstruction would be expected to give localized costovertebral angle tenderness, with fever arising from infection beyond a partially or completely obstructed ureter. IVP early in the course of the process should be diagnostic.

Serial hemoglobin and hematocrit measurements would direct attention to possible occult blood loss. Again, back pain should direct attention to the retroperitoneum and pelvic examination and IVP can help identify the location of the hematoma.

Retroperitoneal drainage of this hematoma through a lower quadrant abdominal incision, extended vertically into the flank, is ideal as tissue planes are easily developed from this approach (1). Blood vessels can be more easily traced and bleeding points identified. Other vulnerable structures such as the ureter can be avoided. Ureteral repair in the event of damage is also more easily accomplished. Finally, long-term negative suction drainage is more practical and comfortable through such an incision rather than through a vaginal approach.

Assuming that the cervical neoplasia has been completely removed, the patient should do well. The Jackson-Pratt drain should be left in place until total drainage in 24 hours is 10 to 15 cc or less. Broadspectrum antibiotic coverage tailored to bacterial cultures and sensitivities should be continued for a full therapeutic course. Should hysterectomy be necessary in the future consideration should be given to prophylactic antibiotics which appear to eliminate the increased morbidity of hysterectomy performed soon after cervical conization (2, 5, 6). If hysterectomy is done after 6 to 8 weeks, scarring might be expected in the right lateral and posterior cervical area.

References

1. Byron RL, Yonemoto RH, Riihimaki DU, et al: Retroperitoneal ligation of the hypogastric arteries for pelvic hemorrhage. *Am Surg* 33:25-28, 1967.
2. Forney JP, Morrow CP, Townsend DE, et al: Impact of cephalosporin proplylaxis on conization-vaginal hysterectomy morbidity. *Am J Obstet Gynecol* 125:100-103, 1976.
3. Krebs HB: Outpatient cervical conization. *Obstet Gynecol* 63:430-424, 1984.

4. Stafl A, Mattingly RF: Cervical intraepithelial neoplasia. In Mattingly RF, Thompson JD (eds): *TeLinde's
   Operative Gynecology*, 6th ed. Philadelphia, JB Lippincott, 1985.
5. Van Nagell JR, Roddick JW, Cooper RM, et al: Vaginal hysterectomy following conization in the treatment
   of carcinoma-in-situ of the cervix. *Am J Obstet Gynecol* 113:948-951, 1972.
6. Wisborg T: The cone biopsy-hysterectomy time interval
   related to wound infection. *Acta Obstet Gynecol Scand*
   51:1-4, 1972.

CHAPTER 83

Postmenopausal Endometrial Hyperplasia

SAUL B. GUSBERG, M.D., D.Sc.

CASE ABSTRACT

A 62-year-old, mildly hypertensive, obese multipara has recently developed bright red, painless postmenopausal genital bleeding. She had been taking 0.625 mg of conjugated estrogen for 5 of every 7 days for the previous 8 years. Although there was some multiparous relaxation, the findings on pelvic examination were otherwise within normal limits. A Pap smear reported as Class I had been obtained 6 months previously, showing good cornification. The uterine cavity measured 9 cm in depth, and an endometrial biopsy was obtained and reported as showing adenomatous hyperplasia of the endometrium without atypia.

DISCUSSION

First, one must clarify several aspects of the case abstract concerning this patient. The term "adenomatous hyperplasia without atypia" indicates a mild degree of this type of hyperplasia; we would call it grade I or possibly II, for we classify adenomatous hyperplasia in grades I, II, and III for increasing order of intensity. We have avoided the term atypia for grade III because of its imprecision and have also avoided the use of carcinoma-in-situ for grade III because the criteria for invasion in the endometrium are so loose and in addition, this lesion is reversible, especially in young women (3). These degrees of intensity are confluent, like dysplasia and carcinoma-in-situ of the cervix.

In addition, one must note the negative Pap smear 6 months prior to the described episode of bleeding. There are hazards of reassurance for the postmenopausal Pap, for its accuracy for endometrial cancer is poor, and its detection rate for adenomatous hyperplasia is negligible. While one can rely on the Pap smear for cervical cancer screening, it is not appropriate for endometrial cancer screening with the usual technique. We must teach the public to understand this difference, for the postmenopausal woman may take false confidence from a negative Pap in the face of uterine bleeding.

Since we learned long ago that obesity was a cofactor for adenomatous hyperplasia and carcinoma of the endometrium, this obese 62-year-old would be at risk in any case without prolonged estrogen administration. We now know that the postmenopausal woman is not devoid of estrogen, for the adrenal prehormone androstenedione is converted peripherally, probably in fat, to the potent estrogen, estrone. This, of course, will constantly stimulate her endometrium without progestational modification. Administered estrogen, if prolonged, can also increase (1) the risk for adenomatous hyperplasia and carcinoma (2), though it does not appear to increase the risk for those with endogenous risk factors. Cycling the estrogen administration does not appear to decrease the risk, although the addition of a progestin, if the dose is appropriate and if the estrogen chosen was appropriate, has been reported to do so (5).

The choice of a diagnostic strategy for this postmenopausal bleeder is very important, for there is a significant coincidence of endometrial cancer in the uteri of those with adenomatous hyperplasia. If aspiration curettage has been used for biopsy, we would be very confident of its accuracy. In any case, the patient with adenomatous hyperplasia has a greater than normal risk for future endometrial carcinoma; this prospective risk has been described as 20 to 25%, a very significant proportion. Therefore, she must be followed carefully.

The technique of endometrium sampling is different for those women in whom infertility is an issue, for the secretory change indicating an ovulatory cycle is general and requires but a few strips of endometrium that can be obtained with a Meigs curette. In the case of screening or diagnosis of cancer and its precursors, a general sample is required for pathologic endometrial histology, and it may vary from one site to another. I have indicated above that the Pap smear taken in the usual cervical fashion is not useful for this problem. There are a variety of endometrial cytologic washing techniques disclosing adenomatous hyperplasia only in accord with the amount of histologic material recovered. Cytologic samples are generally inadequate for this purpose. We have, therefore, preferred a histologic method with proven accuracy for adenomatous hyperplasia and endometrial cancer that obtains a general tissue sample without anesthesia, that is, aspiration curettage (4). It can be used for diagnosis, as stated, and also for screening women at high risk, such as those with the syndrome of obesity, infertility due to failure of ovulation, and dysfunctional uterine bleeding. It is also applicable as an annual screening technique for those on long-term estrogen administration or preliminary to such medication.

Since the probable cause of this patient's adenomatous hyperplasia is prolonged estrogen administration, the withdrawal of this medication should allow the endometrium to revert to its normal postmenopausal quiescent state. If the diagnosis was made by aspiration curettage, we would be satisfied by its accuracy so that formal D&C would not be necessary unless bleeding did not cease. However, all patients should be checked again by endometrial aspiration curettage in 4 months to be certain of the disappearance of the abnormality. This would be especially important in this obese patient who could be producing a significant

amount of estrogen on her own. Those subjects who are 20 to 50 lb overweight have a 3-fold risk for endometrial cancer, while those 50 or more lb overweight have a 9-fold risk. In the usual subject, withdrawal of estrogen will cure the abnormality.

Only in those who refuse to stop estrogen ingestion is there a need for further decision making. With mild adenomatous hyperplasia, a progestin may be added cyclically; in the more severe grades of intensity, we prefer hysterectomy and ask our patients to collaborate in the choice of withdrawal of estrogen versus surgery.

An occasional patient, especially the elderly, may not be sure of the source of the perineal blood, whether vaginal or rectal in origin. In such instances, a vaginal tampon placed high in the vagina can aid in this determination. The diagnostic use of hysteroscopy or hysterography is reserved for the occasional patient whose adenomatous hyperplasia has disappeared but staining continues. All types of endometrial sampling may miss small polyps, and visual surveillance may assist in the discovery.

Adenomatous hyperplasia is a significant cancer precursor that can assist us in the prevention of invasive cancer. But we should not overreact therapeutically when the etiologic agent can be identified.

References

1. Gusberg SB: Precursors of corpus cancer. I: Estrogens and adenomatous hyperplasia. *Am J Obstet Gynecol* 54:905, 1947.
2. Gusberg SB: The changing nature of endometrial cancer. *N Engl J Med* 302:729, 1980.
3. Gusberg SB, Kaplan AL: Precursors of corpus cancer. IV. Adenomatous hyperplasia as stage ō cancer of the endometrium. *Am J Obstet Gynecol* 87:662, 1963.
4. Gusberg SB, Milano C: Detection of endometrial cancer and its precursors. *Cancer* 47:1173, 1981.
5. Hammond CB, Jelousek FR, Lee KL, et al: Effects of long term estrogen replacement therapy. II: Neoplasia. *Am J Obstet Gynecol* 133:537, 1979.

CHAPTER **84**
Breast Cyst

CLYDE L. RANDALL, M.D.
JOHN R. EVRARD, M.D., M.P.H.

CASE ABSTRACT

A 3-cm cystic lesion was palpable in the upper outer quadrant of the left breast of a 38-year-old nulligravida. The remainder of the breast imparted an ill-defined but shotty sensation to the examiner, and the patient mentioned some monthly premenstrual breast pain. Aspiration of the cyst by a 22-gauge needle brought forth 15 cc of grossly blood-tinged fluid.

DISCUSSION

Management of symptomatic benign breast disease is often determined by severity and/or persistence of the woman's complaints. There has been increasing effort to manage symptomatic breast disease as an endocrinologic dysfunction within tissues containing steroid receptors. Since mastalgia and other symptoms are frequently related to the menstrual cycle, often the dysfunctions are related to ovarian or pituitary hormones. Objective criteria for the treatment are difficult to establish, because benign breast disease is not consistently related to a clinically detectable lesion or to predictable histopathologic findings. Consequently, a diagnostic work-up must include procedures to exclude malignancy and secondly to alleviate the patient's symptoms.

Procedures which are useful in establishing the diagnosis and in ruling out malignancy are: history and physical examination, xerography, transcutaneous biopsy using a Lee wire, by insertion of a hooked wire for marking the biopsy site, and by simple open breast biopsy. Use of these techniques have amply been described by Mitchell.

Procedure

Aspiration biopsy of the fluid in the cyst was apparently the first step in the clinician's management. Many clinicians do not examine this fluid histologically or cytologically, but I believe it necessary especially when the fluid is bloody or blood-tinged. Fresh blood could indicate injury from the needle used for the biopsy whereas old blood could be due to necrosis of an intraductal papilloma or other tumor of longer standing. The bulk of the fluid should be centrifuged, and the sediment divided. Half should be suspended for study of cytologic smears and, if there is appreciable sediment, some should be embedded for a histologic study as well. If there is no evidence of malignant cells in the fluid, and the palpable tumor has disappeared after the aspiration, excisional biopsy would be indicated only if mammography suggested a focus of neoplasia; otherwise, the patient should be examined every 6 months and she should be instructed regarding the technique and importance of self-examination of the breast.

Considerations

Huguley and Brown have reported an evaluation of breast examination, as evidenced in their review of histories of 2092 women who developed breast cancer in the state of Georgia between June of 1975 and February of 1979. Among this group, 78% of the lumps in the breast that proved to be cancer were first detected by the woman herself (57% accidentally, 21% during routine self-examination). They also found that frequency of self-examination decreased the percentage of breast cancer found by self-examination. In the women who practiced self-examination, 30% were found in the stages 0 or 1, whereas only 19% of the cancers developing in women who did not practice self-examination were in equally early, favorable stages at the time of diagnosis.

The clinician in the present case apparently made a diagnosis of a cyst of the breast, and she had many other findings to go along with cystic mastitis; consequently, the clinician elected to do an aspiration biopsy of the cyst. As a general rule, 15% of breast masses are malignant, and 20% of breast masses in patients under age 40 years are malignant. Also, malignant tumors tend to be painless and nontender and tend to be hard, irregular, and fixed to the skin or the muscle. Benign tumors, on the other hand, tend to be painful premenstrually, and they are tender to touch. They are mobile and nubby, and tend to be bilateral, fibrous, and grow in cystic tissue. The fluid in the case presented was slightly bloody, and this should point once more toward a malignancy. While many clinicians do not have cystic fluid examined under the microscope, the fact that fluid is blood tinged would suggest injury from the needle during the puncture and aspiration, whereas blood of longer standing would make me suspect a malignant tumor which had broken down. Assuming that the fluid contained no malignant cells and that the mass had disappeared after the aspiration, it is highly likely that this woman is suffering from cystic mastitis and should so be treated. After the patient has been counseled regarding the nature of the cyst and the procedure of cyst aspiration, she should be placed in the supine position, and the cyst aspirated using a 25 gauge needle on a 20-ml syringe. The skin over the mass is stabilized using the left index finger and thumb, and a 4 to 5-mm skin wheal is raised with a 25 gauge needle. The needle is then raised so that it is tangential to the chest wall, and the needle track is infiltrated with one percent lidocaine down to the mass. The 25 gauge needle is then

replaced on the 20 cc syringe with the mass being stabilized between the index finger and thumb, and the needle passed tangentially to the chest wall down to and into the mass. The physician should never point the needle directly at right angles to the skin for fear of penetrating the pleura and producing a pneumothorax. Fluid, if obtained, is generally cloudy, brownish fluid. Surgeons' opinions vary as to whether or not to have the fluid studied for cytology of histology. Certainly, if the fluid is bloody it should be examined cytologically or histologically. After needle aspiration of the cyst, if the fluid contains neoplastic cells either histologically or cytopathologically, or if a tumor mass persists, a histologic diagnosis must be obtained by open biopsy to determine the nature of the tumor. If no fluid is obtained upon aspiration, a thin-needle biopsy may be obtained, a transcutaneous biopsy may be obtained using a Lee needle, or an open biopsy may be utilized. If the lesion is visible on xerography, a bent wire may be passed down to the tumor, and another mammography with the bent wire in place may be obtained. Removal of the tumor along with the wire may then be performed, and another xerography may be performed to be certain that the tumor is included in the specimen with the wire.

In this patient, the benign nature of the mass would be indicated by the premenstrual pain and tenderness in the mass, other evidence of mastitis in the breast, absence of fixation of the mass, and absence of the mass after aspiration of the cyst. Each woman on whom the diagnosis of cystic mastitis is made should be taught the technique and benefits of breast self examination. She should also be examined by her physician every 6 months.

Medical Treatment

Many women experience premenstrual breast soreness and tenderness especially in the upper outer quadrant. The fit of the brassiere is the first thing which should be checked, since many women wear old garments that are not appropriate for the present breast shape. In women who have severe enough mastodynia to require treatment, a course of oral contraceptive pills may be useful in alleviating the symptoms. Especially useful are those progestational agents which contain Norethynodrel, and Norethisterone, and Norgestrel, since these drugs have a higher progestational effect and androgenic effect than the other progestational compounds. Another agent which may be used to relieve the bloating and pain associated with the breast in the last phase of the menstrual cycle is medroxyprogesterone acetate, which should be given daily the last 2 weeks of the menstrual cycle. A synthetic drug which is useful in limiting fibrocystic changes and its symptoms is danazol (Danocrine). This drug should be administered in courses from 3 to 6 months and may be started with doses as low as 100 mg/day. The drug can be increased to 400 mg/day without causing virilizing changes or amenorrhea.

Abstinence from methylxanthines (coffee, tea, cola) may be useful. It has been said to work by interfering with the action of phosphodiesterase which interferes with cyclic adenosine monophosphate. Also, women with persistent nipple discharge, even in the absence of demonstrated pituitary pathology, may benefit from bromocriptine (Parlodel) 2 1/2 mg per day in three doses.

Since carcinoma of the breast is such a common disorder, even following treatment of the patient for benign disease, we are required to teach the patient self examination and meticulously examine the patient monthly for at least 6 months to a year. It might be wise to follow the guidelines of the American Cancer Society of 1983 which recommends that every woman have a baseline mammography between ages of 35 and 40 years, that between ages 40 and 49 years that they have a biennial mammography, and that following age 50 years they have a yearly mammogram performed.

Selected Readings

Baggs WJ, Amor RL: Thermographic screening for breast cancer in a gynecologic practice. *Obstet Gynecol* 54:156, 1979.

Berg JW, Robbins CF: A late look at the safety of aspiration biopsy. *Cancer* 15:826, 1962.

Duguid HLD, Cuschieri A: Reply to editor re Webb's comments 9 & 12. *Br Med J* 2:185, 1979.

Fox S, Baum J, Klos D, Tson C: Breast cancer screening: The underuse of mammography. *Radiology*. 156:607-611, 1985.

Huguley M Jr, Brown L: The value of breast self-examination. *Cancer* 47:989, 1981.

Kline TS, Joshei LP, Neal HS: Fine needle aspiration of the breast: Diagnosis and pitfalls. *Cancer* 44:1458, 1979.

Lyle: Population Council Survey, July 1980.

Mahoney LJ, Bird BL, Cooke GM: The best available screening test for breast cancer. *N Engl J Med* 301:315, 1979.

Mitchell GW Jr: Breast disease. In Nichols DH, Evrard JR (eds): *Ambulatory Gynecology*. New York, Harper & Row, 1985, pp. 99-103.

Peacock E Jr: Management of benign disease of the breast. *Am Surg* 44:626, 1978.

Rubin E, Miller V, Berland LL, et al: Hand-held real-time breast sonography. *AJR* 144:623-624, 1985.

Teixidor HS: The use of ultrasonography in the management of masses of the breast. *Surg Gynecol Obstet* 150:486, 1980.

Webb AJ: Comment to editors: Needle aspiration of the breast with immediate reporting of material. *Br Med J* 2:491-492, 1979.

Weber WN, Sickles EA, Callen PW, et al: Nonpalpable breast lesion localization limited efficacy of sonography. *Radiology* 155:783-784, 1985.

CHAPTER 85

Cystosarcoma Phyllodes

DOUGLAS J. MARCHANT, M.D.

CASE ABSTRACT

A 6-cm painless mass appeared in the inner quadrant of the right breast of a 59-year-old multipara. According to the patient, the tumor was growing rapidly. Physical examination revealed a solid mass and no axillary adenopathy. The lesion was excised, and the final diagnosis was cystosarcoma phyllodes.

DISCUSSION

Cystosarcoma phyllodes is a rare tumor of the breast. It usually is benign and is really not a sarcoma. The name phyllodes was given to the tumor because of the "leaf-like" characteristics noted on microscopic examination. These lesions account for only 2% to 3% of the fibroepithelial tumors of the breast (1). They are seen in older women; however, they may be found in teenagers. Recently, I saw a patient 14 years of age with a large benign cystosarcoma phyllodes. She was referred by her pediatrician because of asymmetry of the breasts and a tentative diagnosis of hypertrophy of one breast. These neoplasms are probably derived from an adenofibroma—again, a common lesion in teenagers.

The stroma may be cellular and made up of cells with hyperchromatic nuclei and many mitoses suggesting a malignant character. The pathologist must make the differential diagnosis between an adenofibroma with a cellular stroma and cystosarcoma. These tumors may appear malignant but rarely metastasize.

As noted in this patient, cystosarcomas tend to grow rapidly; in women with large breasts, they may reach a considerable size before being clinically evident.

As they grow, they push the normal breast tissue away. They have no true capsule but rarely invade adjacent breast tissue. They remain well circumscribed and mobile and often have a nodular feeling. Generally they do not invade the skin, but large tumors may produce ulceration due to pressure.

Because of the rarity of metastasis, most experts favor wide local excision. A major study by Treves and Sunderland (3) 30 years ago recommended radical mastectomy. Norris and Taylor (2) suggested simple mastectomy with low axillary dissection. Local excision is favored because when these lesions metastasize like other mesenchymal tumors, they metastasize through the blood stream and rarely involve the axillary nodes. If local excision is unsuccessful, it can be repeated with a reasonable expectation of cure. Finally, it is not possible to predict from their microscopic features which tumors will metastasize.

The best method to approach these lesions is as follows: Even in the young patient, a mammogram or a xeromammogram is obtained; in my 14-year-old patient I was not absolutely certain that I was dealing with a tumor because of the large size of both breasts. The mammogram clearly revealed the lesion. In another patient two separate lesions were identified. There is no risk to the patient if the films are taken on a dedicated mammographic unit. It is foolish to attempt excision of a 10- to 15-cm tumor through circumareolar incision. Once the lesion has been identified, an incisional biopsy is taken for frozen section diagnosis. If cystosarcoma phyllodes is diagnosed, wide local excision with a rim of normal breast tissue is the most reasonable primary treatment. Once hemostasis has been secured, and this may be a difficult problem since many of these tumors are quite vascular, the breast tissue should be allowed to fall together by itself. Attempts at reconstruction with the patient in the supine position often result in a deformity when the patient is erect. In my experience, particularly in young patients, the breast tissue approximates itself in a very natural manner within a very few days. It is wise to leave a small Penrose drain in for 24 to 48 hours. I employ a pressure dressing that is removed in 24 to 48 hours.

These patients should be followed closely. Breast self-examination must be reinforced, and in patients 50 years of age or older, screening mammography on a yearly basis is reasonable. A local recurrence should be excised removing a generous amount of normal breast tissue.

The key points in managing cystosarcoma phyllodes are as follows:

1. High index of suspicion in young patients and all patients with rapidly growing tumors that are nodular and not attached to the skin.

2. Preoperative mammography (or xero-mammography.)

3. Incisional biopsy and rapid section to determine the diagnosis.

4. Wide local excision employing the lines of Langer.

5. Reapproximation of the breast tissue using a minimum number of sutures.

6. Regular follow-up every 6 months by the physician and reinforcement of breast self-examination.

References

1. Haagensen CD: *Diseases of the Breast,* ed. 2. Philadelphia, WB Saunders, 1971.
2. Norris HJ, Taylor HB: Relationship of histologic features to behavior of cystosarcoma phyllodes. *Cancer* 20:2090, 1967.
3. Treves N, Sunderland DA: Cystosarcoma phyllodes of the breast: A malignant and benign tumor, a clinical pathological study of 77 cases. *Cancer* 4:1286, 1951.

CHAPTER 86
Solitary Breast Nodule

HENRY C. McDUFF, JR., M.D.

CASE ABSTRACT

During routine annual examination of a 42-year-old patient, a 1.5-cm nodule in the outer quadrant of the upper right breast was found. There was no tenderness and no axillary adenopathy was palpable. The patient was scheduled for excisional biopsy in an ambulatory surgical center.

DISCUSSION

The patient described above must be considered suspect for an early stage I breast cancer. Her age is suspect of this disease, and confirmatory family history would be helpful. It must be remembered that the leading cause of death in women ages 45 to 55 years is breast cancer, and early attention to a nodule of these dimensions is imperative. A mammography should be obtained initially to complete survey of the remaining portion of the right breast along with a total radiologic evaluation of the left breast. The sensitivity of mammography at the present time is such that refinements in evaluation are much more accurate, benign versus malignant. A fine needle biopsy of this area could be done as an office procedure using great care in syringe manipulation that the material is not aspirated beyond the confines of the needle. I believe strongly that the mammography should be obtained prior to needle biopsy since the trauma of the procedure could possibly distort the radiologic image. If the needle biopsy is positive for cancer, definitive options for therapy should then be presented to the patient, modified radical mastectomy or wide regional excision, axillary dissection and then radiation. If a needle biopsy is negative, a formal in-hospital excisional biopsy should be performed with wide margins such that the biopsy itself could be considered adequate local treatment if the pathology is benign and adequate local treatment for the first stage of therapy if the histology is malignant, and tyelectomy, axillary dissection, and radiation is the option selected by the patient for cure.

An excisional breast biopsy for a small lesion in the upper outer quadrant of breast can be handled very adequately in an ambulatory surgical setting. Ideally, a wide margin 2-cm specimen should be removed. This specimen should be sent as a fresh specimen to pathology for histologic evaluation so that estrogen and progesterone receptor studies could then be performed if the diagnosis is malignant. If the histologic diagnosis is positive for malignancy, axillary node sampling/dissection is imperative if the patient elects to be treated by local excision and radiation. This is performed to confirm or deny the clinical staging, to identify a prognostic index, and to determine whether or not adjuvant chemotherapy should be used in support of the local excision and the planned radiation treatment. This patient's age, 42 years and premenopausal, has a high potential for negative estrogen receptor studies and the converse would be true if the patient were in a menopausal age group. Should the histology be malignant, and if regional excision and radiation is the option chosen by the patient, an axillary dissection is mandatory, and this can be handled best through a separate transverse incision in the lower aspect of the axilla. The incision for primary tumor removal should be crescentic in direct relationship to the tumor location and would probably not provide adequate exposure for removal of axillary contents. The axillary dissection should be performed by a gynecologist or surgeon trained and totally familiar with the anatomy of the axilla. It is now considered that a specimen which would allow evaluation of 10 to 14 lymph nodes should be removed. If the histology is positive and if one or more lymph nodes are reported as positive, further consultation with the patient and her family in reference to treatment options is very important. Modified radical mastectomy can be offered and regional tyelectomy plus radiation can also be offered, but adjuvant therapy is imperative, and in the premenopausal woman triple agent chemotherapy should be instituted for minimum of 2 years.

At the present time, we do not have any superb markers for breast cancer, but frozen plasma evaluation should be suggested for titrations of CEA and LASA-P. Should this patient be found to have malignant breast disease with axillary involvement, bone and liver scans should be obtained initially and should be repeated at 6 month intervals for 2 years along with follow-up mammography. At the end of 2 years, these studies should be repeated yearly.

Clinical examination by the operating surgeon and by the medical oncologist should be carried out at 3-month intervals for a period of 2 years, 6-month intervals for an additional 3 years, and one a year beyond 5 years. Seventy-five percent of the lymphatic drainage of breast goes to axilla, the remaining 25%, mostly inner quadrant lesions, drain into the internal mammary chains. If this lesion were geographically in the inner quadrants of the breasts, I would strongly recommend modified radical mastectomy as the primary surgical approach since appropriate cosmesis is difficult to achieve in inner quadrant lesions. I feel that retroareolar tumors which prove to be malignant should also be managed by modified radical mastectomy since nipple sacrifice would often be necessary.

CHAPTER 87

Microcalcification in Breast

DOUGLAS J. MARCHANT, M.D.

CASE ABSTRACT

Screening xeromammography had been performed on a 59-year-old postmenopausal multipara. In the upper inner quadrant of the left breast, a focal concentration of six microcalcifications was identified in a breast that was otherwise mammographically normal. No mass was palpable in the breast nor masses in the axillae. The patient was told of this report and she asked what she should do about it.

DISCUSSION

The management of the occult lesion provides a challenge both to the radiologist and to the operating surgeon. Apparent guidelines from a variety of sources suggest that a baseline mammogram be performed at age 35 years and that annual mammography be performed on a yearly basis. As a result of these recommendations a number of patients are referred because of the finding of an occult lesion, either asymmetric density or the presence of microcalcifications. In this particular case we are dealing with the presence of a geographic cluster of microcalcifications.

The first issue to be resolved is to be certain that the calcifications are located in the breast parenchyma. The occurrence of an isolated cluster of punctate microcalcifications located in the skin is not a rare phenomenon. We have recently reported our experience with the extramammary location of geographic microcalcifications. Confirmation of the extramammary location is accomplished with a superficial marker and an optimal tangenitial view.

Assuming that the geographic cluster is intramammary and assuming that this is the patient's first mammogram the question arises: Is biopsy necessary? This depends upon the exact configuration of the microcalcifications, the presence or absence of other microcalcifications in the same breast or the opposite breast, and ultimately, the experience and confidence of the radiologist. Frequently additional or magnified film screen mammography is re-

quired. We have seen a number of patients referred for the evaluation of "isolated microcalcifications" only to discover that a careful review of all films indicates multiple areas of microcalcification in both breasts suggesting the benign process sclerosing adenosis.

When multiple areas of microcalcification are present in the same breast in the absence of a palpable lesion, the decision to biopsy any one of the areas is certainly an arbitrary one and we prefer to follow these lesions to assess their stability. The films will be repeated in 3 to 6 months depending upon the configuration of the microcalcifications and the degree of suspicion reported by the radiologist.

Biopsy is recommended if a single group of microcalcifications is found.Clearly this requires a localization technique. We have recently reported our experience with the needle wire system utilizing a tough, pseudo-elastic alloy which permits reposition of the needle if necessary. The needle is so constructed that the option of injecting dye is available and the size of the needle prevents transection during surgery. The needle and the wire can be left in place to permit easier dissection during the biopsy.

We discuss the implication of the film and the biopsy with the patient and we demonstrate the microcalcifications in the mammogram. We point out that in our experience 80% of these lesions are benign, but that we cannot eliminate the possibility of an early nonpalpable cancer. Our biopsies are performed on a Day Surgery basis under local anesthesia. This option is discussed with the patient. She is given a permit explaining the procedure and a small booklet describing the operation of the Day Surgery area.

Clearly, the localization of the occult lesion requires the utmost in cooperation between the radiologist and the operating surgeon. The patient is scheduled for localization with the curved and retractable wire as previously described. This is inserted using local anesthesia. Appropriate films are taken. If the radiologist is dissatisfied with the localization process, the wire is withdrawn partway through the needle and reinserted until an accurate localization has been achieved. These films are reviewed both by the radiologist and the surgeon. The wire or the needle and the wire are taped to the patient's skin and she is taken to the Day Surgery area for biopsy.

I prefer to mark my incisions with the patient in the sitting position to achieve the best cosmetic result. A circumareolar incision is employed when practical. In some cases the incision incorporates the needle. In others it is made at a distant point to intersect the needle during the dissection. Prior to the prep, in addition to marking out the location of the incision, I take measurements from the localization film and transfer them to the patient's skin, marking the approximate position of the needle relative to the incision. The breast is carefully prepared and draped, 1% Xylocaine without Adrenaline is used. I prefer to control bleeding as it is encountered with fine plain catgut ligatures. As the area in question is reached, the needle or wire is stabilized using an Allis clamp and the tissue in the general location of the microcalcifications as localized by the needle tip are excised by sharp dissection. The entire specimen including the wire and needle is sent for specimen radiography to confirm the presence of the microcalcifications. If only some of the microcalcifications have been removed, additional tissue is taken. This is an important step since the biopsy may, in fact, be an integral part of the surgical treatment of the disease.

Hemostasis is obtained using fine ligatures of plain catgut and the breast tissue is loosely reconstructed. I prefer to close the skin with vertical mattress suture of 5-0 nylon. When the last suture has been placed, I inject some ad-

ditional 1% Xylocaine along the incision. This markedly decreases postoperative discomfort. No drains are employed. The incision is covered with Telfa and a generous amount of "fluffs" and the entire dressing held in place with an Ace bandage incorporating both breasts more or less as a tube brassiere. This is left in place for 48 hours. Discomfort is minimal and there is far less ecchymosis during the postoperative period. This is important since, as mentioned above, the biopsy may be an integral part of the surgical procedure and the appearance of marked ecchymosis or hematoma greatly interferes with the definitive surgical treatment. The patient is seen in 1 week for evaluation of her incision, additional treatment, planning and removal of sutures.

In our experience, 80% of these lesions are benign, as previously stated. In other words, we perform 5 biopsies to detect one cancer. We believe this is a conservative and reasonable approach. Others recommend a ratio of 20:1. We believe this is excessive and unnecessary surgery. In our experience performing this procedure on a Day Surgery basis under local anesthesia, we are successful 96% of the time in removing the microcalcifications on the first attempt. In 4% of the cases, repeat biopsy has been performed. All (100%) of these have been successful. In some cases, these are performed under general anesthesia because of the scarring associated with previous biopsy. Again, this procedure is performed on a Day Surgery basis.

In summary, we believe that the management of the occult lesion requires considerable judgment and experience and the utmost in cooperation between the radiologist and the operating surgeon.

Selected Readings

Homer MJ: Breast imaging: Pitfalls, controversies and some practical thoughts. *Radiol Clin North Am* 23:459, 1985.
Homer MJ: Nonpalpable breast lesion localization using a curved and retractable wire. *Radiology* 157:259-260, 1985.
Homer MJ, Marchant DJ, Smith TJ: The geographic cluster of breast calcifications. *Surg Gynecol Obstet* 161:532-534, 1985.
Homer MJ, Smith TJ, Marchant DJ: Outpatient needle localization and biopsy for nonpalpable breast lesions. *JAMA* 252:2452, 1984.

CHAPTER 88
Pneumothorax During Mastectomy

HERBERT EBNER, M.D.

CASE ABSTRACT

A radical mastectomy was being performed on a 42-year-old patient with a large medullary carcinoma of the breast that was attached to the pectoral fascia. While both pectoralis muscles were being removed from the chest wall, it was observed that one of the perforating intercostal vessels was bleeding furiously. An assistant stabbed at the bleeding site with a hemostat, but unable to secure the vessel stabbed a little deeper with another hemostat. A sucking sound was immediately evident, and it was apparent that the tip of the second hemostat had penetrated the pleural cavity.

DISCUSSION

A "loss of cool," a panic reaction, and misguided aggressive zeal were the harbingers of this unfortunate complication. Instead of stabbing at the bleeding site, the intercostal vessel should have been grasped with the hemostat placed parallel to the chest wall.

The sucking sound is an absolute indication that air now has direct access to the pleural space—a traumatic, open pneumothorax. A further complicating factor is the possibility of shed blood accumulating within this pleural cavity. The source of this bleeding may be the large vessels of the chest wall. We have witnessed this occur following a "simple" thoracentesis with the needle encountering an intercostal artery or a vein. The ensuing hemorrhage may be sufficiently profuse to induce shock. Blood in the pleural space, a hemothorax, has the propensity to remain liquid for some time. This is due to the movement of the heart and lungs inducing early defibrination, and in addition, fibrinolytic substances are liberated from the pleural mesothelium.

A further alarming feature of an hemothorax is its ability to increase in volume even after the bleeding has been controlled. The extravascular osmotic pressure is increased by hemolysis and the enzymatic breakdown of protein. This results in increased transudation from the subpleural capillaries into the hemothorax. If

therapy is not expeditiously initiated, pulmonary venous and cardiac tamponade can ensue.

The special situation of tension pneumothorax, one of the most critical of medicosurgical emergencies, can occur with a sucking chest wound or with a lung leak produced by a laceration with a sharp instrument. Lung laceration is the more common etiologic factor. Large volumes of air enter the pleural space during inspiration. This air is prevented from escaping during expiration by collapse of soft lung tissue, which occludes the laceration. Sucking chest wounds that produce tension pneumothorax are less frequent. Air enters the hemithorax during inspiration because of the intrapleural negative pressure. This air cannot escape during expiration because of the one-way flap valve effect of the injured chest wall tissue. This positive pressure in the pleural space produces some collapse of the ipsilateral lung and some compression of the contralateral lung, and obstruction of blood flow in the great veins and pulmonary vessels. This derangement is, of course, compounded if a hemothorax coexists. If allowed to progress, the larger veins of the mediastinum are compressed, and the diastolic filling of the heart is impeded, with a resultant decrease in the cardiac output.

Another potential deleterious effect of traumatic pneumothorax is the phenomenon of mediastinal flutter. During inspiration the mediastinum is displaced toward the sound side, and the reverse occurs with expiration. This pendulum effect drastically interferes with the mechanics of ventilation and has an adverse effect on gas exchange. The expired gases from the sound side flow up the trachea but are also diverted in part into the bronchial tree on the injured side; with the next inspiration, they are then drawn back again to the sound side. The end result is an increase in the functional dead space and carbon dioxide retention.

We have run the gamut of the dire consequences of this therapeutic misadventure to stress the need for immediate and definitive treatment. The degree of physiologic derangement depends, of course, on the age of the patient, her prior ventilatory reserve, the size of the chest wound, the presence or absence of pleural adhesions, and the thickness of the mediastinum.

Treatment

The alert anesthesiologist who is carefully monitoring the patient during surgery will detect increased airway resistance and diminished tidal volume as early signs of tension pneumothorax. If the radical mastectomy is being conducted under endotracheal anesthesia, as it should be, the situation is rapidly obviated. Otherwise an endotracheal tube must be inserted with dispatch and controlled respiration initiated. Controlled respiration is the most effective technique to ensure adequate oxygenation and elimination of carbon dioxide. In addition, the chest is rendered more compliant by the use of relaxants so that less positive pressure need be used to inflate the lung, with less resultant air leak.

Controlled respirations can be achieved in three different ways: (a) paralysis of the respiratory muscles, (b) depression of the respiratory center, or (c) removal of the carbon dioxide stimulus to the respiratory center by actively hyperventilating the patient. A combination of the above three modalities can be utilized, but in actual practice the apnea is usually arrived at by the use of muscle relaxants together with the intermittent, intravenous administration of narcotics. The narcotics help to maintain controlled respiration by their central depressant action, and the total dosage of the muscle relaxants is thereby reduced. They also contribute a degree of postoperative analgesia.

Although needle aspiration of hemothorax or small pneumothorax is occasionally satisfactory, it is generally safer to institute basal drainage with an underwater seal. The pleural wound is closed and the catheter for an underwater seal is placed through a separate stab wound placed in a more caudal position. Many surgeons insist on this technique routinely whenever the pleural cavity is opened. Blood will not accumulate in the pleural cavity, and continued blood loss can be readily monitored. The amount of blood loss is assessed quickly and simply by examining the contents of the drainage bottle, and the need for further surgical intervention is evident earlier. In addition, the anesthesiologist can force air out of the pleural space after the skin has been closed. Postoperatively, the patient will accomplish this by coughing. Normal spontaneous breathing is allowed to resume as soon as skin suturing is started. On the occasion when the chest is closed without drainage, controlled respiration is continued until after the skin has been sutured. In this situation the chest is not considered airtight until the skin suturing has been completed. Should spontaneous breathing start prior to this, the lung might collapse and prove difficult to re-expand.

Blood volume and electrolyte balance must be restored. The decision intraoperatively for transfusion or infusion with blood, crystalloids, or colloids will depend upon the careful assessment and interpretation of a number of parameters. Each parameter alone has significant limitations in this respect, and all must be correlated and evaluated in the decision-making process. The vital signs include the blood pressure, the pulse rate, the heart sounds, the urinary output, and the body temperature. In addition, the general appearance of the skin and the degree of capillary refill of the mucous membranes and the nail beds should be considered in this assessment. The patient should be under continuous electrocardiographic monitoring, and it is advisable to have a central venous line in place. A word of caution is in order in regard to this central venous pressure (CVP) measurement. Monitoring of the CVP is a procedure of great value and, when intelligently used, serves as an important adjunct in the management of hemorrhage. It is useful in providing an early warning of reduced venous return associated with hypovolemia. It is firmly established as a simple method of estimating the ability of the right side of the heart to tolerate and to eject a fluid load, and it may also be a guide to the onset of occult bleeding. Its results, however, require careful interpretation and observer flexibility. It is not per se an indicator of the circulating blood volume, nor does it demonstrate the functional efficiency of the left side of the heart (1). In most cases, however, CVP readings, when taken in the total context and correlated with other mentioned parameters, are of great value in determining the need for volume replacement. Patients having marginally adequate cardiac function can be more precisely monitored by using a pulmonary artery (Swan-Ganz) catheter than by relying on CVP measurements. This applies particularly in the presence of pulmonary hypertension, right heart disease, and chronic lung disease.

The anesthesiologist and the surgeon must be fully cognizant of each other's problems and techniques and must work together in a coherent manner. Only a concerted approach will result in proper managment of this unfortunate and challenging complication.

Reference

1. DeLaurentis DA, Hayes M, Matsumoto T, et al: Does central venous pressure accurately reflect hemodynamics and fluid volume patterns in the critical surgical patient? *Am J Surg* 126:415, 1973.

CHAPTER 89
Modified Radical Mastectomy

DOUGLAS J. MARCHANT, M.D.

CASE ABSTRACT

A modified radical mastectomy was recommended for an obese 45-year-old nulligravida. During the dissection, the thoracodorsal nerve was preserved, but the long thoracic nerve was not identified until after it had been cut. It was not involved with tumor.

DISCUSSION

Primary operable breast cancer is defined as mammary adenocarcinoma which, on the basis of routine clinical evaluation, appears confined to the mammary tissue and ipsilateral lymph nodes and has received no prior therapy (6). Operations for invasive breast cancer include radical mastectomy and modified radical mastectomy, or "partial" mastectomy and radiotherapy. Radical mastectomy includes removal of the entire breast including the nipple and most of the overlying skin in continuity with the pectoralis major and minor muscles, the axillary contents, and frequently the thoracodorsal nerve (1).

Modified radical mastectomy developed by Patey (4) includes a wide range of operations that have in common total excision of the breast with an axillary node dissection while preserving the pectoralis major muscle. This operation leads to improved comestic results and less impairment of upper extremity function when compared with a standard radical mastectomy. When the operation has been performed correctly, the extent of the axillary node dissection is not affected by retention of the pectoralis major muscle. A number of modifications of this procedure have been described (2–5, 7). These techniques leave the pectoralis minor intact. Scanlon has recommended dividing it at its origin. Survival rates of total mastectomy with the several varieties of axillary lymph node dissection apparently equal those after the more extensive radical mastectomy. Unfortunately, lesser procedures which include a simple mastectomy and axillary sampling often have been confused with the modified radical mastectomy.

In this particular case, the type of modified radical mastectomy is not described, but for the purpose of discussion let us assume that it is the Patey modification with removal of the pectoralis minor muscle and complete axillary dissection.

To permit better exposure of the axilla, I prefer to have the arm suspended, producing relaxation of the pectoralis major muscle. When the arm is abducted at right angles to the trunk as in the radical mastectomy, it is more difficult to retract the pectoralis major muscle. In the Willy Meyer standard American technique for radical mastectomy, the axilla is dissected *before* the muscles and the breast are removed from the chest wall. I prefer to do the chest wall dissection first and then proceed with the axillary dissection either following removal of the pectoralis minor muscle as in the Patey modification or retraction of this muscle as in the Madden. Some have suggested that excising the breast and muscles prior to the axillary dissection increases the chance of distant metastasis. This is unlikely to be the case since we now recognize that in many if not the majority of cases of early cancer, there is already distant metastasis that must be treated by some form of adjuvant therapy.

Assuming that the pectoralis minor muscle has been removed from the coracoid process, dissection is begun by excising the costocoracoid fascia over the brachial plexus parallel and just above the axillary vein. I prefer to do the dissection with forceps and the knife, occasionally employing the "beaver blade" which presents a cutting surface at right angles to the shaft of the scalpel. While some employ the cautery for the chest wall dissection, I do not believe it should be used in the axilla. Using this technique, small vessels are identified and appropriately ligated. The yield of nodes identified in the specimen will increase markedly with the use of meticulous sharp dissection.

Following dissection of the axillary vein, attention should be turned to the apex of the axilla. The tissue must be dissected from the medial portion of the axillary vein to where it passes beneath the subclavius muscle. This mass of tissue in the cleft between the chest and the axillary vein contains the highest axillary lymph nodes. These should be marked as such. We use small sterile brass "buttons" marked 1, 2, and 3 to indicate the level of the axillary dissection. These are sutured to the tissue as it is removed.

As one continues laterally, the lateral thoracic artery is identified, clamped, and cut. As the dissection of these tissues is carried further laterally, the thoracodorsal vessels are reached. It is at this point that the surgeon must identify and preserve the long thoracic nerve of Bell. This is found in the cleft between the serratus muscle and the fascia overlying the axilla. The nerve is in the fat just beneath the medial surface of this fascia.

In the present case, in spite of the distortion produced by the large amount of fat in the axilla, the thoracodorsal nerve was identified, but the long thoracic nerve was cut. Cutting this nerve produces a "winged scapula." Many surgeons deliberately sacrifice the thoracodorsal nerve. This is encountered as it comes across the subscapular muscle from beneath the axillary vein to join the thoracodorsal vessels. Anatomically the nerve presents among the lymph nodes of the central and scapula group. It is for this reason that the nerve often is sacrificed. Paralysis of the latissimus muscle that results from cutting this nerve produces a slight weakness of adduction and internal rotation and is seldom noted by the patient.

Trauma to the long thoracic and thoracodorsal nerves can be prevented by meticulous accurate sharp dissection in the axilla. Sharp dis-

section identifies even the smallest vessel which can then be clamped and tied. The combination of a bloody field and significant amounts of fatty tissue is almost certain to result in trauma to the axillary contents. By doing the chest wall dissection first, one is presented with a clean entry into the axilla, and appropriate retraction of the pectoralis major muscle by elevating the arm identifies the coracoid process and the pectoralis minor muscle. Thus, with proper exposure and sharp dissection, the long thoracic nerve will not be injured. The decision regarding the thoracodorsal nerve is a philosophic one. If one believes that the lymph nodes adjacent to this nerve may be involved, the nerve can be sacrificed without significant loss of function; however, the division of the long thoracic nerve of Bell results in an ugly deformity for which there is no known treatment.

In the event that the long thoracic nerve of Bell has been unexpectedly or inadvertently transected, it is probably worth the trouble for the initial surgeon to bring the severed ends of the nerve together using a few interrupted fine sutures. If axons have been fortuitously aligned, salvage is possible. If a defect to be bridged exists between the nerve ends, each end should be marked with a metal clip, and at some future date referral may be made to a suitable specialist in microsurgery for anastomosis or nerve transplantation.

References

1. Haagensen CD: *Diseases of the Breast*, ed. 2. Philadelphia, WB Saunders, 1971.
2. Madden JL, Kandalaf TS, Bourque R: Modified radical mastectomy. *Ann Surg* 175:624, 1972.
3. Maier WP, Leber D, Rosemond GP, et al: The technique of modified radical mastectomy. *Surg Gynecol Obstet* 145:69, 1977.
4. Patey DH, Dyson WH: The prognosis of carcinoma of the breast in relation to the type of operation performed. *Br J Cancer* 2:7, 1948.
5. Pickren JW, Rube J, Auchincloss H: Modification of conventional radical mastectomy. *Cancer* 18:942, 1969.
6. Regional Cancer Control Committee: In Marchant DJ (ed) *Primary Breast Cancer Recommendations for Diagnosis and Treatment*, Hagerstown, MD, Harper & Row, 1981.
7. Scanlon EF, Caprini JA: Modified radical mastectomy. *Cancer* 35:710, 1975.

CHAPTER 90
One Positive Axillary Lymph Node

HENRY C. McDUFF, JR., M.D.

CASE ABSTRACT

This 36-year-old multipara presented to her physician with a 2-cm mass in the upper outer quadrant of her right breast. Treatment involved excisional biopsy, frozen section, and, sequentially under the same anesthesia, a modified radical mastectomy with removal of the pectoralis minor muscle. The frozen section evaluation identified infiltrating ductal carcinoma, and the formal pathology report defined no residual tumor in the breast and the recovery of 26 lymph nodes, one of which was positive for metastatic tumor.

Her preadmission testing was confined only to a chest x-ray, peripheral blood studies, blood chemistry, and urinalysis; all were reported to be within normal limits.

DISCUSSION

Carcinoma of the breast is the most common cancer affecting women in the United States and the most common cause of cancer death in women. In the age group of 45 to 55 years, it is the most common cause of all deaths. It is estimated that this year there will be approximately 100,000 new cases diagnosed, with 36,000 deaths due to breast cancer. The current incidence of breast cancer in the United States is approximately 80 per 100,000 women. A newborn female child runs a 10% risk of developing breast cancer in her lifetime (7, 10).

Ninety percent of abnormal breast masses are patient discovered, and for the most part, the size of the mass at the time of identification is 2 cm or larger (9). The limit of cognizance of breast cancer by palpation seems to be approximately 1 cm in diameter. The doubling time for breast cancer lesions is approximately 90 days. This would mean that a patient with a 2-cm lesion has probably had the disease for 8 to 10 years, 30 doubling times being required to achieve a 2-cm size, and probably would have had a detectable breast mass for a period of approximately 10 to 12 months.

The type of operation performed, which involved removal of the pectoralis minor muscle, is classical in definition of modified radical mastectomy, and the identification of 26 lymph nodes indicates the completeness of axillary dissection. We may then state that this patient received optimal treatment for her disease in an attempt to effect local control (3, 13). It should be further stated that the performance of excisional, rather than incisional, biopsy was highly appropriate and protective in reference to intraoperative dissemination of tumor.

One could argue that a preoperative xeromammogram would be helpful in identifying occult lesions in the contralateral breast and that a bone scan would be helpful in identifying disseminated disease, which might then lead to a different primary approach to the breast lesion. Clinically, this patient should be stage I, T-1, N-0, M-0, and the pathologic stage would be stage I, T-1, N-lai (micrometastasis).

The patient's one positive node is important, and it is the responsibility of the pathologist to define whether the node itself is involved, whether there is extranodal extension, and whether this is a micrometastasis (less than 2 mm.). The work of Fracchia (8) and Fisher (4) indicates that micrometastasis, involving one to three nodes, does not change the prognosis. Macrometastasis, on the other hand, greater than 2 mm, is associated with a decreased survival at 5 years for stage I, 95% versus 80%. Older material from Monroe (12) of Chicago indicates that one positive node would change the survival at 5 years from 74% to 56%.

In general, the identification of any positive lymph nodes in breast cancer carries a more grave prognosis, particularly if more than four nodes are involved. The patient under discussion has one positive lymph node. Statistically, there would be a 13% incidence of recurrence at 18 months, a 50% incidence of recurrence at 5 years, and a 60% recurrence rate at 10 years (6). This is opposed to a 5% recurrence rate at 18 months where no nodes are involved, an 18% recurrence at 5 years, and a 24% recurrence rate at 10 years, again where no nodes are involved (5, 14). The survival rate for N0 disease at 10 years is 65%, and for positive nodes, N+, the survival rate at 10 years is 38%.

This patient most certainly should have the benefit of a contralateral mammogram and a bone scan for baseline studies. Liver scans are not as yet sufficiently sophisticated to be of great help in the evaluation of breast cancer. This patient's excisional biopsy specimen should be appropriately cleaned and prepared for estrogen receptor studies (11). The clinical response of breast cancer patients to endocrine therapy can be predicted with some accuracy on the basis of positive binding of estrogen to cytosol receptors in breast cancer tissue. Positive estrogen receptor assays have been correlated with a favorable prognosis and a prolonged disease-free interval, and this is considered by some authorities to be independent of axillary node metastasis, tumor size, or menopausal status (19). It is not yet totally defined whether receptor assays will also serve to predict response to chemotherapy. New work is underway concerning nuclear as well as cytoplasmic receptors, and the quantitation of estrogen receptors reported in femtomoles per gram is considered increasingly important. This indicates that the estrogen receptor (ER) status of the primary tumor is a useful marker for the biologic aggressiveness of the disease.

Compared to older patients, premenopausal patients are more likely to have ER− tumors, and those younger patients who do have ER+ tumors usually demonstrate a lower quantitative concentration.

Receptor assays also give a definite idea for long-range treatment planning in case there is disease relapse. Current work has also indicated that ER− patients, and they are generally premenopausal, will respond favorably to

chemotherapy as opposed to attempts to modify the hormonal environment (15).

I believe that this patient should receive the benefits of multiple agent chemotherapy, and the proposed effectiveness of this therapy will in some way be influenced by the results of the estrogen receptor assay studies. It has been shown that tumors with the most rapid doubling time are the most sensitive to chemotherapy, and it would suggest that ER− tumors should be most responsive to chemotherapy. Certainly recent studies have indicated that hormonal therapy in ER− patients is not outstandingly effective (2, 16).

Variable figures have been quoted from many large institutions concerning the value of contralateral breast biopsy at the time of definitive breast removal. Some investigators have reported figures as high as 40% positive for tumor. It should be borne in mind that, for the most part, this refers to lobular carcinoma-in-situ, and here we are dealing with infiltrating ductal carcinoma. I believe that the enthusiasm for contralateral mirror image biopsy is waning at the present time in all cell types except lobular disease.

There would appear to be no indication for the use of radiation therapy in this patient. Everything possible has been done to control her local disease, and multiple drug chemotherapy is of much greater benefit in managing potential tumor extension. If tylectomy plus axillary sampling was elected as the primary method of treating this patient, then radiation *would* play a very important role in support of the limited type of surgery.

At the present time, radiation therapy is reserved for biopsy-proven local recurrence (18). In this instance, receptor assays should again be obtained because the receptors in recurrent disease are not always the same as the receptors in the primary disease. If a recurrent chest wall lesion should be ER+, then oophorectomy should be advised if the patient is premenopausal. If it is negative, then supposedly hormonal alteration will not be helpful and radiation should be chosen.

There is very little indication for the performance of contralateral mastectomy until or unless disease is later identified in this breast. The opposite breast is always a favored site for recurrence, but at the present time, the prophylactic removal of that breast for this reason seems totally unjustified. There are certain patients whose breasts are of such dimensions that the removal of one results in an unstable posture and extreme difficulty in effecting cosmetic recovery. A prophylactic contralateral simple mastectomy for purposes of patient comfort can occasionally be justified on these grounds.

Ultimate consideration here involves whether or not bilateral ovarian removal should be carried out in a 36-year-old patient with one positive node (1). If we were to assume that this patient has a negative bone scan, a negative contralateral breast xeromammogram, and normal liver enzymes, then her only objective evidence of disease extension would be the solitary node recovered in her axillary dissection. If we were to again assume that this patient's estrogen receptor study is negative, which it very probably could be in her age group, then we would have clear indication that alteration of the hormonal environment should be deferred certainly until there was any future evidence of recurrence. Years ago, sequential oophorectomy following primary mastectomy was considered to be appropriate therapy (17), and patients so managed seemed to have a prolonged disease-free interval. Careful follow-up of these patients, however, identified the fact that their total survival was not extended when compared to a group of patients where therapeutic oophorectomy was performed at the time of recurrence. There is, at the present time, excellent evidence that adjunctive chemotherapy in the ER− premenopausal woman is far superior to prophylactic castration. A patient such as this should be followed extremely carefully, both during and following her adjunctive chemotherapy. Chest x-rays should be performed yearly and contralateral mammography, bone scan, and liver enzymes every 2 years.

Summary

This 36-year-old patient with one positive lymph node, whether it be a micro- or macrometastasis, and most certainly if it is extra-nodal as well, *should be studied* for estrogen-binding receptors. *She should* receive multiple drug chemotherapy, because there is significant statistical evidence at the present time to indicate its benefits. She *should not* be given prophylactic radiation therapy, since the primary disease has been well handled by modified radical mastectomy, and contralateral biopsy does not appear to be indicated in consideration of the cell type involved, infiltrating ductal. There appears to be *no evidence* for contralateral mastectomy *nor* for prophylactic castration.

Since it is here recommended that chemotherapy be added to the primary surgery, the decision concerning type of drug and the duration of treatment is important, and certainly the follow-up of a patient on chemotherapy should include her potential for the development of soft tissue tumors, i.e., Hodgkin's, lymphoma, or leukemia. There is generous evidence in the literature to support this possibility when phenylalanine mustard is used as the adjunctive chemotherapy agent.

Educational Philosophy Regarding Breast Surgery

It is difficult to obtain figures indicating how many or what percentage of operating gynecologists today have training in and permission to perform major breast surgery. The majority of obstetric and gynecologic residency programs do not include major breast surgery in the content of their core curriculum, and very few of the newly established fellowships in gynecologic oncology allow for this exposure. There is no doubt that obstetrician-gynecologists now clearly function as primary physicians to women, and in this capacity, they have the opportunity to detect breast lumps in a far greater ratio than most general surgeons, family practitioners, or internists. The credentials committees of many hospitals allow obstetrician-gynecologists to perform incisional or excisional breast biopsies with general surgical stand-by in case sequential major mastectomy procedures are to be carried out. This allows for the patient's personal obstetrician-gynecologist to continue in the identification role and to then participate "as an assistant" in the performance of mastectomy in the event that this procedure appears indicated and appropriate patient consultation has been explored.

The practicing obstetrician-gynecologist and residents in training both participate in office evaluation of breast masses and consultations in reference to the appropriate method of breast self-examination. The obstetrician-gynecologist also is frequently the first person either to identify or confirm the presence of an abnormal breast mass, and he is frequently the first one to suggest diagnostic studies, such as mammography, thermography, ultrasound, fine needle biopsy, breast cyst aspiration, or recommendations for formal biopsy. All physicians dealing with female patients with breast lumps are committed to the full disclosure of treatment options, which would include: (a) formal excision biopsy, followed immediately by mastectomy after positive frozen section identification of cancer, (b) formal excisional biopsy only, to be then followed by further patient discussion and then the subsequent performance of definitive therapy, or (c) tylectomy with axillary sampling, followed by radiation.

It is now fairly well established that, in properly selected cases, mastectomy or tyelectomy plus radiation is of equal value in controlling local disease. Follow-up studies cannot mention cure, *only control of local disease*. Unfortunately, breast cancer is not always a local disease, and indeed many authorities at the present time consider breast cancer to be a systemic disease from its inception.

I believe that a study group should be formed, which would address itself to the problem of the diagnosis and treatment of breast disease, which could then be incorporated in the core curriculum of an obstetric-gynecologic residency. This would more appropriately then lead to a sequential continuum of patient care that does not exist today.

References

1. Binder SC, Flynn WJ, Katz B, et al: Endocrine ablative therapy of metastatic breast cancer. *CA* 27:354, 1977.
2. Bonadonna G, Brusamolino E, Valagussa P, et al: Combination chemotherapy as an adjuvant treatment in operable breast cancer. *N Engl J Med* 294:405, 1976.
3. DeVita V: Multimodal treatment of primary breast carcinoma. *Am J Med* 70:844, 1981.
4. Fisher B: Cancer of the breast: Size of neoplasm and prognosis. *Cancer* 21:1071, 1969.
5. Fisher B: Number of lymph nodes examined and the prognosis of breast carcinoma. *Surg Gynecol Obstet* 131:79, 1970.
6. Fisher E: Detection and significance of occult axillary node metastases in patients with invasive breast cancer. *Cancer* 42:2025, 1978.
7. Fisher E.: Pathologic findings from the National Surgical Adjuvant Breast Project. *Am J Clin Pathol* 65:439, 1976.
8. Fracchia A: Axillary micrometastasis and macrometastasis in carcinoma of the breast. *Surg Gynecol Obstet* 144:839, 1977.
9. Haagensen CD (ed): The symptoms of mammary carcinoma. In *Diseases of the Breast*. Philadelphia, WB Saunders, 1971, p. 466.
10. MacMahon B, Cole P, Brown J: Etiology of human breast cancer: A review. *J Nat Cancer Inst* 50:21, 1973.
11. McGuire WL, Carbone PP, Sears ME, et al: Estrogen receptors in human breast cancer: An overview. In McGuire WL, Carbone PP, Vollmer EP (eds): *Estrogen Receptors in Human Breast Cancer*. New York, Raven Press, 1975.
12. Monroe C: Lymphatic spread of carcinoma of the breast. *Arch Surg* 57:479, 1948.
13. Moxley JH, Allegra JC, Henney J, et al: Treatment of primary breast cancer. *JAMA* 244:797, 1980.
14. Nealon TS, Jr: The treatment of early cancer of the breast (T1-N0-M0-T2-N0-M0) on the basis of histological character. *Surgery* 89:279, 1981.
15. Packard RA: Selection of breast cancer patients for adjuvant chemotherapy. *JAMA* 238:1034, 1977.
16. Packard RA, Prosnitz LR, Bobrow SN: Selection of breast cancer patients for adjuvant chemotherapy. *JAMA* 238:1034, 1977.
17. Peetz M, Awrich AE, Moseley HS, et al: Results of oophorectomy by menstrual and estrogen receptor states in patients with metastatic breast cancer. *Am J Surg* 141:554, 1981.
18. Valagussa P, Bonadonna F, Veronesi U: Patterns of relapse and survival following radical mastectomy. *Cancer* 41: 1170, 1978.
19. Wittliff JL: Specific receptors of the steroid hormones in breast cancer. *Semin Oncol* 1:109, 1974.

CHAPTER **91**
Procidentia in an Elderly Multipara

J. GEORGE MOORE, M.D.

CASE ABSTRACT

A chronically hypertensive 88-year-old multipara, no longer able to wear a supportive pessary, has developed a total procidentia. The patient was moderately hypertensive, 190/110, though had been taking hydrochlorithiazide and methyldopa daily for a number of years. She lived alone, managing her own affairs, and seemed alert and in otherwise good health.

DISCUSSION

It is generally agreed that age alone is not a contraindication to indicated surgical procedure. Medical complications certainly influence the choice of procedures that will correct the clinical problem. In this instance, one must ensure that blood electrolytes are in proper balance and that maximal cardiovascular stability has been attained.

In a patient on hydrochlorithiazide and methylodopa, plasma potassium must be maintained between 3.5 and 4.5 mg/dl. Electrocardiography should ensure that cardiac irregularities are minimized and a lidocaine intravenous infusion should be used to maintain stability of cardiac rhythm postoperatively. Hypertension must also be controlled postoperatively, especially during periods of pain. An arterial line should be placed intra-operatively and maintained postoperatively. If hypertension exceeds 200 mm Hg systolic or 125 mm Hg diastolic, vasodepressive medication should be employed, using hydrolazine or even nitroprusside if necessary.

The surgical procedure chosen to correct the procidentia depends on the condition of the patient. Ideally a vaginal hysterectomy, correction of the enterocele, and a complete colpectomy (total colpocleisis) is the procedure of choice for a complete procidentia. Adding the colpectomy to the procedure generally secures a lasting correction of the prolapse. If the patient will not consent to vaginal obliteration and if a total colpectomy is not elected, a careful repair of the endopelvic supports such that a narrow, deep vagina with a well-supported, high perineum is indicated to preclude a subsequent prolapse of the vagina. If the maintenance of a functional vagina is required, a sacrospinous colpopexy (and enterocele repair) is likely to give the best functional result. An abdominal hysterectomy or uterine suspension will *not* correct the procidentia!

Minimally in a debilitated patient, a LeFort procedure (1, 2) (partial colpocleisis) under local anesthesia might be considered. This latter procedure can be done quickly, with minimal blood loss and it maintains reasonable uterine support with a very low recurrence rate. The partial colpocleisis does have drawbacks. Recurrence is likely if an enterocele is left unrepaired, and stress incontinence will ensue unless a urethral plication is done and unless the perineum is built up close to the urethra. In the LeFort procedure, the relatively strong posterior vaginal wall, when sutured to the anterior wall, has a tendency to pull the urethra down, resulting in incontinence with minimal increase in intra-abdominal pressure. Modification of the LeFort procedure to provide a functional vagina is generally not indicated because of poor satisfaction and the increased chance of recurrence. Another undesirable feature of the LeFort procedure is the difficulty in investigating subsequent uterine bleeding, in that a D & C is virtually impossible.

Total procidentia implies that the entire uterus (including corpus) is outside the vagina. In most cases, the complete uterine prolapse is accompanied by a cystocele, rectocele, and enterocele, and correction of each of these defects is required. This entails correction of the enterocele (high ligation of the enterocele sac, preferably with nonabsorbable suture material and careful approximation of the uterosacral ligaments) along with an anterior and posterior colporrhaphy. If a vaginal hysterectomy is carried out (and it should be) a total colpectomy (complete colpocleisis) almost certainly precludes recurrence. Even with a complete colpocleisis, repair of the enterocele and reconstruction of the pelvic support is essential. If the enterocele is not corrected, a vaginal evisceration can occur in the late postoperative course.

References

1. LeFort L: *Bull Gen de Therap* 92:337, 1877.
2. Spiegelberg O: Colporraphia mediana. *Berl Klin Woch* 9:249, 1872.

CHAPTER 92

Endocrine Problems of the Acute Surgical Menopause

BURTON V. CALDWELL, M.D., PH.D.

CASE ABSTRACT

A total abdominal hysterectomy and bilateral salpingo-oophorectomy had been performed on a 36-year-old multipara because of chronic menorrhagia associated with adenomyosis interna. Hospitalization and convalescence were uneventful, but 6 months later the patient complained of disabling "hot flashes" and nocturnal sweating, dyspareunia, obesity, and the progressive loss of libido. All of these have in her view altered unfavorably the quality of her life and collectively are of more bother to her than her previous menorrhagia.

DISCUSSION

In making the final decision as to whether or not a surgical menopause is advisable, certainly the overriding considerations relate to the prevention and/or treatment of any underlying utero-ovarian pathology that the surgeon has detected. However, there are many instances where a decision must be made at a relatively early age of life, for example, under the age of 35 years, whereby the long-term effects of the removal of the ovaries must be given adequate considerations as well. Clearly, there are endocrine effects of removing the gonads that have been well-established in the last decade, and it is the responsibility of the physician to make the patient aware of the potential long-term consequences of estrogen depletion and to detail in advance the risk factors and the therapies which must be instituted in order to prevent some of the more severe consequences of surgical castration and to provide a recommendation for therapeutic modalities which should be considered in the treatment of all patients undergoing early menopause.

Surgical Castration and Coronary Vascular Disease

It is well recognized that throughout the normal reproductive life-span women seem to be protected from serious cardiovascular disease.

Studies to elucidate the mechanisms for this phenomena have centered on the role of estrogens secreted by ovarian tissue as the most likely agent imparting this decreased susceptibility. It is true that the gonads secrete other steroids, notably progesterone and a small amount of androgens, but is is unlikely that these classes of steroid hormones have any major impact on specific long-term disease processes. From the onset of puberty through the initiation of menopause, women make 10- to 100-fold more estrogen than their male counterparts, and it is only after this level of estrogen in the blood has returned to relative equivalence with males that the risk of coronary vascular disease begins to approach that of the male. Precisely how estrogens retard the pathogenesis of artherosclerosis and myocardial infarction has never been clearly established despite the concentrated effort over decades to unravel this association. Most workers have concentrated on the effects of estrogens on lipid metabolism and have noted that there are clear differences in pre- and postmenopausal women and men. The rise of serum cholesterol levels following bilateral oophorectomy is similar to that seen following menopause, although surgical castration appears to promote the rise in cholesterol levels over a much shorter period of time. This elevation in serum cholesterol seems to be caused by a rise in *all* the lipoprotein fractions, namely, high density, low density, and very low density. Also, a decrease in the *ratio* of high-density (HDL) to low-density lipoprotein (LDL) has been described, and it is this ratio of HDL:LDL that is thought to be directly related to added risks or susceptibility to cardiovascular disease. No other known atherogenic factors have ever been shown to change significantly at the time of menopause, whether induced surgically or occurring in the natural sequence. Few believe that these lipid changes in themselves are the only factors accounting for the increased coronary heart disease seen with cessation of ovarian function, but most view these changes as suggesting that there are key metabolic differences that are regulated by ovarian secretions.

Table 92.1
Changes in Lipid Metabolism after Menopause

1. Cholesterol levels increase.
2. Increases in high-density, low-density, and very low-density lipoproteins.
3. Decrease in ratio of HDL:LDL.

Table 92.1 shows the changes in detail, while Table 92.2 outlines the most salient features of all of the factors which may be related to menopause and coronary heart disease as contained in the complete analysis conducted by the Framingham study. It is worth noting the salient points of this study. (a) Prior to the onset of menopause, most coronary heart disease in women occurs in the form of uncomplicated angina pectoris. (b) After the age of approximately 54 years, there is a marked increase in the incidence of coronary heart disease, and most importantly, the type of heart disease seen in women shifts to the more serious myocardial infarction. (c) No premenopausal women developed myocardial infarctions in the Fra-

mingham study or died of coronary heart disease despite approximately 8500 premenopausal subject-years reported in this group. (d) Coronary heart disease incidence rates for women having surgical menopause were substantially higher than for premenopausal women, especially if the surgical menopause was performed before the age of 44 years. It should be noted that other studies have also looked at the effect of hysterectomy and bilateral oophorectomy and found insignificant differences in coronary heart disease and concluded that surgical menopause did not lead to an increased risk. The differences between the two populations of patients and the methods of anylysis are considerable, and at the present time most are swayed by compelling evidence produced in the Framingham study. (e) The comparative incidence rate between premenopausal women and men of the same age for coronary heart disease is approximately 1 to 15. This changes more rapidly in the perimenopausal period, suggesting that the impact of menopause is not only substantial, but it is also relatively abrupt and then progresses very slowly after the first 5 or 10 years, if at all.

This and other studies have also looked at the effects of hysterectomy and suggested that removal of the uterus alone may also impart an increased risk to the development of coronary heart disease. The data from all the surgical castration patients from the Framingham study are of most concern to gynecologists faced with the decision to remove these organs, and the relative risk-benefit ratios must be carefully considered.

Other observations from the Framingham study and similar cooperative studies are of some interest. For example, it has been shown that women who smoke cigarettes go through natural menopause earlier than women who do not. It has been suggested that this may account for some of the earlier findings that menopause was

Table 92.2
Framingham Study Findings on Coronary Heart Disease

	Primary Form	Female to Male Incidence
Premenopause	Angina pectoris	Lower than male (1:15)
Perimenopause	Angina pectoris	Rapidly approaches male
Postmenopause	Myocardial infarction	Equal to male (1:1)
Surgical menopause	Myocardial infarction	Rapidly approaches male
Hysterectomy	Myocardial infarction	Higher than age-matched control woman

associated with increased coronary heart disease risk. Most coronary heart disease in women under the age of 54 years is, however, angina pectoris, and the Framingham study found no association between cigarette smoking and this manifestation, while the clear association of cigarette smoking with myocardial infarction as it pertains to menopausal women has been established. It is, therefore, important that, in the surgical castration of a patient, she be even more strongly advised not to smoke since she will have the added pressure of early estrogen withdrawal and tobacco as increased risk factors for developing myocardial infarction. Other studies have shown that women who develop coronary heart disease go through the menopause earlier, but the difference is not statistically significant. The relatively high coronary heart disease incidence in women in the perimenopausal interval would indicate the incidence rate rises before the complete cessation of menstruation, although proof of this possibility will require study of considerably greater numbers of women examined over a shorter period of time.

Adding to the difficulty in trying to determine the exact nature of the changes occurring in menopause that might be associated with cardiovascular disease is the finding that sex differences are particularly absent in certain populations throughout the world, for example, Japanese, Bantus, and black Americans, all groups in whom the incidence of atherosclerosis is less common than that seen in the white American population.

From these epidemiologic studies, the most important factor that should be taken into consideration is that premature castration before the age of 40 years can place women into an added risk category for coronary vascular disease. Serum cholesterol and triglycerides of these women will be significantly higher than in women who continue to menstruate until the normal menopause, and their incidence rate of coronary heart disease will increase as will the severity, i.e., the type of the disease itself. None of the studies thus far conducted is able to shed much light on the reason for the abrupt loss of protection after ovarian secretion ceases, but it is clear that merely replacing the estrogens of these patients is not the therapeutic answer. Estrogen use after menopause was accompanied in the Framingham cohort by coronary heart disease incidence about twice that observed in

Table 92.3
Effects of Estrogen Therapy at Menopause

Finding	Incidence
Angina Pectoris	Double (age-matched controls)
Myocardial Infarction	No change
Mortality	No change

women not receiving such therapy (Table 92.3). The type of increase in heart disease noted with estrogen therapy was primarily for angina pectoris, and it is important to notice that there was no increase in total mortality nor was there a significant association between estrogen use and myocardial infarction. These findings have been previously reported by other workers. It should also be noted that an increase in the risk of cardiovascular disease was seen when estrogen was given to men, although the dose given to men was two to ten times higher than that usually given to women for relief of postmenopausal symptoms. Indeed, with a dose of estrogen equivalent to that given postmenopausal women, there was no difference in incidence of cardiovascular disease between men treated with estrogen and those untreated.

Although the menopause is clearly a period of major changes in the risk of developing heart disease in normal women, in the presence of hypertension, a menstruating woman has approximately the same risk of coronary heart disease as her male counterpart. This elimination of the dominant male-female ratio in the presence of hypertension may explain the fact that coronary heart disease in black women in the southern United States is not significantly different from their male counterparts, since hypertension is common in these same women. It also brings up another potential risk factor that must be considered when contemplating surgery for castration since, if a woman in the premenopausal era has hypertension, there is an even greater risk to the removal of the ovaries and its impact on cardiovascular disease.

In summary, then, of the cardiovascular changes associated with surgical menopause, it is clear that there is an increased risk for the development of serious heart disease, and that estrogen replacement therapy does not substantially reduce this risk. From this consideration alone it would, therefore, be wisest to maintain normal ovarian secretions through the approximate age of the natural menopause unless specific disease is present that places the patient at an even greater risk.

Surgical Castration and Bone Disease

The removal of estrogens prior to the menopause significantly alters the metabolic processes regulating bone mineralization. Up to the age of approximately 25 years in women, bone formation predominates, but after this age and through the time of menopause there is a slow loss of bone mineral content. This loss is both of cortical and medullary bone content and proceeds at a rate approximately the same as that seen in the male. At the time of menopause, there is an abrupt increase in the loss of bone seen in women that occurs over a period of 5 to 10 years and may reduce the bone content in women to the threshold level, placing her at risk for developing osteoporosis and the crush fractures associated with this disorder. In men, the rate of demineralization continues at a slow rate, and it is not until about the age of 65 to 70 years that men will approach the potential for osteoporosis that is seen in women 20 years earlier. Surgical castration merely changes the age at which this abrupt loss of bone begins. Since women generally live longer than men, there is a significantly higher incidence of osteoporosis and hip fractures in women; this incidence is merely doubled if menopause has occurred prior to the age of 40 years.

The mechanisms by which estrogens protect against bone demineralization are more clearly understood than are the mechanisms by which estrogens seem to protect against cardiovascular disease. Estrogens act on the bone and on the gut not only to increase absorption of calcium but to slow the destructive process that occurs as a natural sequence of bone demineralization. The level at which estrogen interacts in the bone on the osteoblast and osteoclast and its antagonism of bone demineralization is not known, but most feel that it imparts its protection to the bone by permitting a normal process of bone mineralization rather than actively reducing demineralization. Estrogens may be important for regulating all of the calcium metabolism, and there is evidence for an effect of estrogen on the kidney and its important role in the metabolism of vitamin D to more active forms. Vitamin D's interaction with parathy-

roid hormone may also be at multiple levels, including gut, kidney, and bone. It is not the purpose of this chapter to deal with the biochemistry of the metabolic changes, but merely to detail the risk factors associated with estrogen withdrawal and to suggest the replacement therapy indicated.

Unfortunately, at the present time there is no way to determine exactly which patient is at major risk to develop premature osteoporosis; therefore, it is recommended that all patients undergoing premature menopause, whether natural or surgical, be treated for prevention of premature osteoporosis. Although it is possible to investigate calcium metabolism, generally the urinary calcium to creatinine ratios, vitamin D and its metabolite measurements, and/or parathyroid hormone levels do not add to our ability to assign relative risks for the development of bone demineralization. X-rays of the spinal column are generally of little use except for making the diagnosis of osteoporosis, but the newly developed methods of computerized axial tomography (CAT) of the wrist and forearm may provide more definitive information for the future management of these cases. Treatment for young patients (under age 45 years) following surgical castration is simply conjugated estrogen (Premarin) for 25 days and 10 mg of Provera for the last 10 days of each 25-day therapy. Women will have a moderate amount of menstrual flow, and the therapy is reinitiated after 5 days of menses. We recommend continuing this therapy monthly at least to the age of 45 years and perhaps longer, since recent evidence suggests that the protection against demineralization of the bone continues through the age of 50 years. The action of estrogen in this regard is specifically to retard the time at which active bone demineralization occurs, and it does not in any way repair osteoporotic lesions once they have occurred. Therefore, it must be used as a *preventative*, rather than a treatment of previously discovered osteoporosis, to be fully effective. We also favor the use of calcium supplements in these women who have an added risk to osteoporosis until the same age of approximately 50 years. When the entire reproductive tract has been removed, we continue to favor the use of progesterone since it is uncertain whether replacement alone imparts an added risk to the development of estrogen-sensitive tumors in other areas of the body which are known to respond to estrogen, notably the breasts and vagina. In the absence of the uterus, therefore, we recommend using Provera for 10 days at least every third month as a means of opposing the constant estrogen stimulatory action of the reproductive tissues.

Other Endocrine Consequences of Estrogen Withdrawal

Early withdrawal of estrogen may significantly alter other hormone-regulated events, in particular: libido; hair texture, quantity, and distribution; and vaginal mucosal integrity. The well-known association of the menopause and hot flashes is frequently thought as a frivolous disorder in women, but it is a serious enough consequence in some women to demand the physician's attention. When the hot flashes occur in the evening and throughout the night, they may very well disrupt the normal sleep pattern and create a constant fatigue and susceptibility to emotional lability. There are other therapeutic modalities which may decrease "hot flashes," e.g., propanolol (Inderal), 20 mg HS (hour of sleep). However, when atrophic vaginitis, decreased libido, and dry skin are also concerns, then oral or vaginal estrogens are preferred. The lowest dose that "works" is recommended with attempts to withdraw hormones each 6 months. Frequently, in younger castrate women, it is this constellation of symptoms that brings the patient to her gynecologist's attention, and the opportunity to initiate estrogen therapy for *prevention* of all hypoestrogenic risks can be seized upon.

Summary

Women undergoing surgical castration such as the patient identified in the case abstract should be treated with replacement estrogen and progestins at least until the age of 45 years. Although this treatment does not reduce all the risks of estrogen withdrawal at an early age, there are sufficient benefits that outweigh the risks. Clearly maintaining ovarian function for as long as possible is a worthy goal for physicians to consider when contemplating surgical procedures which may be delayed.

Risks of Estrogen Replacement Therapy

Volumes have been written about the potential risks associated with estrogen replacement therapy, and the reader is referred to the recommended literature for details of the ongoing controversy. These risks may or may not be real, but the risks of *not* initiating therapy are genuine and any dilution of the recommendation to initiate therapy in young castrated women is not justified. Suffice it to say that when progestins are added to cycling estrogen replacement, little or no evidence has been presented to argue favorably against their use. The need to prevent premature osteoporosis is sufficient to compel its recommendation, while other benefits may appear more frivolous—libido, vaginitis, emotional lability, etc—but they too are worthy of the concerned physician's attention.

Selected Readings

Gordon F, Kannnel WB, Hjortland MC, et al: Menopause and coronary artery disease: The Framingham study. *Ann Intern Med* 89:157, 1978.

Hammond CB, Jelovsek FR, Lee KL, et al: Effects of long-term estrogen replacement therapy. *Am J Obstet Gynecol* 133:537, 1979.

Jick H, Watkins RN, Hunter J, et al: Replacement estrogens and endometrial cancer. *New Engl J Med* 300:218, 1979.

Lindsay R, Hart DM, MacLean A, et al: Bone response to termination of estrogen replacement treatment. *Lancet* 1:1325, 1978.

Mosler BA, Whelan EM: Postmenopausal estrogen: A review. *Obstet Gynecol Surv* 36:467, 1981.

Petitti DB, Wingerd J, Pellegrin F, et al: Risks of vascular disease in women: Smoking, oral contraceptives, noncontraceptive estrogens, and other factors. *JAMA* 242:1150, 1979.

Schiff I, Ryan KJ: Benefits of estrogen replacement. *Obstet Gynecol Surv* 35:400, 1980.

CHAPTER 93
Surgical Patient with History of Previous Thrombophlebitis

ROBERT E. ROGERS, M.D.

CASE ABSTRACT

Vaginal hysterectomy with colporrhaphy has been recommended for 350-lb, 62-year-old, multiparous, normotensive black female with a progressive and symptomatic genital prolapse including a second degree prolapse of the uterus, a large cystocele, enterocele, rectocele, and perineal defect. She has been unable to retain a pessary. Following a cholecystectomy 12 years previously, the patient developed a pulmonary embolus on the fifth postoperative day, which was treated by 3 months of anticoagulant therapy. There is no history of previous phlebitis or of varicose veins.

DISCUSSION

The patient with an increased risk for thromboembolism is becoming a more common problem than previously. This is because we are operating on older patients, frequently with medical and surgical problems that would have been absolute contraindications for surgery in earlier years.

The incidence of thromboembolism is variable and it depends on the age, the medical condition of the patient, and the operative procedure performed. The incidence of thromboembolism in a large series of gynecologic patients is approximately one in 1000 operations. A number of factors influence the incidence: (1) surgical or nonsurgical trauma, (2) obesity, (3) age over 40 years, (4) varicose veins, (5) previous thromboembolic disease, (6) estrogen use, (7) atherosclerotic cardiovascular disease, (8) cardiac failure, (9) immobilization. It is important to realize that 95% of pulmonary emboli arise from thrombi in the deep venous system of the pelvis and lower extremities. The gynecologic surgeon must be alert to the fact that every patient is a possible candidate for thrombosis and thromboembolism.

The patient presented here has at least three of the risk factors mentioned above, therefore, she must be considered at high risk for a repeat thromboembolic event. The only risk factor under either the patient's or the physician's control is the patient's obesity. The possibility of the patient making any meaningful reduction in weight is doubtful. All patients with this risk factor should be counseled and helped to reduce obesity. Our success in this area has been limited.

Two approaches to this problem must be considered, mechanical and medical. The mechanical approaches include ambulation, the compression of superficial veins with fitted elastic hose, stimulation of the calf muscles to act as a blood pump, intermittent compression of the leg, and proper protection of the legs at the time of surgery.

Three mechanical approaches are recommended in the patient presented. The first of these is fitted elastic hose. In the morbidly obese patient an adequate fit of these garments is difficult and requires prior planning. Most often the garment is not available "off the shelf" and must be ordered. The hose should be available at the time that the patient is admitted to the hospital and the patient should wear them at the point that her usual activity is limited, generally the day of admission.

A second mechanical factor is the placement of the patient in stirrups. The greatest care must be given to avoiding point compression of the lower extremities in stirrups. For this reason the orthopaedic stirrup or the "hanging stirrup" should be chosen. The leg should be arranged in the stirrup so as not to compress any portion of the extremity. The antiembolism hose must be in place, elevated on the thigh and unwrinkled through the procedure.

The third mechanical consideration is early ambulation, within hours of surgery. The patient may start by simply standing at the bedside and breathing deeply. Early and frequent ambulation must be encouraged. Meticulous attention must be given to the elastic hose to make certain that they are properly pulled up on the thighs. Occasionally in the morbidly obese patient it may be necessary to tape the hose to the upper thigh.

Medical measures involve the alteration of the patient's blood coagulability. Several approaches are available, low- and full- dose heparin, low dose heparin with dihydroergotamine, oral anticoagulation, intravenous Dextran, and preoperative aspirin therapy.

In the patient presented, one might consider the possibility of operating using the mechanical methods and not altering coagulability. Most surgeons weighing the risk of altering coagulability against the risk of operating without anticoagulants will choose to alter the patient's clotting function.

Operating under full anticoagulation is possible, but in most surgical situations particularly when the vaginal route is chosen, it is not recommended. The best solution would be limited alteration of clotting ability during the surgery and immediate postoperative period.

Dextran 70 or Dextran 40 has occasionally been used for prophylaxis. It is generally given in volumes of at least 500 ml over a 4- to 6-hour period starting at the time of the operation and then repeated daily for 2 to 5 days. Dextran may be associated with a slight increase in bleeding. In elderly patients it carries a danger of fluid overload.

Low dose aspirin is said to reduce the incidence of thrombophlebitis and thromboembolism. There is no documentation of its usefulness in pelvic surgery.

Subcutaneous low-dose heparin given in a dose of 5000 units 2 hours pre-operatively and then every 8 to 12 hours postoperatively has been shown to be effective prophylaxis in many studies. When this agent is used there is an increase in intraoperative and postoperative bleeding and wound hematomas prove to be significantly increased.

A combination of heparin sodium, 5000 units, and dihydroergotamine mesylate 0.5 mg has become available for prevention of deep vein thrombosis. This combination appears to inhibit at least two of the factors which lead to phlebitis: hypercoagulability and stasis. Dihydroergotamine has been shown to exert a selective constrictive effect on the veins and venules and to some degree a constricted effect on the arterioles and arteries. Venous return appears to be accelerated and venous stasis prevented. The combination of heparin sodium and dihydroergotamine mesylate is available as "Embolex" (Sandoz).

At the time of the planned vaginal hysterectomy and colporrhaphy the patient should be carefully positioned with particular attention to the support of the legs. The planned operation should be carried out in a routine fashion but particular attention must be given to hemostasis. In this situation an electrocautery is useful to coagulate small vessels that one might ignore in the course of most vaginal operations. A vaginal pack is advisable after the operation is complete, even if the surgeon does not customarily use one. Pressure on small bleeding vessels will control bleeding and prevent vaginal hematomas. The surgeon must be aware that delayed bleeding and wound hematomas are most common, even with low dose heparin.

Selected Readings

Hirsch J, Genton E, Hull R: A practical approach to the prophylaxis of venous thrombosis. In: *Venous Thromboembolism*. New York, Grune & Stratton, 1981, pp. 108 -121.

Mosier K: Pulmonary thromboembolism. In: *Harrison's Principles of Internal Medicine*. New York, McGraw Hill, 1983, pp. 1561-1567. 1561-67.

CHAPTER 94

Hysterectomy in the Morbidly Obese Patient

CLYDE L. RANDALL, M.D.

CASE ABSTRACT

A 44-year-old, para 2 gravida 2, 280 lb in weight and 5 ft 1 inch in height, has suffered from chronic recurrent menorrhagia "refractory to curettage and to hormone manipulation" and hysterectomy has been advised.

DISCUSSION

Consideration of the management of this patient's problem must begin with at least two assumptions: first, it is assumed that within the past 6 months a curettage was employed in a manner adequate to rule out carcinoma in the endocervix as well as the uterine fundus, and that no malignancy was found.

Should the curettings have been reported to show adenocarcinoma and: (a) the operator is certain that the material did not come from the endocervix, (b) that he "curetted out all that was there," and (c) the pathologist reported a mature type adenocarcinoma he would call grade I, the findings would warrant the diagnosis of adenocarcinoma of the uterus stage I, grade I. Under those circumstances a total hysterectomy by either a vaginal or suprapubic operation would be adequate treatment of that carcinoma (7).

Removal of the adnexa would be optional; if this could be accomplished easily it should not add significantly to the operating time or the risks involved. If the operator does not believe that prophylactic removal of the ovaries at age 44 years is in the woman's best interests, only total hysterectomy would be adequate treatment of the bleeding and a stage I grade I adenocarcinoma.

A second essential assumption would be that previous observation of this patient has convinced us that she cannot be expected to tolerate the loss of menstrual blood during the time necessary to lose enough weight to make any significant improvement in her "operability." We must assume also the medical efforts to minimize her anemia due to blood loss have not been effective, so that hysterectomy has seemed necessary and has been accepted by the patient.

Body weight of 280 lb in a woman only 5 ft 1 inch in height suggests a markedly obese and pendulous abdominal wall and massive thighs. It is hoped that the surgeon contemplating a hysterectomy on this very obese woman is a gynecologist equally familiar and experienced with the techniques of vaginal as well as transabdominal surgery. To an experienced vaginal surgeon this degree of obesity would not contraindicate the vaginal approach. To an experienced abdominal surgeon the incision necessary to reach the uterus through this markedly obese and pendulous abnormal wall would not only be a time consuming and troublesome part of the surgery but, postoperatively, the incision would be likely to account for or contribute to complications which, at best, would prolong the patient's hospitalization and recovery.

In the patient's best interests the surgeon's choice of operation should be the procedure likely to be followed by fewer and less major complications. If there were no advantages to the vaginal operation except the avoidance of a large complication-prone abdominal incision, the operator would be justified in preferring a vaginal hysterectomy (3, 6). However, before the approach to hysterectomy is to be decided there are considerations which should be taken into account whenever major surgery is being contemplated and the patient is markedly obese (1).

The morbidity associated with obesity not relative to the eventuality of surgery has been repeatedly documented. Cardiovascular disease, including hypertension, arteriosclerosis, cerebral hemorrhage, coronary or peripheral thrombosis, all are risks frequently accounting for the decreased life expectancy which obesity assures. Increasing age and increasing body weight are both associated with increasing diabetes. Gall bladder disease and gall stones are frequently associated with obesity and heavy deposits of mesenteric and omental fat as well as fatty peripheral musculature contribute to habitual hypoventilation. Reduced diaphragmatic excursion disposes to hypostatic congestion, and accounts for reduced cardiopulmonary capacity unless the risks are realized and remedial measures are encouraged.

Obviously it is of the utmost importance that the significantly obese patient being considered for surgery be subjected to a thorough preoperative appraisal fo health and habits (9, 10). A thorough history, including an evaluation of organ-system-function, a thoughtful and complete physical examination and finally, adequate laboratory studies, including routine biochemical profiles, should all be a part of the preoperative survey. Unless the indication for surgery is an emergency, the preoperative discovery of such anemia as this patient will probably show should be investigated although the cause seems obvious. Remedial measures may be planned for the convalescent period even though the immediate problem can be remedied by blood transfusions to carry the patient through surgery. More comprehensive management may be indicated, and could be an important factor in the long-term evaluation of the benefits of the operation.

It may also be important for the physicians considering the risks versus the expected gains an operation would provide to remember that many obese individuals have deep and long standing emotional problems which may effect the patient's desire to get well—even the desire to live. Evaluation and counseling before surgery could make a significant difference in the patient's postoperative motivation, the length of hospitalization and the degree of improvement the patient will be willing to attribute to the operation. Only when all such information is considered can the physician weigh the risks

versus the probable benefits of the surgery he may advise.

Many studies of the characteristics of the obese and the effects of obesity on health and longevity have been based on objective studies using adequate controls and following a prospective protocol. Reports of the complications following surgery on the obese, however, have usually been retrospective surveys of what happened (5, 6). Even though "matching controls" may have been considered, undocumented factors may have contributed to the outcome. In spite of the possibility that the recommendations made and the conclusions drawn by the authors quoted may be questioned, it is our conviction that the observations which have been reported warrant the attention of the clinicians responsible for advising a significantly obese patient to undergo abdominal or pelvic surgery.

We are told that preoperative pelvic examination of this patient provides the following information; there is minimal genital relaxation, the uterus is slightly enlarged and movable, the cul-de-sac is free, and the uterosacral ligaments are palpable, with firm traction the cervix can be brought down by an inch.

In consideration of those findings on examination, when the patient is this markedly obese, we believe the experienced vaginal surgeon would have several good reasons to recommend a vaginal rather than a transabdominal approach to the uterus when a hysterectomy is indicated.

Marked vaginal relaxation and/or uterine prolapse is usually considered to make the technique of vaginal hyesterectomy no easier than when relationships are normal, hence the lack of decensus in this instance does not contraindicate a vaginal hysterectomy.

Since the uterus is movable and the cul-de-sac also seems free of adhesions, the fact that the uterosacral ligaments are palpable and probably contribute to the lack of uterine descent on traction should not discourage the vaginal approach. Actually the vaginal surgeon will be pleased to find palpable, substantial uterosacrals because this obese patient will have need of good vaginal support after a hysterectomy. With the help of good uterosacral ligaments, closure of the vagina can be accomplished through the vagina with better maintenance of the vaginal axis, better appreciation of the potential for a postoperative enterocele and obliteration of any such weakness than could have been accomplished by an operator working through the distance and difficulties of a deep abdominal incision through an obese abdominal wall.

There are other advantages to be realized in the choice of the vaginal operation when hysterectomy is indicated for an obese patient. Anesthesia need not be so "deep," abdominal packing will not be displacing the omentum and mesentary and decreasing the excursion of the diaphragm. The head of the operating table need be lowered only to the degree desired by the anesthesiologist. Considering the blood loss incident to opening a large and obese abdomen, the vaginal and parametrial dissections and vaginal removal of the uterus should not result in greater blood loss than usually experienced during a suprapubic total hysterectomy through an obese abdominal wall.

There is one point upon which all reports agree regarding the complications likely to follow abdominal surgery in the significantly obese patient. All too frequently such an abdominal incision as an obese patient requires heals poorly or develops a degree of infection which jeopardizes the integrity of the scar. Complications in the incision during convalesance are not as serious as cardiopulmonary, intra-abdominal, or intravascular complications, but it is generally agreed that an unsatisfactory condition of the abdominal incision is the most frequent and predictable of the problems which prolong the obese patient's hospital stay.

We recognize that abdominal surgeons and many gynecologists simply prefer the suprapubic approach for hysterectomy, largely we suspect because of the frequency with which they open the abdomen and the confidence they develop in their ability to deal with the problem encountered. We believe, however, that for this patient the often emphasized advantage of opening the abdomen and being able to explore the abdomen and detect an unsuspected risk to the patient's future health does not warrant the risks of the complications so frequently developed in the incision through an obese abdominal wall. The obvious risks inherent in this degree of obesity favor a choice of operative procedure that will subject this patient to the risks of as few as possible of the recognized complications of the operation itself.

Even if the surgeon contemplating a hysterectomy on this patient had accomplished panniculectomy successfully at the time of other indicated abdominal surgery for other obese women, I believe for this patient, the operator should not consider the addition of a panniculectomy to the operative procedure. Certainly the thought of accomplishing an excision of the panniculus at the same time should not wisely be regarded as a point favoring the transabdominal approach. Incision through an abdominal wall of this type will, at best, be time-consuming and account for blood loss that certainly would be increased by extension of an already large abdominal incision in order to accomplish an elective panniculectomy. Then after hysterectomy was accomplished, the time required to close such a huge abdominal wound would add considerably to the total operating time.

Except for the individual surgeon's preference for doing a suprapubic rather than a vaginal hysterectomy, for a patient this obese, we fail to see a significant advantage to opening this patient's abdomen. We do recognize, however, that many abdominal surgeons will prefer the suprapubic approach, in which case there might be question as to the relative merits of a vertical or a transverse incision. While the majority of abdominal surgeons prefer a vertical incision (particularly in the upper abdomen) many gynecologic surgeons prefer a low transverse incision for pelvic laparotomy.

Data comparing abdominal wound healing in obese patients does not provide convincing evidence of fewer wound complications with any one of the several types of incision which could be used. The accuracy of hemostasis or the development of hematomata, the presence or the development of infection, the technique of wound closure and the suture material used —all are variables which are certain to obscure the possible merits of the type and location of the incision itself. However, published reports do seem to have established that better results can be expected when large laparotomy wounds in an obese abdomen are closed by special suture techique and suture material.

The Smead-Jones type of hidden retention suture was emphasized by Jones et al (4) and, more recently, by Morrow et al (5) and Gallup (2). Delayed on nonabsorbable suture material was recommended by each group reporting improved results, most recently polyglycolic acid, polydiaxonone (PDS or Maxon) or Prolene have been used. Because of the probability of potential space superficial to the fascia, drainage should be assured by placement of a suction drain, the tube brought into the wound through a skin puncture lateral to the incision. This precaution is particularly important when the patient is diabetic, for a wound infection is almost a certainty if effective drainage is not employed.

While the surgeon contemplating abdominal or pelvic surgery on a significantly obese patient has reason to expect a technically difficult operation, and a postoperative course prolonged by complications, the patient's satisfactory recovery will be no less dependent upon the interest, discernment, and efforts of the anesthesiologist. A patient this obese often proves to be a severe test of the anesthesiologist's skills (8). Maintaining intravenous channels may be difficult due to thin-walled invisible veins in areolar tissue. A fatty neck may make it difficult to maintain an adequate airway. Obese patients frequently have a low gastric acidity and large residual gastric volume, both of which add to the risk of aspiration, atelectasis, and/or pneumonia.

The patient's preoperative cardiorespiratory status is likely to have indicated marginal ventilation. Anesthesia, almost any degree to which the head of the table may be lowered, and particularly the surgeon's retractor-held packing, are likely to limit still further diaphragmatic excursion. More than expected blood loss may call for increased intravascular fluids when the patient's enlarged heart has already been compromised by poor respiratory excursion and hypoventilation. While forced closed ventilation during anesthesia may provide increased pulmonary perfusion, it has been shown such effort may provide adequate ventilation of only the superior chest and upper lobes, leaving the base of the lungs poorly aerated, congested, and liable to postoperative atelectasis.

Regional anesthesia has not been shown to be an easily employed relatively safer alternative. Dosage required for the significantly obese cannot safely be determined by the formula established for bodies whose weight includes substantially less fat. Circulatory characteristics of the obese make the diffusion levels less predictable. Overdosage and the problems of a ''high spinal'' may be experienced. Even with a variety of problems, intravenous and inhalation anesthesia will usually be the anesthesiologist's choice.

Following surgery, the obese patient must be carefully monitored as to fluids, oxygen, intermittent positive pressure breathing, semirecumbent position and early voluntary movement. The surgeon and all attendants must watch for any one of the variety of postoperative complications the obese patient may experience.

The advantages of a vaginal hysterectomy are more apparent during the postoperative convalescence. Without the wound of an abdominal incision the patient will move more readily, breathe more easily deeply and will be agreeable to being propped up higher in bed. She will be out of bed sooner, move about more readily and be less inclined to resist early ambulation. With unsplinted, deeper inspirations there will be fewer postoperative pulmonary problems and with earlier ambulation, a decreased risk of thrombosis in veins of the lower extremities and pelvis.

Even when pulmonary and circulatory functions have seemed adequate and there is no question of an intraperitoneal problem, in the obese patient an abdominal incision warrants careful and daily attention. The relatively poor vascularity in a large incision in a fatty abdominal wall makes for slow and poor healing. Voluntary movements of the patient involve movement of a heavy abdominal wall and significant pulling on an incision poorly or incompletely healed. Some separation may be noted but then prove to be insignificant, or sudden dehiscence may be discovered. Fortunately, the latter does not occur often and has been reported no more frequently in the obese, even though it would seem a more likely complication in a patient whose large abdominal wound may be healing slowly and show pockets of separation.

If the risk of lower extremity and/or deep pelvic vein thrombosis is decreased by early and frequent ambulation the value of prophylactic activity is certainly greater in the obese patient. Often the obese are not naturally active and must be motivated repeatedly. The value of prophylactic heparin is not questioned, but its use does not relieve the patient of the need for frequent movement. Some patients must even be convinced that helpful nursing is not provided to relieve the patient of having to move about and help herself as much as possible.

We have long believed it advisable to insist

on a few precautions that have seemed to reduce the risks of deep vein thrombosis. The leg of the patient while in Trendelenburg position should be adjusted in the supports until it appears there is no compression along the inner thighs or the popliteal space. While she is still on the operating table, before taking the patient's legs down out of stirrups, wide elastic bandages should be applied from the sole of the foot to above the knee. Unless this prophylactic routine is followed, some patients will develop an alarming degree of hypotension within a very few minutes after the lower extremities are lowered to the level of the head and body. The leg wraps are not removed until voluntary movements and skeletal muscle tone seem normal. Another rule, because we have been impressed by the occurence of pulmonary embolism when a bed patient who had been relatively inactive has been encouraged to have a bowel movement on a bed pan, we say "early ambulation," and when the patient is bedfast we recommend enemas for a bowel movement; *no straining on a bedpan.*

Faced with a patient with this degree of obesity and an indication for hysterectomy, we would emphasize that no routine management would be likely to assure the best result we would hope to achieve. Taking all the possibilities into account, we should be able to handle

any problem that develops, but this type of patient needing a hysterectomy may require our best perceptions and certainly will require our best efforts.

References

1. Buckwalter JA: Nonsurgical factors important in the success of surgery for morbid obesity. *Surgery* 91:113-114, 1982.
2. Gallup DG: Modifications of celeiotomy techniques to decrease morbidity in obese gynecologic patients. *Am J Obstet Gynecol* 150:171, 1984.
3. Howkins J, Stallworthy J: *Bonney's Gynaecological Surgery,* 8th edition, p. 223, Baltimore, Williams & Wilkins, 1974.
4. Jones TE, Newell ET Jr, Brubaker RE: The use of alloy steel wire in the closure of abdominal wounds. *Surg Gynecol Obstet* 72:1056, 1941.
5. Morrow CP, Hernandez WL, Townsend DE, et al: Pelvic celiotomy in the obese patient. *Am J Obstet Gynecol* 127:335, 1977.
6. Pitkin RM: Abdominal hysterectomy in obese women. *Surg Gynecol Obstet* 142:532-536, 1976.
7. Pratt JA: Common complications of vaginal hysterectomy: Thoughts on prevention and management. *Clin Obstet Gynecol* 19:645-659, 1976.
8. Putman L, Jenicek JA, Allen CR, et al: Anesthesia in the morbidly obese patient. *Soc Med J* 67:1411-1417, 1974.
9. Strauss RJ, Wise L: Operative risks of obesity. *Surg Gynecol Obstet* 146:286-291, 1978.
10. Williams SV: Preoperative management of the overweight patient. In: Goldman D, et al (eds): *Medical Care of the Surgical Patient.* Philadelphia, JB Lippincott, 1982, Chap 13, pp. 174-187.

CHAPTER 95

Adnexal Abscess After Vaginal Hysterectomy

DAVID H. NICHOLS, M.D.

CASE ABSTRACT

Vaginal hysterectomy without repair was performed shortly following menstruation upon a 42-year-old multipara with chronic menorrhagia. No "preventive" antibiotic was given because of a history of allergy to penicillin. A low grade afternoon fever was noted on the 3rd day, which responded within 48 hours to gentamicin and clinda-mycin therapy. Hospitalization was otherwise uneventful, and the patient was discharged the morning of the 6th postoperative day. Because of fever and left lower abdominal pain, the patient was re-admitted on the 8th postoperative day, and a vagi-nal cuff abscess diagnosed, incised and drained of 10 cc of purulent material from which a culture grew out antibiotic resistant *Enterococci* and *Bacteroides fragilis*. The patient was discharged 2 days later and the Penrose drain removed from the vagina a week later. On the 20th day postoperative from the original surgery, the patient was re-hospitalized because of severe left-sided lower abdominal pain. An ill-defined tender 5-cm cystic left adnexal mass was palpated and its presence confirmed by sonography.

DISCUSSION

Because the ovaries often are brought closer to the vaginal cuff with peritonealization following vaginal hysterectomy than following total abdominal hysterectomy, they are perhaps more vulnerable to postoperative infection in the premenopausal patient, particularly in the presence of a vaginal cuff infection (1). This might be related to their vulnerability around the time of ovulation, or the presence of a culture medium within the ovary from a postovulatory corpus hemorrhagicum (Fig. 95.1). This patient must be considered to have an adnexal abscess or oophoritis until proven otherwise, as, for example, by laparoscopic examination. Although certain antibiotics (clindamycin, cefamandol, cefoxitin, and metronidazole) are believed to have superior qualities of abscess penetration, ovarian abscess may be resistant to such therapy. By the location of the ovary higher within the pelvis than the tubes, it may be inaccessible to safe transvaginal postopera-tive drainage, and require a transabdominal oophorectomy or salpingo-oophorectomy for resolution. This may be in contrast to the clinical resolution of salpingitis during conservative or nonsurgical treatment by rest and appropriate antibiotic administration. Posthysterectomy ovarian abscess, occasionally subsequent to ovulation, characteristically becomes clinically evident a week or two following the patient's discharge from an apparently uneventful post-hysterectomy hospital course. The patient may call and describe an onset of fever with a severe noncramping often unilateral pelvic pain. If an adnexal abscess is identified, the presence or absence of hydronephrosis or retroperitoneal hematoma may be studied by sonography. If ovarian abscess cannot be excluded, a diagnostic laparoscopy should be performed. If the diagnosis is confirmed, the ovary and usually the tube should be excised by transabdominal laparotomy.

Prevention of this problem is achieved by meticulous hemostasis during surgery, the use

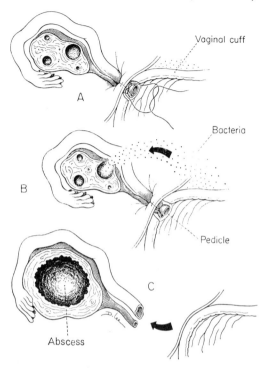

Figure 95.1. Possible mechanism for the development of an adnexal abscess after vaginal hysterectomy is shown diagramatically. *A*. The close proximity of the adnexal structures to the vaginal cuff after vaginal hysterectomy is depicted. *B*. Postoperative ovulation exposes the stroma of the ovary to bacterial invasion from the infected vaginal cuff. *C*. Disintegration of suture holding the pedicle to the vaginal cuff permits retraction of adnexal abscess high into the pelvis. Reproduced with permission from Ledger WJ, et al: Adnexal abscess as late complication of pelvic operations. *Surg Gynecol Obstet* 129:973-978, 1969.

of an appropriate preoperative antibiotic or antibacterial, and possibly by burying the adnexal stump beneath the vaginal wall during the operative procedure, though leaving a finger-tipped size opening in the posterior portion of the vaginal vault for drainage.

In the patient described, laparoscopy confirmed the diagnosis, and a transabdominal left salpingo-oophorectomy was performed. Recovery was uneventful.

Reference

1. Ledger WJ, Campbell C, Taylor D, Wilson JR: Adnexal abscess as late complication of pelvic operations. *Surg Gynecol Obstet* 129:973-978, 1969.

CHAPTER 96
Psychiatric Consequences of Gynecologic Surgery

ANDREW E. SLABY, M.D., Ph.D., M.P.H.

CASE ABSTRACT

Total abdominal hysterectomy with elective bilateral salpingo-oophorectomy was performed upon a maiden 39-year-old school teacher to relieve discomfort associated with a large fibroid uterus. Surgery was uncomplicated and convalescence smooth. An incidental finding at surgery was superficial ovarian endometriosis.

Following discharge from hospital, the patient gradually became despondent and depressed over her lost reproductive capacity and progressively withdrawn and resentful. She was brought to the hospital Emergency Room some 6 months after surgery, unconscious following an alleged overdose of sleeping tablets.

DISCUSSION

Reactions to hysterectomy vary but, in all cases, are present to a greater or lesser degree. Most frequent responses to hysterectomy and loss of reproductive capacity in the premenopausal years are depression, anger, anxiety, and psychosomatic complaints (4, 8, 9). Loss of uterus, even by women with several children or by women who do not posit any immediate desire to have a child—such as nuns, individuals vowing never to marry and have children, and lesbians not desiring children or marriage to man is difficult. Reactions to hysterectomy as to elective sterilization (1, 2, 6, 7, 10) are dependent on age, marital status, religion, ethnic background, social class, previous psychiatric status, number of children borne, reason for surgery (e.g., cancer), social support, husband or partner's response, and plans for divorce or remarriage (unpredictable events in many cases). True prevalence of regret after sterilization is reported to be 3.6% to 20% (10). Both premenopausal and postmenopausal women perceive hysterectomy as mutilation of their bodies. The organ historically defining their roles as potential mothers and women has been removed. Prior to menopause, loss of uterus surgically represents irreversible foreclosure of

ability to have children. It is the end of an era...the end of the reproductive era. The younger the woman, the greater the possibility of such a reaction. If a hysterectomy takes place near the anticipated time of menopause, there may be less dramatic response. Nevertheless, the reality remains that an organ has been removed that defines women to be different from men. In addition, the fear exists that organs are removed unnecessarily or removed because of medical indications (e.g., cancer) not revealed to the patient. In the former instance, a woman may feel that she is one of many people she reads about in the popular press who have undergone unnecessary surgery. Patients have become medically sophisticated. Many feel that the decision to undergo surgery should be one of both surgeon and patient, educated as to consequences both of having and not having surgery. If a malignancy is suspected, what is the possibility that a clinical laboratory test such as a Pap smear or a biopsy may be in error? Frank discussions with patients and their significant others prior to an operation of the indications and contraindications of surgery and of limitations of tests and of projected outcomes with and without surgery can serve to reduce anxiety prior to surgery and anger and depression afterward. It also serves to minimize instigation of unproductive litigation if indications for a surgical procedure seem more ambiguous.

Depression is a normal response to the loss of the uterus, much as it is to menopause and loss of a breast by surgery. Patients with a family or past personal history of affective illness are at higher risk to develop the signs and symptoms of a depression at such times (9). In one study (4) of 102 women who underwent hysterectomy, the incidence of depression was higher before surgery than afterward. Risk factors for posthysterectomy depression included prior history of affective illness, lower socioeconomic status, and high preoperative scores on anxiety. Fears of cancer and of adverse sexual effects were the main sources of anxiety. Divorced women, regardless of surgery, are at eight times the risk for psychiatric problems requiring hospitalization (7). Divorce, in fact, is rated nearly as stressful as death of spouse on Rahe and Holmes Life Events Scale. Psychologic consequences of gynecologic procedures are reduced when women learn more about their problems and are supported by their families and others with similiar problems (1).

The first step in management of depression as a complication of hysterectomy is to anticipate it and discuss the possibility with patient, spouse (or spouse-equivalent), and family if she so desires. Women referred to gynecologists, when compared to controls, report more psychiatric problems, especially if divorced, separated, widowed, or complaining of pelvic pain (3). Included in the discussion should be description of early symptoms of depression. In the case summarized at the beginning of this chapter, it was apparent that the patient was slipping into depression. She was portrayed as "despondent and depressed" and becoming more withdrawn and resentful. These symptoms and signs suggest to a clinician or family that expected depression has become greater than anticipated and psychiatric consultation is necessary to commence treatment and evaluate risk for self-destructive behavior. The patient was a single woman living alone. In such instances, follow-up visits must be scheduled such that a depression may be identified sufficiently early so that the morose mood does not cause a patient to cancel appointments and slip unrecognized into a suicidal state.

Prior to surgery, the full meaning of a hysterectomy and loss of reproductive capacity, if in the premenopausal years, should be discussed and the patient allowed to participate in the decision to pursue surgery, given the reality of the psychologic and medical consequences of having surgery. An alternate surgical approach to hysterectomy, such as myomectomy, may be elected. As with so many choices in life, loss of a uterus and reproductive capacity is ambivalent. While it represents the end of a reproductive era and mutilation of a woman's body, it also ironically allows a greater equality with a man. A woman is no longer burdened with the vicissitudes of the menstrual cycle and has, without fear of medical complications of birth control, the freedom to have sexual liaisons without fear of pregnancy. Some women may focus more on this, especially if professional and more androgynous in their orientation than others who may feel their uniqueness is lost or that some men may reject them because they cannot give them children. The fear of being barren may be particularly great if a woman is young and unmarried at the time of hysterectomy and would like to bear children or feels a potential husband will reject her because she cannot have children. A comparable response may occur with women who are married to men who to some degree determine their virility by fathering children for the world to see to validate their heterosexual orientation and manhood. Finally, a young woman in an unhappy marriage considering a divorce and a remarriage to a more suitable partner may feel her chances are compromised if she is not able to offer a man the possibility of fathering a child (7). Sexual satisfaction is reported as improved by women undergoing elective sterilization. When difficulty arises, it is usually anticipated by disturbances at initial assessment (6). Tubal ligation is not analogous to the mutilation and irreversible impact of hysterectomy, but the assumption of sterility was prior to microsurgical corrective techniques.

Most women have strong emotional bonds to their gynecologists because of the intimacy entailed in discussion of gynecologic problems and sexual life and of the physical examination. This is so even if a gynecologist is a woman, appears aloof, or is not consciously "liked" by the patient. Intimacy alone serves to bond, and choices may be made out of fear or vulnerability in a bonded relationship rather than rationally. It is, therefore, all the more imperative that all aspects of an anticipated procedure be presented as objectively as possible and a patient allowed to participate to the greatest degree possible in decisions made.

Early signs of depression that should be discussed with a patient are significant sleep disturbance (difficulty falling asleep, awakening in the middle of the night, and early morning awakening or the antipode, hypersomnia), appetite and weight disturbance, decreased libido, increased "blues", diurnal variation in mood with feeling worse in the morning, tearfulness, feelings of worthlessness, pessimism about the future, and suicidal thoughts. If a patient does not know if she has lost weight because of failure to have weighed herself, ask if her clothes are fitting loosely. Family history of depression, suicide, alcoholism, mania, bankruptcy (as an indicia of mania), and sociopathy suggest vulnerability to affective illness in the face of stress, even if the patient herself has not yet had a depressive episode.

Incidence of depression increases with each decade of life (1). Hysterectomy performed prior to menopause is not at that time of greatest risk for depression under usual circumstances so that a history of depression would be found less likely in a premenopausal woman undergoing hysterectomy than it would be in a postmenopausal woman who, in fact, may have experienced her first depression at menopause. Women who, in fact, experience depression at menopause or following the birth of a child would be anticipated to experience another at the time of hysterectomy. This would obviously not be due to a foreclosure of opportunity to have children in a postmenopausal woman, since that has already occurred, but rather because of another mutilation of the image of womanhood and because of fear of cancer if the hysterectomy was performed because of the presence of a malignancy.

Evaluation of suicidal potential is an integral part of the evaluation of a depression by a physician who has identified it. Suicide risk is increased in women who have a personal or family history of suicide, are currently depressed, or are divorced, separated, or widowed. Suicide risk among the depressed is 80-500 times that of the general population (8). Other factors increasing suicide risk are a history of schizophrenia or of borderline personality disorder, lack of social supports, and predominant homosexual orientation (2, 3, 5).

Loss of a uterus is always ambivalent. As stated earlier, it represents both the end of an era as well as the ultimate in sexual freedom. A man seldom experiences that which a woman does prior to menopause, when she becomes aware that she can never again produce a child. Men, even in their 80s and 90s, may father a child with a woman in their reproductive period if they so wish. A woman after menopause or hysterectomy cannot. There is both the feeling of rage at not being able to do so as well as, in this era of androgyny, some potential for happiness at the feeling of freedom and ability to compete with men without the hindrance of confrontation of womanhood in the form of menses and the reality that pregnancy can be avoided without the artificial means of birth control. Some equality with men is ironically achieved at a core level when a woman may elect to have a sexual liaison for pleasure without the fear of pregnancy or the need to avoid it by artificial means. Life is complex and what may appear to be a solely or predominantly negative event is ambivalent, and in this ambivalence exists tension that enhances conflict and anxiety.

Use of groups for women who have undergone hysterectomy, either self-help or more formalized groups, allows women to explore the many facets of such surgery together and to provide support to each other at a time of stress. Women in posthysterectomy groups discuss the issues around hysterectomy such as the implications concerning identity as women, fear of occult cancer, and fear— sometimes real— that men may see them as barren and, therefore, not wish to pursue them as marital partners or wish to divorce them because of their inability to have children. They also discuss the ambivalences.

Hysterectomy is a complicated procedure, both surgically and psychologically. As with so many other things in life, the responses to it are complex and not always easily predictable. Problems can be minimized, however, by exploring preoperatively with a woman the risks and benefits of such surgery and by allowing her to participate, as she should, in the decision as to what will happen to her body. Early identification of possible areas of conflict and ambivalences allows patient and gynecologist the opportunity to develop plans of management that obviate more destructive consequences. All gynecologists should be aware of the early signs of depression and of how to evaluate self-destructive potential. Whenever there is doubt as to whether a depression is present or of the severity of suicidal potential, a psychiatrist should be consulted to help manage the case. Management includes both psychotherapy and sociotherapy, in addition to the use of antidepressants in doses indicated where endogenous signs of a depression (e.g., sleep and appetite disturbance) accompany the affective change.

The author wishes to thank Mr. Ari Solomon and Ms. Kimberly Durand who, respectively, participated in research for and presentation of this chapter.

References

1. Baker M, Quinkert K: Women's reactions to reproductive problems. *Psychol Reports* 53:159-166, 1983.

2. Blendin KD, Cooper JE: The regrets of sterilized women. *Lancet* 2:578-579, 1984.

3. Byrne P: Psychiatric morbidity in a gynecology clinic: An epidemiologic survey. *Br J Psychol* 144:28-34, 1984.

4. Lalinec-Michaud M, Engelmann F: Depression and hysterectomy: a prospective study. *Psychosomatics* 7:550-558, 1984.

5. Lieb J, Lipsitch II, Slaby AE: *The Crisis Team.* New York, Harper & Row, 1974.

6. Psychological sequelae of female sterilization. *Lancet* 2: 144-145, 1984.

7. Renshaw D: Divorce. *Ob Gyn Annu* 13:313-330, 1984.

8. Slaby AE, Tancredi LR, Lieb J: *Clinical Psychiatric Medicine.* Philadelphia, Harper & Row, 1981.

9. Slaby AE, Lieb J, Tancredi LR: *The Handbook of Psychiatric Emergencies,* ed. 3. New York, Medical Examination Publishing Company, 1985.

10. Wright AF: The regrets of sterilized women. *Lancet* 2:578, 1984.

CHAPTER 97

Medicolegal Complications Consequent to Unauthorized Surgery

DAVID LANDEL NICHOLS, ESQ., B.A., M.A., J.D.

CASE ABSTRACT

A 28-year-old nullipara with a history of previous unilateral salpingectomy 4 years previously for ectopic pregnancy was hospitalized because of moderately severe crampy lower abdominal pain and tenderness, accentuated by motion of the cervix. A pregnancy test was positive, and another ectopic pregnancy was suspected. Written operative consent was obtained for "laparoscopy and possible laparotomy," and the patient was taken to surgery the day following admission, where laparoscopy confirmed the presence of an unruptured pregnancy in the remaining tube. Laparotomy was performed, and the tube and uterus were removed, followed by an "incidental appendectomy."

The postoperative abdomen was distended, but bowel sounds were initially present. By the third postoperative day, the patient was febrile, the abdomen was diffusely painful and tender, and bowel sounds were absent. A diagnosis of peritonitis was established, and at repeat laparotomy it was found that the tie around the appendiceal stump had slipped, and there was full communication between the cecal lumen and the abdominal cavity with spillage of intestinal contents.

Following appropriate treatment and a long stormy postoperative course, the patient some months later brought suit against her surgeon alleging grave damages, and complained that no consent had been given for either the hysterectomy or appendectomy.

DISCUSSION

The medicolegal issues here relate in the United States to both the unauthorized "incidental" appendectomy and the hysterectomy. In an unauthorized appendectomy without complications the patient may have positive or neutral feelings postoperatively concerning the appendectomy, but should an untoward event take place the culpability falls squarely upon the shoulders of the surgeon. The lack of specific surgical consent or informed consent concerning the possibility of incidental surgery may be a grave and serious omission from the preoperative discussions with the patient. If it is the surgeon's practice to remove the appendix routinely, the patient deserves to know it, as well as the possible consequences of additional surgery.

The unauthorized removal of the uterus which the physician may consider a useless and potentially dangerous organ is also open to question. In the case presented the patient might feel that her rights have been violated, taking the position that in this day and age her uterus might have served as the future respository for an embryo resulting from an in vitro fertilization! Should the surgeon even *remotely* consider preoperatively an "incidental hysterectomy," he is well-advised to share his views with the patient, that she may participate in the decision as to what might be done, and she will have been informed of the projected benefits and risks to her health and welfare.

Most surgeons know well that full and adequate disclosure of the risks of anticipated surgery is a responsibility that the law very clearly places on them. Perhaps not quite so many know also that to be able to sustain an effective defense to a lawsuit for surgical complications or unauthorized surgery they must be able to show that before the surgery the patient was made to know of several things, including the need for surgery, that there existed a risk of certain specific complications or undesirable results, and that the surgery would probably be beneficial despite the risks. The surgeon should also be able to show that the patient voluntarily accepted these particular risks as a predicate to treatment. Relevant medicolegal complications arise typically in two areas: when the surgeon fails to observe these requirements formally in what is most often an informal discussion with the patient, and when the surgeon fails to document adequately his execution of these responsibilities. The problems may be mutually exclusive, as in the not uncommon case of the systematic and conscientious surgeon who makes full disclosure but who is now sued by an ungrateful patient whose real motivation in commencing a malpractice action is an attempt to vindicate her inability or unwillingness to pay the surgeon's fee. Some suggestions will be offered as to how to deal with these shortcomings anticipatorily; but first we shall take a look at the legal nature of the allegations of wrongdoing we would be seeking to rectify.

The essential legal basis of the dealings between doctor and patient lies in contract law. For there to be a valid contract there must be a meeting of the minds of the contracting parties. Here, the doctor agrees to perform certain health care services on the patient's body without guaranteeing the results, and the patient agrees to compensate the doctor and gives consent to the treatment (3). The "consent" part of the contract is the focus of the issue we know as "informed consent." Because the doctor is an expert, in order to equalize the position of the parties to the contract (as the law tends to want to do), the doctor is given the reaffirmative responsibility to disclose all material risks reasonably foreseeable (4). The question of which risks are "material" and "reasonably foreseeable" has been addressed by legal decisions which have provided only sketchy answers, but by considering those cases together we might infer the emergence of a trend. Some states have adopted a "reasonable patient" disclosure standard, in which disclosure of risks ought to be made by a physician when a reasonable person, who knows what the physician knows about a patient's circumstances, would likely attach significance to the risks (1). Other states have applied to disclosure responsibilities the "community standard" language familiar to medical negligence cases: to show a lack of informed consent, the plaintiff must prove by expert medical evidence what a reasonable medical practitioner of the same discipline and same or similar circumstances would have disclosed about the risks incident to a proposed diagnosis or treatment (9). This is known as the "professional disclosure standard" (2).

Irrespective of this difference in disclosure standards, in a scholarly analysis McCallum has interpreted the law to suggest that a risk disclosure is advisable where the probability of maloccurrence exceeds 1% (3, p. 373). He goes on to say that "Even more remote contingencies should be disclosed if the result is extreme in comparison to the elective nature of the surgery." Alternatives for treatment should be discussed including any ongoing academic debates concerning efficacy or propriety of the treatment (1). Many doctors feel that they are protecting themselves by blanket consent forms, but these have been uniformly rejected by the courts (7). They do not show the "meeting of the minds" discussed earlier.

A better idea is to use detailed consent forms, unique for each operation, spelling out the attendant risks with particularity. Variable sections tailored to a patient's needs might better evidence actual discussion between the doctor and patient. This, in turn, would demonstrate that the patient actually assumed the risks of treatment—the best defense against a suit for failure of informed consent (1). McCallum suggests that a good source of consent forms reflecting "community standards" could be a blue ribbon committee of the local or state medical association in conjunction with the association's legal counsel (3, p. 372). In response to precisely this sort of suggestion, the Texas legislature established in 1977 the Texas Medical Disclosure Panel to issue standard information sheets stating what it is that the patients in that state ought to be told about different treatment available (8). Readers of the advertisements in medical magazines and journals may have considered another possible source for detailed consent forms: commercial form companies. One might suppose himself to be adequately protected if he has the patient sign a veritable "grocery list" of consent, risk disclosure, and disclaimer forms for every conceivable complication, but courts would probably look upon this practice in the same way that they view the blanket consent forms, to-wit, that these impersonal forms simply do not necessarily evidence a "meeting of the minds." Instead, the surgeon might be better advised to consult with his own lawyer and have him draft one brief disclosure form for each complication (or group of commonly associated complications). Individual bits of information can also be stored and conveniently retrieved on a personal computer. In each event, the patient would then be asked to sign a little package of disclosure and consent forms tailor-made for her particular surgery. The surgeon would know in advance what forms to put in the little packet by using a checklist for that general surgical concern, and he could conveniently make additions and deletions to suit the case at hand. As he goes through the forms with the patient he discusses each orally, checking off entries on the checklist as he goes. To document in writing the act that each written risk disclosure and consent form was discussed with the patient orally, the doctor might designate a special column on his checklist for the patient to initial. Besides the specific prepared forms, other things could be included on the checklist to ensure that appropriate preoperative oral disclosure has not been overlooked. Some relevant issues that gynecologists might include were suggested by Belinson (personal communication):

1. Expected diagnosis
2. The expected surgical procedure
3. The risk of bowel injury
4. The risk of "ostomy" potential
5. Castration
6. Possible hysterectomy
7. Sexual function
8. Estrogen replacement
9. Convalescence—how much and how long

Additionally, it is advisable for the disclosure-and-consent form to mention the names of the doctors whom the patient authorizes to operate on her (5) and should reflect who it is that is granting the consent. If it is not the patient granting the consent, the form should state the legal basis for the consent, (i.e., general power of attorney in the husband). Again, oral disclosure to reinforce and supplement the brief forms might be documented by having the patient initialing each item in a separate column. The patient's assent and signature should be witnessed by a third party, and the surgeon should then retain the original while giving the patient a carbon copy.

Admittedly, having one's lawyer draft special brief disclosure and consent forms for each material or reasonably foreseeable maloccurrence will entail some expense. Yet, as much money as doctors spend on malpractice insurance, it is astounding that many still do not seem to appreciate the cost-effectiveness of a personalized disclosure package such as this. Disclosure and consent would be documented; and, with the convenient checklist format, the surgeon would know at a glance whether he might have overlooked something in his preoperative discussions with the patient. Use of the checklist should be as automatic as Miranda warnings are to the policeman. One ought not to operate unless the patient has been informed of her rights.

To the disclosure responsibilities discussed here, the law provides exceptions where: (a) a true emergency exists, patient consent is impossible, and efforts to obtain the consent of a relative are unreasonable under the circumstances; or (b) risk disclosure itself would pose a significant psychologic barrier to effective therapy (although the physician must not lie to a direct question). These exceptions are not addressed extensively here because they are beyond the scope of the focal issue of informed consent where the doctor alleges a contractual meeting of the minds. It is this latter issue that has sparked the greatest amount of malpractice litigation, the plaintiff typically complaining: "I would not have let the doctor operate on me had I only known what the risks were!" By the use of a formal disclosure-and-consent checklist two things are accomplished: the physician protects himself legally through documentation; and, perhaps more importantly, he is less likely to overlook the disclosure of what are to him routine facts of life that may be perceived very differently by the patient. Good medical practice makes no allowance for such misunderstandings.

Although the law differs greatly from state to state, the advice offered here should be generally invaluable throughout the United States. Also, if your state sets forth statutory disclosure requirements as Texas does, for example, doctors are cautioned against mere statutory compliance. The better practice is to take such requirements as additions to the disclosure mandated by traditional legal standards in your state (6).

Recommended Surgical Resolution of Factual Hypothetical

The *surgical* problem here relates to peritonitis resulting from fecal leakage from the cecum after slippage of an appendiceal tie. This might have been prevented by double ligature of the appendiceal stump. Similar leakage can develop from intestinal perforation by necrosis following spillage from phenol used to "cauterize" the appendiceal or tubal stump. For this reason, we long ago abandoned the routine use of phenol and alcohol for this purpose, substituting local swabbing with povidone-iodine (Betadine). Once the catastrophe was recognized in the patient described above, the proper treatment was laparotomy with religation of the stump, drainage, and the general intensive supportive treatment of peritonitis (ed.).

References

1. Canterbury vs. Spence, 464 F. 2d 772 (D.C. Cir., 1972).
2. LeBlang TR: Informed consent--duty and causation: A survey of current developments. *The Forum* 18:280, 1983.
3. McCallum RD: Gynecological errors and medical malpractice. In JH Ridley (ed): *Gynecologic Surgery*, 2nd ed. Baltimore, Williams & Wilkins, 1981, p. 367.
4. Perna vs. Pirozzi, 442 A. 2d 1016 (1983), aff's in 457 A. 2d 431 (1983).
5. Natanson vs. Kline, 350 P. 2d 1093 (1960).
6. Richards EP, Rathbun KC: The law of patients' rights in Texas. *Tex B J* 44:1059, 1981.
7. Tex. Rev. Civ. State. Ann., Art 4590 (F) 6.03.
8. Richards EP, Rathbun KC: Informed consent and the Texas Medical Disclosure Panel. *Tex B J* 46:349, 1983.
9. Wilson vs. Scott, 412 S.W. 2d 299, 302 (1967).

Index

Page numbers in *italics* denote figures; those followed by "t" denote tables.